Respiratory Care:
National Board Review

Publishing Director: David Culverwell
Acquisitions Editor: Richard Weimer
Production Editor/Text Design: Sandra Tamburrino
Art Director/Cover Design: Don Sellers, AMI
Assistant Art Director: Bernard Vervin
Manufacturing Director: John Komsa

Copy Editor: Jeanne Carper
Typesetter: Compolith Graphics, Indianapolis, IN
Printer: R. R. Donnelley & Sons Co., Harrisonburg, VA
Typefaces: Baskerville (text), Benguiat (display)

Respiratory Care:
National Board Review

C. A. Brainard, BA, RRT

Associate Professor, Allied Health Technologies
Crafton Hills College, Yucaipa, California

with the assistance of

Michael J. Wirth, BS, RRT

Formerly: Respiratory Therapy Instructor
Crafton Hills College, Yucaipa, California
Currently: Staff Member, Pulmonary Physiology Laboratories
Loma Linda University Medical Center, Loma Linda, California

and contributions by

Arnie L. Kosmatka, PhD, RRT

Associate Professor, Allied Health Technologies
Director, Respiratory Therapy Programs
Crafton Hills College, Yucaipa, California

Brady Communications Company, Inc.
Bowie, MD 20715
A Prentice-Hall Publishing Company

Respiratory Care: National Board Review

Library of Congress Cataloging in Publication Data

Brainard, C. A., 1947-
  Respiratory care.

  Bibliography:p.
  1. Respiratory therapy—Problems, exercises, etc.
  2. Respiratory therapy—Examinations, questions, etc.
  I. Wirth, Michael, J., 1949-   II. Title. [DNLM:
  1. Respiratory therapy—Examination questions. WB 18 B814r]
  RC735.I5B73   1984   615.8'36'076   84-6410

ISBN 0-89303-816-4

Prentice-Hall International, Inc., London
Prentice-Hall Canada, Inc., Scarborough, Ontario
Prentice-Hall of Australia, Pty., Ltd., Sydney
Prentice-Hall of India Private Limited, New Delhi
Prentice-Hall of Japan, Inc., Tokyo
Prentice-Hall of Southeast Asia Pte. Ltd., Singapore
Whitehall Books, Limited, Petone, New Zealand
Editora Prentice-Hall Do Brasil LTDA., Rio de Janeiro

Printed in the United States of America

88 89 90 91 92 93 94 95   3 4 5 6 7 8 9 10

to

Susan and Kevin

and to

respiratory care practitioners
everywhere who know that
good patient care is its own
reward

Contents

xi

Foreword

Approximately twenty-five years ago an apparition arose, out of the basements of hospitals, when a group of uneducated artisans, who carried pipe-wrenches and looked like plumbers, suddenly appeared on the wards and participated in the medical care of patients. They had been asked to come by physicians and nurses because the beneficial effects of oxygen had just been recognized and no other group had the expertise to ensure that the gas would be administered safely and effectively. They were ambitious people who recognized an opportunity, and they were quick to develop new and improved methods for the administration of oxygen and to search for the education and recognition which would allow them to enter as members of the health care team. Thus, a new allied health profession evolved—"Respiratory Therapy."

As their presence became more and more evident, Respiratory Therapists were regarded by many as a threat to the traditions of ethical Medicine. It appeared that another cult of entrepreneurs, with little education or ethical motivation and with no scientific background, but with their miraculous "cures," were about to exploit the field for economic gain.

This threat has never materialized. Instead, Respiratory Therapy has developed to become recognized as an essential component in the mainstream of modern medical and nursing practice. Members of the profession are now highly educated, well motivated professionals. They are recognized experts in a highly specialized field of Medical Care, they have proven their professional integrity, and they are true allies of the physicians who supervise their practice.

There have been two reasons for this development. First is the fact that Respiratory Therapy has recruited intelligent students, carefully selected under guidance of Medical Advisors, in full conformity with the traditional standards of organized Medicine. Second is the fact that many physicians and qualified educators have recognized the need for this allied health profession and have dedicated themselves to the education of its members.

It seems that this book achieves a happy marriage of these two endeavors. First, it sets forth and adopts in comprehensive detail the standards and the body of knowledge which have been prescribed by physicians—through the National Board for Respiratory Care, the Joint Review Committee for Respiratory Therapy Education, and other organizations. Secondly, it provides students with "directions" by which they can benefit from every item in the prescription.

The magnitude of the prescription is considerable and, to the dilettante, it will be overwhelming. But to serious students it will be a challenge. In meeting this challenge, the students will gain the confidence which allows them to demonstrate their proficiency, and they will gain the inspiration which supports them in the life-long process of education.

Bruce M. Shepard, MD
Associate Medical Director
School of Respiratory Care, Crafton Hills College

Preface

This textbook grew out of a series of National Board for Respiratory Care (NBRC®) Examination Review Seminars offered in conjunction with the California Society of Respiratory Care, Chapter II, and the Department of Allied Health at Crafton Hills College. The modest syllabus, first developed in 1980, has undergone numerous revisions in response to suggestions from both students and colleagues. Since 1980 the percentage of participants who pass their board examinations has risen steadily and now it is approximately twice the national average (80–100% Crafton Hills as opposed to 40–50% national).

The experience of these seminars has identified the following weaknesses that candidates typically have when taking the examinations:

1. Unfamiliarity with examination content and questions
2. Poor mathematics skills
3. Weak patient assessment skills
4. Inability to interpret pulmonary function and hemodynamic data

This book presents a successful program for correcting these weaknesses. However, it must be emphasized that without a thorough knowledge of the scientific basis for respiratory therapy, this book will not have the desired effect. This reservoir of knowledge can only be developed through years of education, tempered by a mature commitment to improving professional skills. For the individual who has a solid foundation of basic knowledge, an examination review tool such as this can often make a critical difference.

The major goal of this instructional guide is, of course, to help the candidate gain NBRC credentials. It is hoped, however, that in some way this book will help keep that spark of intellectual curiosity alive long after the letters RRT are placed after the successful candidate's name.

Acknowledgments

This book could not have been written without the help of many individuals. Foremost among these is Joan Holtke, who patiently and expertly guided the manuscript through the maze of drafts and proofs. In a similar light, this project could not have thrived without the generous support of Charles Q. Simcox, PhD. Special thanks are also in order for Kenith Bryson, RRT, who gave me the opportunity to conduct the original seminars. To my contributing authors, colleagues, and students, I offer my gratitude for inspiration, hard work, editorial commentary, and valued friendship. Finally, these acknowledgments would not be complete without tribute to my friends and mentors, Ross N. Giem, MD, Bruce M. Shepard, MD, and Michael J. Wirth, RRT, who have spent many years trying to help me understand what they mean when they say, "When dealing with the critically ill, knowing what kind of disorder the patient has is frequently less important than knowing what kind of patient the disorder has."

Introduction

A. How to Use This Book

An alarmingly large number of candidates for the National Board for Respiratory Care® (NBRC®) examinations fail to pass by a frustratingly few percentage points. These individuals probably had the necessary background to pass, but something just did not "click" right on examination day. This situation is best avoided with the proverbial ounce of prevention. This book is no panacea, but it can provide the following two useful functions: (1) to jog your memory and (2) to teach you how to take the NBRC Examination.

When was the last time you used the Fick equation? How about a Beckman analyzer? Calculated an FEF_{25-75}? If you are like most candidates, you are clutching your chest right now, thinking, "They would not *really* ask about those things, would they?" Suddenly, a hideous scenario flashes across your mind. You are sitting on a park bench, unemployed and penniless. You hear yourself say to the unfortunate soul sitting next to you, "One point! I missed passing by one point. If I had only been able to remember what an OR/NOR gate was, I would be rich today."

Levity aside, all of us could use a good jog in the memory department from time to time. Want a good start? Turn to the Mathematics Review and Pretest and look up some of your least favorite equations. If that does not work, try the case histories in the Hemodynamics Review and Pretest. If that does not work, save your money and go out and have a night on the town compliments of me.

When taking a test, some people answer the question at hand and then, like efficient little test-taking machines, move confidently to the next question and so on, until they have finished the test. Others find themselves getting bogged down right from the start. Awash in a sea of confusion, they waste their time trying to figure out what the question is asking, rather than trying to determine the correct answer. They cannot get beyond the technical details to see how the problem at hand relates to actual patient care. How does one learn not to get hung up on the mechanics of the NBRC Examination? Well, usually a little extra practice is all that it takes to fine tune those test-taking instincts. With over 1400 NBRC type questions, this book should provide ample opportunity for that.

Text Structure

This text is divided into a Pretest and Review Section and a Posttest and Mastery Section. Section I contains four pretest and review units. Unit I is a complete review of the mathematics of respiratory care. From tank factors to sophisticated hemodynamic calculations, 34 separate mathematics pretest modules are presented along with a brief discussion of their clinical significance. Unit II contains 20 situational sets of the type found on the Entry Level Examination. Most candidates are unfamiliar with these types of questions because they have not appeared in the respiratory therapy examination review literature prior to this publication. Unit III is a review of hemodynamics for the advanced practitioner candidate. An increasing number of questions on this examination require an understanding of such concepts as the pulmonary wedge pressure and pulmonary vascular resistance (see reference 98). This section should prove very informative because much of this material has never been presented in this context before. Unit IV contains 40 separate pretests, one for each NBRC Entry Level and Advanced Practitioner Examination category. For the really serious candidate, this unit represents the heart of the book. The more than 700 questions are designed to assess each one of the 398 specific competencies listed in the NBRC Composite Examination Matrix (see reference 80).

Section II contains one full-length Entry Level Examination (Unit I) and one full-length Advanced Practitioner Examination (Unit II). These posttests are constructed according to specifications outlined in the NBRC Composite Examination Matrix (see references 80, 45, and 98). Posttests, especially when taken under examination-like conditions, are a reliable way of assessing a candidate's mastery and overall preparedness for the NBRC Examination.

Important

Before you begin to review the pretest sections, please examine the remainder of this introductory section carefully. It contains valuable information regarding examination content, type of question, and so on. Some of the information can also be found in your NBRC Candidate Handbook (which you should also read carefully). Much of it, such as the description of each individual examination category, can only be found here and will allow you to use this text much more efficiently.

B. Examination Content

In March, 1983, the NBRC began its new credentialing system by administering the first Entry Level Examination. The new Advanced Practitioner Examination is also part of that system. These examinations were developed on the basis of a national job analysis survey (see reference 45) completed in 1981. The survey identified the job description of the respiratory therapy practitioner as being composed of 398 separate tasks. Additionally, the study specifically delineated which tasks were performed by practitioners entering the profession (entry level) and which were performed by the advanced practitioner. Armed with this information, the NBRC constructed a Composite Examination Matrix (see reference 80). This matrix provided the specifications from which Entry Level and Advanced Practitioner Examinations have been constructed.

The goal of NBRC examinations is to determine whether the candidate possesses cognitive skills necessary to practice respiratory therapy on an entry level or an advanced level. The idea of constructing allied health profession national board examinations around a comprehensive job description is not a new one. The NBRC has, however, done an outstanding job with its examinations, and those concerned with the respiratory therapy profession are in debt to its leadership.

However, putting all well-deserved gratitude aside, those of us who have earned our credentials should perhaps feel a little bit lucky. These are the most complex and difficult examinations ever designed by the NBRC. Their content outlines contain hundreds of competencies for which the candidate is responsible.

To use your time most effectively, you must first know which topics are going to be assessed on a given examination. For instance, should a candidate spend a considerable amount of time studying chest physical assessment while preparing for the Advanced Practitioner Examination, valuable time would be wasted because this is assessed *primarily* on the Entry Level Examination (see references 45, 80, and 98). *This is not to say that the advanced practitioner candidate should not have a thorough understanding of the principles of chest physical assessment or any of the topics emphasized in the Entry Level Examination.* For example, the advanced practitioner's decision to recommend chest tube placement for a patient with a tension pneumothorax could not possibly be made without the ability to assess chest physical data. In examining the Entry Level and Advanced Practitioner Examination category descriptions on the next few pages, you will note that many topics are assessed on one examination only. This should not prove confusing if you remember the following statement:

> *The entry level candidate need concern himself or herself only with the topics described in the Entry Level Examination category section. Advanced practitioner candidates should concern themselves with Advanced Practitioner Examination category topics in particular but must also be able to demonstrate a general understanding of basic concepts.*

The latter should not prove difficult because these individuals are already Certified Respiratory Therapy Technicians.

It is of highest importance that you determine what is on the examination before you begin studying. To do this, please read the next pages very carefully, since they present a detailed account of the content of each examination. Should you have further questions regarding an examination category, please refer to the pretest module for that particular content area as presented in Unit IV of Section I.

C. Entry Level Examination Matrix

The following is the Entry Level Examination matrix. It lists the number of items assessed on each performance level. These represent the hierarchy of cognitive (intellectual) skills in order of complexity.

Table 1. Entry Level Examination Content Outline Matrix.

		Number of Items at Each Complexity Level			
		Recall	Application	Analysis	% Per Category
I.	Clinical Data (60 Items)				30
A.	Review patient records	2	5	2	4.5
B.	Collect and evaluate clinical information	8	13	0	10.5
C.	Recommend and obtain diagnostic procedures	1	4	1	3
D.	Perform and evaluate laboratory procedures	3	7	2	6
E.	Assess therapeutic plan	2	7	3	6
II.	Equipment (50 Items)				25
A.	Select, assemble, check, and correct malfunctions of equipment	13	26	3	21
B.	Ensure the cleanliness of all equipment	3	5	0	4
III.	Therapeutic Procedures (90 Items)				45
A.	Educate patients	0	2	1	1.5
B.	Control infection	1	3	1	2
C.	Maintain airway	3	5	0	4
D.	Mobilize and remove secretions	2	5	2	4.5
E.	Ensure ventilation	2	7	2	4.5
F.	Ensure oxygenation	2	7	2	5.5
G.	Assess patient response to therapy	2	7	2	5.5
H.	Modify therapy	2	6	2	5
I.	Recommend modifications in therapy	1	5	2	4
J.	Initiate cardiopulmonary resuscitation	2	7	2	5.5
K.	Maintain records and communication	1	2	0	1.5
	Totals (200 Items)	50	123	27	100

1. *Recall.* These questions test the ability to recall or recognize specific information. For example, a question may ask that the candidate recognize the average length of the adult trachea.
2. *Application.* These questions ask that the candidate be able to relate knowledge or facts to a new or changing situation. For example, if the candidate is informed that a 70-kg patient has a

minute alveolar ventilation of 2.5 L/min, it could safely be
assumed that the patient is hypoventilating.

3. *Analysis.* This is the most complex of the performance levels. As
    such it is built on a foundation of the first two. These questions
    ask that a large body of often complex information be analyzed to
    arrive at a solution. For example, the candidate may be asked to
    correctly evaluate a patient's pulmonary status or, having done
    so, to recommend that therapy be modified.

D. Entry Level Examination Categories

The preceding examination matrix lists 21 content areas. The following is a brief description of each of these. These descriptions are designed
to provide an overview to help map out a study plan. For a more
detailed explanation, please refer to the Table of Contents and look up
the specific examination category in Unit IV of Section I.

I. Clinical Data
    A. Review patient records. Questions in this category assess the
        candidate's ability to interpret existing clinical data, progress
        notes, patient history, and respiratory therapy orders. Most
        of the questions in this area are concerned with the candi-
        date's knowledge of medical terminology and normal labora-
        tory values.
    B. Collect and evaluate clinical information. Questions in this
        category assess the candidate's ability to:
        1. Perform a chest physical assessment
        2. Conduct a patient interview
        3. Perform bedside pulmonary function tests
        4. Interpret a chest roentgenogram on a *basic* level
    C. Recommend and obtain diagnostic procedures. Questions in
        this category assess the candidate's ability to:
        1. Obtain sputum and arterial blood samples
        2. Recommend other bedside and/or laboratory procedures
    D. Perform and evaluate laboratory procedures. Questions in
        this category assess the candidate's ability to:
        1. Perform arterial blood analysis
        2. Perform and evaluate basic pulmonary laboratory tests
    E. Assess therapeutic plan. Questions in this category assess the
        candidate's ability to:
        1. Determine pathophysiologic state (e.g., infant respira-
            tory distress syndrome, chronic obstructive pulmonary
            disease, croup)
        2. Evaluate all respiratory care plans to determine appro-
            priateness

II. Equipment
In the clinical setting, the respiratory therapy practitioner must
select, assemble, check proper function, and correct existing malfunctions for the following types of respiratory therapy equipment:
A. Medical gas storage, delivery, metering, and analyzing
devices
1. Medical gas cylinders
2. Regulators and reducing valves
3. Flowmeters
4. Oxygen analyzers
B. Oxygen administration devices (all oxygen administration
devices *except* portable liquid oxygen administration devices)
C. Humidity and aerosol therapy devices (humidifiers and aerosol generators of all types)
D. Airway care and resuscitation devices
1. All emergency and nonemergency airways
2. All resuscitation devices
E. Intermittent positive pressure and incentive breathing devices
F. Continuous mechanical ventilator devices (all continuous
mechanical ventilator devices except external negative pressure devices on a *basic* level)
G. Cardiopulmonary function monitoring devices
1. Spirometers
2. Respirometers
3. Blood gas analyzers
Also included in this Equipment category are questions assessing
the candidate's ability to:
H. Ensure cleanliness and/or sterilization of all equipment
III. Therapeutic Procedures
A. Educate patients. Questions in this category assess the candidate's ability to explain respiratory therapy clinical goals in
simple and understandable terms so as to achieve an optimal
therapeutic outcome.
B. Control infection. Questions in this category assess the candidate's ability to protect the patient from nosocomial infection
and assess his/her understanding of the principles of infection
control.
C. Maintain airway. Questions in this category assess the candidate's ability to:
1. Use humidity therapy
2. Maintain proper cuff inflation and position
D. Mobilize and remove secretions. Questions in this category
assess the candidate's ability to:
1. Use aerosol therapy
2. Use chest physical therapy
3. Perform suctioning techniques
4. Administer aerosolized drugs
E. Ensure ventilation. Questions in this category assess the candidate's ability to:
1. Use intermittent positive pressure breathing (IPPB)
therapy

2.   Use incentive spirometry therapy
3.   Place a patient on a ventilator
F.   Ensure oxygenation. Questions in this category assess the candidate's ability to:
1.   Administer oxygen therapy
2.   Administer positive end-expiratory pressure (PEEP) and continuous positive airway pressure (CPAP) therapy to prevent hypoxia
G.   Assess patient response to therapy. Questions in this category are designed to test the candidate's ability to:
1.   Note hazardous and adverse reactions to all forms of therapy
2.   Monitor effectively all parameters necessary to evaluate a patient's cardiopulmonary status on a *basic* level
H.   Modify therapy. Questions in this category are designed to assess the candidate's ability to:
1.   Terminate therapy based on patient's adverse response
2.   Modify effectively all respiratory therapy modalities based on the patient's response
I.   Recommend modifications in therapy. Questions in this category are designed to assess the candidate's ability to recommend modifications in respiratory therapy based on the patient's response on a *basic level.*
J.   Initiate cardiopulmonary resuscitation. Questions in this category are designed to assess the candidate's ability to initiate, modify, or conduct basic cardiopulmonary resuscitation (CPR) techniques in an emergency setting.
K.   Maintain records and communication. Questions in this category are designed to assess the candidate's ability to:
1.   Chart results of all respiratory therapy procedures
2.   Note and interpret the patient's objective and subjective responses to therapy

E.   Advanced Practitioner Examination Matrix

The following is the Advanced Practitioner Examination matrix. It lists the number of items assessed on each performance level. These represent the hierarchy of cognitive (intellectual) skills in order of complexity.

1.   *Recall.* These questions test the ability to recall or recognize specific information. For example, a question may ask that the candidate recognize normal values for the physiologic shunt fraction ($\dot{Q}_S/\dot{Q}_T$) for various patients.
2.   *Application.* These questions ask that the candidate be able to relate knowledge or facts to a new or changing situation. For example, the candidate is informed that a patient whose oxygen

consumption is normal has a $C(a-\bar{v})o_2$ of 7.5 vol%. Given this information, the practitioner should be able to determine that the cardiac output is decreased.

3. *Analysis.* This is the most complex of the performance levels. As such it is built on a foundation of the first two. These questions ask that the candidate take a large body of often complex information and analyze it to arrive at a solution. For example, the candidate may be asked to evaluate a patient's pulmonary status or, having done so, recommend that therapy be modified.

Table 2. Advanced Practitioner Examination Content Outline Matrix.

		Number of Items at Each Complexity Level		
		Recall	Application	Analysis	% Per Category
I.	Clinical Data (25 Items)				
A.	Review patient records	2	6	2	10
B.	Collect and evaluate clinical information	1	3	1	5
C.	Perform and evaluate laboratory procedures	2	6	2	10
II.	Equipment (10 Items)				
A.	Select, assemble, check, and correct malfunctions of equipment	3	3	0	6
B.	Ensure cleanliness, calibration, and quality control	1	2	1	4
III.	Therapeutic Procedures (65 Items)				
A.	Maintain airway	0	2	1	3
B.	Ensure ventilation	1	2	4	7
C.	Ensure oxygenation	0	1	2	3
D.	Assess patient response to therapy	4	12	4	20
E.	Modify therapy	1	4	2	7
F.	Recommend modifications in therapy	4	5	13	22
G.	Assist physician with special procedures	0	2	1	3
	Totals (100 Items)	19	48	33	100

F. Advanced Practitioner Examination Categories

The preceding examination matrix lists 13 content areas. The following is a brief description of each of these. These descriptions are designed to provide an overview to help map out a study plan. This is only an overview. For a more detailed explanation, please refer to the Table of Contents and look up the specific examination categories in Unit IV of Section I.

I. Clinical Data
   A. Review patient records. Questions in this category assess the candidate's ability to interpret existing clinical data, progress notes, patient history, and respiratory therapy orders. Most of the questions in this area are concerned with the candidate's knowledge of medical terminology and normal laboratory values.
   B. Collect and evaluate clinical information. Questions in this category are designed to assess the candidate's ability to interpret chest roentgenograms on an *advanced* level.
   C. Perform and evaluate laboratory procedures. Questions in this category are designed to assess the candidate's ability to perform and evaluate pulmonary laboratory tests on an *advanced* level.
II. Equipment
   In the clinical setting, the advanced respiratory therapy practitioner must select, assemble, check proper function, and correct existing malfunctions for the following types of respiratory therapy equipment:
   A. Airway care and resuscitation devices
      1. Laryngoscope and intubation devices
      2. Suctioning equipment
   B. Continuous mechanical ventilator devices
      1. External negative pressure devices
      2. Fluidic devices (on an *advanced* level)
      3. Advanced pneumatically powered/electronically controlled devices
   C. Cardiopulmonary function monitoring devices
      1. Spirometers
      2. Transducers and pneumotachometers
      3. Cardiovascular monitoring devices
      4. Blood gas analyzers
   Also included in the equipment category are questions assessing the candidate's ability to:
   D. Monitor effectiveness of sterilization procedures
   E. Perform calibration and quality control procedures on all respiratory therapy equipment

III. Therapeutic Procedures
  A. Maintain airway. Questions in this category are designed to assess the candidate's ability to:
    1. Perform endotracheal intubation and extubation
    2. Select appropriate endotracheal tubes
  B. Ensure ventilation. Questions in this category are designed to assess the candidate's ability to:
    1. Select ventilator
    2. Initiate and adjust continuous mechanical ventilation
    3. Initiate and adjust intermittent mandatory ventilation (IMV), synchronized intermittent mandatory ventilation (SIMV), and other weaning procedures
  C. Ensure oxygenation. Questions in this category are designed to assess the candidate's ability to:
    1. Initiate and adjust PEEP and CPAP therapy
    2. Initiate and adjust combinations of IMV, SIMV, and PEEP therapy
  D. Assess patient response to therapy. Questions in this category are designed to assess the candidate's ability to:
    1. Note hazardous and adverse reactions to all forms of therapy
    2. Monitor all parameters necessary to evaluate the patient's cardiopulmonary status on an *advanced* level
  E. Modify therapy. Questions in this category are designed to assess the candidate's ability to:
    1. Terminate therapy based on patient's adverse response
    2. Modify all respiratory therapy modalities based on patient response
  F. Recommend modifications in therapy. Questions in this category are designed to assess the candidate's ability to recommend modifications in respiratory therapy based on the patient's response.
  G. Assist physician with special procedures. Questions in this category are designed to assess the candidate's ability to assist the physician in performing:
    1. Bronchoscopy
    2. Insertion of chest tubes
    3. Tracheotomy
    4. Other invasive diagnostic and therapeutic techniques

G. NBRC Type Questions

There are three specific types of questions used on NBRC written examinations. Unfortunately, many candidates may only be familiar with the first one or two of these types.

  I. Simple Multiple Choice
     Question:

Which of the following most accurately represents the Pa_{O_2} for a healthy 60-year-old patient?
A. 50 mm Hg
B. 60 mm Hg
C. 70 mm Hg
D. 80 mm Hg
E. 90 mm Hg
Answer: D

This type of question requires the selection of the *one best response* from five plausible choices. To make guessing difficult, most NBRC questions are written so that all five of the choices are *possible*. In addition, two or even three of the choices may be *very nearly correct*. However, *for each question there is only one correct answer.* There are other methods of increasing the difficulty of these questions. One is to bait the candidate with fashionable therapeutic modes. For example, the candidate may be asked to select between a volume- or pressure-cycled ventilator for use in providing continuous ventilatory support. Clinically, the candidate may never have even *seen* a pressure-cycled ventilator used for this purpose. However, if the settings presented for the volume ventilators are obviously wrong, no other choice would be reasonable and thus correct.

II. Multiple True-False Type Questions
Question:
Three days post total-hip-replacement surgery, a 50-kg, 73-year-old woman experiences pleuritic pain, tachypnea, and tachycardia. Bedside examination reveals grossly distended neck veins and a cough productive of a small amount of blood-streaked sputum. The following laboratory and bedside data are made available at this time:

FI_{O_2}	0.21
Pa_{O_2}	58 mm Hg
Pa_{CO_2}	42 mm Hg
pH	7.37
HCO_3^-	24 mEq/L
Base excess	+0.6 mEq/L
Minute ventilation	26 L/min
V_D/V_T	0.78

Which of the following statements is (are) true regarding this patient's status?
I. The patient's hypoxemia is due to hypoventilation.
II. A blood gas laboratory error is present.
III. Ventilatory support is indicated.
IV. Pulmonary embolus is a likely cause of distress.
A. II and III
B. I only
C. II and IV

D.   III and IV
E.   II, III, and IV

Answer: D

Many candidates find these questions difficult. This may be due either to the large amount of information they contain or to a lack of familiarity with this type of question. Whatever the reason, these questions generally become simpler once a systematic approach is employed, such as follows:

A.   Evaluate the information presented in the question's open statement.
B.   Go down the list of presented choices and make a mark beside the statements that are true.
C.   Select the corresponding combinations of choices.
D.   If still in doubt, make an educated guess. Remember, *there is no penalty for guessing on NBRC written exams.*
E.   Practice taking as many of these questions as possible. This book contains hundreds of them. More will be found in the candidate handbook. Study them all very carefully until comfortable with their format.

III.   Situational Sets

According to the NBRC, situational set type questions are used only on the Entry Level Examination.

Situational sets are mini case histories. They consist of a scenario followed by three to five questions. Like a clinical simulation, they place the candidate in charge of a patient management problem. An example of a situational set appears below.

Directions: Each group of questions below concerns a certain situation. In each case, first study the description of the situation. Then, choose the one best answer to each question following it.

A 64-year-old man with a history of chronic obstructive pulmonary disease (COPD) is brought to the emergency department after several days of increasing distress that did not respond to his home respiratory care program. Arterial blood gas data on room air and 2 L nasal oxygen are as follows:

	Room Air	2 L O$_2$
Pao$_2$	36 mm Hg	65 mm Hg
Paco$_2$	68 mm Hg	65 mm Hg
pH	7.28	7.35
HCO$_3$	35 mEq/L	37 mEq/L

1.   Based on the above information, the respiratory therapy practitioner should now recommend which of the following?
A.   Increase oxygen to 3 L/min
B.   Leave oxygen flow unchanged
C.   Place on continuous ventilatory support
D.   Decrease oxygen to 1 L/min
E.   Place patient on a 35% air entrainment mask

Answer: B

2. Which of the following is (are) most likely to be responsible for this patient's arterial hypoxemia?
   I. Low V/Q
   II. Physiologic shunting
   III. Hypoventilation
       A. I only
       B. I and III
       C. II only
       D. II and III
       E. III only
   Answer: B

3. This patient has a long history of bronchiectasis. Which of the following would be the most valuable adjunct in helping maintain bronchial hygiene?
   A. Aerosol therapy
   B. Continuous ventilatory support
   C. Breathing retraining
   D. Postural drainage techniques
   E. Bronchodilator therapy
   Answer: D

4. Seven days later, the patient is beginning to improve. Acid-base and blood gas data obtained at this time are as follows:

FI_{O_2}	0.21
Pa_{O_2}	63 mm Hg
Pa_{CO_2}	69 mm Hg
pH	7.60
HCO_3^-	37 mEq/L
Base excess	+16 mEq/L

Based on the above data, which of the following is the most correct interpretation of this patient's acid-base status?
A. Acute respiratory alkalosis and metabolic alkalosis exist.
B. An overcompensated respiratory acidosis exists.
C. A laboratory error exists.
D. Fully compensated metabolic alkalosis exists.
E. Fully compensated respiratory acidosis exists.
Answer: C

With the exception of the branching-logic clinical simulation, these situational sets are the most complex devised by the NBRC. Many candidates find them even more difficult than the multiple true-false type. Performance on these questions can be improved by using the following approach:
A. *Read the questions very carefully.* Read and reread the scenarios until you grasp the intent of the situation. Often, the set will follow a particular patient throughout his/her hospitalization. In this case, information presented in each succeeding question must be considered before selecting an answer.

B.   *Practice taking situational set type questions.* Like branching-logic clinical simulations, these questions can be very confusing. Fortunately, this problem is usually alleviated with a little practice. This book contains many such sets. The candidate handbook will contain more. Study them all very carefully.

H. References

Every attempt has been made to reference each question in this book to the latest edition of sources that are part of a candidate's library. In the next few pages there are 104 sources listed that were used in developing these test items. Please note in particular that most of the questions herein have been referenced to sources 1 through 5 with the belief that these texts would most likely form the core of the candidate's library. Unfortunately, for some topics, such as interpretation of sophisticated hemodynamics data, I have had to turn to applied physiology texts and even more recent medical literature. References 25, 38, 41, 42, 46, 49, 61, and 65, in particular, contain much common sense as well as "state of the art" information and are recommended to the advanced practitioner candidate.

Throughout the text the questions are referenced using the following representative format:

(3:321–323) (88:Chap 1)

Each set of parentheses gives the reference number on the left of the colon and the pages or chapters on the right.

Reference Numbers

1.   Shapiro BA, et al: *Clinical Application of Respiratory Care,* 2nd ed. Chicago, Year Book Medical Publishers, 1979.

2.   Burton GG, et al: *Respiratory Care.* Philadelphia, JB Lippincott, 1977.

3.   Spearman CB, et al: *Egan's Fundamentals of Respiratory Therapy,* 4th ed. St. Louis, CV Mosby, 1982.

4.   McPherson SP: *Respiratory Therapy Equipment,* 2nd ed. St. Louis, CV Mosby, 1981.

5.   Shapiro BA, et al: *Clinical Application of Blood Gases,* 2nd ed. Chicago, Year Book Medical Publishers, 1977. 1989

6.   Martz KV, et al: *Management of the Patient-Ventilator System.* St. Louis, CV Mosby, 1979. 1984

7.   Morrison MD: *Respiratory Intensive Care Nursing,* 2nd ed. Boston, Little, Brown & Co, 1973.

8. Rau JL, et al: *Fundamental Respiratory Therapy Equipment.* Glenn Educational Medical Service, 1977.

9. Lough MD: *Newborn Respiratory Care.* Chicago, Year Book Medical Publishers, 1979.

10. Blodgett D: *Manual of Pediatric Respiratory Care Procedures.* Philadelphia, JB Lippincott, 1982.

11. Farzan S, et al: *A Concise Handbook of Respiratory Diseases.* Reston, VA, Reston Publishing, 1978.

12. Robbins SL, et al: *Basic Pathology,* 2nd ed. Philadelphia, WB Saunders, 1981.

13. Lough MD, et al: *Pediatric Respiratory Therapy,* 2nd ed. Chicago, Year Book Medical Publishers, 1979.

14. Mitchell RS: *Synopsis of Clinical Pulmonary Disease,* 2nd ed. St. Louis, CV Mosby, 1978.

15. Korones SB: *High-Risk Newborn Infants,* 3rd ed. St. Louis, CV Mosby, 1981.

16. Ruppel G: *Manual of Pulmonary Function Testing,* 2nd ed. St. Louis, CV Mosby, 1979.

17. Cherniack RM, et al: *Respiration in Health and Disease,* 2nd ed. Philadelphia, WB Saunders, 1972.

18. West JB: *Respiratory Physiology,* 2nd ed. Baltimore, Williams & Wilkins, 1979. 1984

19. Slonim HB, et al: *Respiratory Physiology,* 3rd ed. St. Louis, CV Mosby, 1976.

20. Comroe JH: *Physiology of Respiration,* 2nd ed. Chicago, Year Book Medical Publishers, 1975.

21. Comroe JH, et al: *The Lung,* 2nd ed. Chicago, Year Book Medical Publishers, 1962.

22. Rau JL: *Respiratory Therapy Pharmacology.* Chicago, Year Book Medical Publishers, 1981. 3RD ED 1989

23. Mauss MK: Increased intracranial pressure: An update. *Heart and Lung* 1976;5:6.

24. Kacmarck RM, et al: *The Essentials of Respiratory Therapy.* Chicago, Year Book Medical Publishers, 1979.

25. McIntyre KM, et al: *Advanced Cardiac Life Support.* New York, American Heart Association, 1981.

26. Goodman LS and Gilman A (eds): *The Pharmacological Basis of Therapeutics,* 4th ed. New York, Macmillan, 1970.

27. Ziment I: *Respiratory Pharmacology and Therapeutics.* Philadelphia, WB Saunders, 1978.

28. Rushmer F: *Cardiovascular Dynamics,* 4th ed. Philadelphia, WB Saunders, 1976.

29. Klaus MH, et al: *Care of the High-Risk Neonate,* 2nd ed. Philadelphia, WB Saunders, 1979.

30. Bendixen HH, et al: *Respiratory Care.* St. Louis, CV Mosby, 1965.

31. Hedley-Whyte J, et al: *Applied Physiology of Respiratory Care.* Boston, Little, Brown & Co, 1976.

32. Moser KM, et al: *Respiratory Emergencies.* St. Louis, CV Mosby, 1977.

33. Hudak CM, et al: *Critical Care Nursing,* 2nd ed. Philadelphia, JB Lippincott, 1977.

34. Taylor JP: *Manual of Respiratory Therapy,* 2nd ed. St. Louis, CV Mosby, 1978.

35. Mathewson HS: *Respiratory Therapy in Critical Care.* St. Louis, CV Mosby, 1976.

36. Applebaum EL: *Tracheal Intubation.* Philadelphia, WB Saunders, 1976.

37. Effron DM: *Cardiopulmonary Resuscitation,* 2nd ed. New York, American Heart Association, 1980.

38. Pontoppidan H, et al: *Acute Respiratory Failure in the Adult.* Boston, Little, Brown & Co, 1973.

39. Heironimus TW, et al: *Mechanical Artificial Ventilation.* Springfield, IL, Charles C Thomas, 1977.

40. Darin J: The mode of action of cyclic AMP. *Respiratory Care* 1981;26:228–240.

41. Stevens PM: Assessment of acute respiratory failure: Cardiac versus pulmonary causes. *Chest* 1975;67:1–2.

42. Weil MH, et al: Colloid osmotic pressure and pulmonary edema. *Chest* 1977;72:692.

43. Rogers EJ: Physics vs. physiology in infant ventilation. *Respiratory Therapy* 1972;Sept/Oct.

44. Mullins E, et al: Patient and family education in respiratory care. *Respiratory Care* 1974;19:273.

45. O'Donohue WJ, et al: Development of an entry level examination for respiratory care practitioners. *Respiratory Care* 1982;27:1058.

46. Stevens PM: Positive end expiratory pressure breathing. *Basics of RD* 1977;5:1.

47. Suter PM: Optimum end-expiratory airway pressure in patients with acute pulmonary failure. *The New England Journal of Medicine* 1975;292:284.

48. Miller WF: Fundamental principles of aerosol therapy. *Respiratory Care* 1972;17:295.

49. Rogers RM: Physiologic considerations in the treatment of acute respiratory failure. *Basics of RD* 1975;3:1.

50. Demmers RR: Use of the concept of ventilator compliance in the determination of static total compliance. *Respiratory Care* 1981; 26:644.

51. Bageant RA: Oxygen analyzers. *Respiratory Care* 1976;21:410.

52. Literature available from the National Catheter Corporation.

53. Bergerson BS: *Pharmacology in Nursing,* 14th ed. St. Louis, CV Mosby, 1979.

54. Safar P: *Respiratory Therapy.* Philadelphia, FA Davis, 1965.

55. Cournard A, et al: Physiological studies of effects of intermittent positive pressure breathing on cardiac output in man. *American Journal of Physiology* 1948;132:162.

56. Young J, Crocker D: *Principles and Practice of Respiratory Therapy,* 2nd ed. Chicago, Year Book Medical Publishers, 1976.

57. Literature available from the Bennett Corporation.

58. Hessel EA: Monitoring the patient in acute respiratory failure. *Respiratory Therapy* 1976;p 27.

59. Jones NL, et al: *Clinical Exercise Testing.* Philadelphia, WB Saunders, 1975.

60. Literature available from the Bourns Corporation.

61. Swan HJ: Balloon flotation catheters: Their use in hemodynamic monitoring in clinical practice. *Journal of the American Medical Association* 1975;233:865.

62. Luce JM: Intermittent mandatory ventilation. *Chest* 1981;76:678.

63. Petty TL: *Intensive and Rehabilitative Respiratory Care.* Philadelphia, Lea & Febiger, 1971.

64. Cullen P, et al: Treatment of flail chest. *Archives of Surgery* 1975; 110:1099.

65. Walkinshaw M, et al: Use of volume loading to obtain preferred levels of PEEP. *Critical Care Medicine* 1980;8:81.

66. Demmers RR: Rational and irrational approaches to weaning, editorial. *Respiratory Care* 1976;21:601.

67. Fairley BH: The mechanical ventilation sign is a dodo, editorial. *Respiratory Care* 1976;21:1127.

68. Literature available from the Bird Corporation.

69. Literature provided by the manufacturers of these specific products.

70. Demmers RR: Mechanical ventilation wave patterns. *Current Reviews in Respiratory Therapy* 1980; lesson II, vol 2.

71. Desautels DA, et al: Methods of administering IMV. *Respiratory Care* 1974;19:189.

72. Brainard CA: Calculating I:E ratios, letter. *Respiratory Care* 1978;23:846.

73. Bernhard WN, et al: Adjustment of intracuff pressure to prevent aspiration. *Anesthesiology* 1979;50:363.

74. Shapiro BA, et al: Complications of mechanical aids to lung inflation. *Respiratory Care* 1982;27:467.

75. American Thoracic Society Statement on Intermittent Positive Pressure Breathing. *Respiratory Care* 1979;24:698.

76. Tyler ML: Complications of positioning and chest physiotherapy. *Respiratory Care* 1982;27:458.

77. Benson MS: Ventilator wash-out volume: A consideration in endotracheal suction preoxygenation. *Respiratory Care* 1979; 24:832.

78. Stauffer JL, et al: Complications of endotracheal intubation, tracheostomy and artificial airways. *Respiratory Care* 1982;27:47.

79. Nunn JF: *Applied Respiratory Physiology.* London, Butterworth & Co, 1969.

80. National Board for Respiratory Care Composite Examination Matrix, National Board for Respiratory Care, 1983.

81. Mushin WW, et al: *Automatic Ventilation of the Lungs,* 2nd ed. Philadelphia, FA Davis, 1969.

82. Shapiro BA, et al: *Clinical Application of Blood Gases,* 3rd ed. Chicago, Year Book Medical Publishers, 1982. 1989 4th ed

83. Heimlich HJ: A life saving maneuver to prevent food choking. *Journal of the American Medical Association* 1975;234:398.

84. Mohler JG: Should we correct blood gas values for the patients' reported temperature? California Thoracic Society Proficiency Testing Update, November 1982.

85. Lagerson J: The cough, its effectiveness depends on you. *Respiratory Care* 1973;18:434.

86. Miller WT: An introduction to chest radiology. *Respiratory Care* 1973;18:304.

87. Sugerman HJ, et al: Gram-negative sepsis. *Current Problems in Surgery* 1981;18(No. 7).

88. Mullins E, et al: Patient and family education in respiratory care. *Respiratory Care* 1974;19:273.

89. Stedman TL: *Stedman's Medical Dictionary,* 23rd ed. Baltimore, Williams & Wilkins, 1976.

90. Nelson EJ, et al: *Critical Care Respiratory Therapy.* Boston, Little, Brown & Co, 1983.

91. Pierce A, et al: Bacterial contamination of aerosols. *Archives of Internal Medicine* 1973;131:156.

92. US Department of Health, Education and Welfare: *Isolation Techniques for Use in Hospitals,* 2nd ed. Washington, DC, US Government Printing Office, 1975.

93. Ransohoff J: Head injuries. *Journal of the American Medical Association* 1975;234:861.

94. Boedeher EC, et al: *Manual of Medical Therapeutics,* 21st ed. Boston, Little, Brown & Co, 1974.

95. Bates B: *A Guide to Physical Examination.* Philadelphia, JB Lippincott, 1974.

96. Shepard BM, Medical Director, Respiratory Therapy Department, St. Bernardine's Hospital, San Bernardino, California: Personal communication, 1983.

97. Grey H: *Anatomy of the Human Body,* 29th ed. Philadelphia, Lea & Febiger, 1973.

98. Dunne P: Development of the written registry examination for advanced respiratory care practitioners. *Respiratory Care* 1983; 28:1147–1172.

99. Mishoe SC: A review of physiology, measurements, and clinical significance of colloid osmotic pressure. *Respiratory Care* 1983; 28:1129–1142.

100. Rattenborg CC: *Clinical Use of Mechanical Ventilation.* Chicago, Year Book Medical Publishers, 1981.

101. Armstrong PW, et al: *Hemodynamic Monitoring in the Critically Ill.* Philadelphia, JB Lippincott, 1980.

102. Shoemaker WC, et al: *Textbook of Critical Care.* Philadelphia, WB Saunders, 1984.

103. Rarey KP, et al: *Respiratory Patient Care.* Englewood Cliffs, NJ, Prentice-Hall, 1981.

104. Fishman AP, et al: *Pulmonary Diseases and Disorders.* New York, McGraw-Hill, 1980.

I

Examination Pretest and Review

UNIT I

Mathematics Review and Pretest

There is a bewildering array of formulas and equations for which the respiratory therapy practitioner is responsible. A glance at the NBRC Composite Examination Matrix (see reference 80) confirms this. From tank factors to sophisticated hemodynamic measurements, the practitioner may, at times, feel overwhelmed by an avalanche of laboratory and clinical data.

This need not be the case. With a sound knowledge of the metric system and the ability to organize and solve basic algebraic equations, the calculations used in respiratory care can be done correctly and with confidence.

Important

According to the NBRC Composite Examination Matrix, the Entry Level Examination candidate should be familiar with all but the following calculations contained in this mathematics review section.

1. Q_S/Q_T determinations
2. $C(a-\bar{v})o_2$ calculations
3. Fick equation
4. a/A ratio and respiratory index calculations
5. Pulmonary vascular resistance calculations
6. Spirometry calculations
7. Residual volume determinations

The candidate for the Advanced Practitioner Examination should be familiar with all the material in this section in general and the preceding calculations in particular.

Part I
Medical Gas Therapy Calculations

Contents

A. Conversion Factor Pretest

Questions in this category are designed to assess the practitioner's ability to use important medical gas therapy conversion factors. For example, being able to convert cubic feet of gaseous oxygen to liters of gaseous oxygen would be beneficial in helping the therapist determine actual cylinder contents.

The following pretest was developed to help the candidate become proficient in this area.

1. The respiratory therapy practitioner is asked how many liters of oxygen are contained in 1 cubic foot of gaseous oxygen. Which of the following represents the most correct answer?
   A. 14.7
   B. 7.52
   C. 13.4
   D. 28.3   *P. 360 - K*
   E. 24.9
   (3:428)

27

2. An E cylinder of medical oxygen, when full, contains which of the following number of liters of gaseous oxygen?
    A. 620
    B. 687
    C. 590
    D. 486
    E. 930
        (3:432)

3. An H cylinder of medical oxygen, when full, contains approximately which of the following number of liters of gaseous oxygen?
    A. 9600
    B. 5300
    C. 7400
    D. 6900
    E. 4700
        (3:432)

4. The respiratory therapy practitioner is asked how many cubic feet of gaseous oxygen are contained in 1 cubic foot of liquid oxygen. The most correct answer would be which of the following?
    A. 920
    B. 283
    C. 314
    D. 860   × 28.3 = 24,338 cu' in 1 cu' of liquid O_2
    E. 750
        (3:434)

B. Cylinder Duration Pretest

Questions in this category are designed to assess the practitioner's ability to determine the amount of time that a particular medical gas cylinder will run before going dry under the clinical conditions stated in the question. In solving these questions, the candidate must be able to recall that the so-called tank factors for E-, G-, and H-size oxygen cylinders are 0.28, 2.41, and 3.14, respectively. These factors must then be inserted into the following equation:

$$\text{Cylinder Duration in Minutes} = \frac{\left(\begin{array}{c}\text{Actual Cylinder}\\\text{Gauge Pressure}\\\text{psig}\end{array}\right)(\text{Tank Factor})}{\text{Actual Delivered Liter Flow (L/min)}}$$

As can be seen, the equation gives cylinder duration in minutes. This means that the value must be divided by 60 to convert it to hours of cylinder duration.

The following pretest was developed to help the candidate become proficient in this area.

1. The respiratory therapy practitioner is asked to set up a full E cylinder of oxygen to deliver 3 L/min to a patient with chronic

do we calculate

obstructive pulmonary disease. How long will it take for the cylinder to run empty at the above liter flow?

A. 3 hours and 55 minutes
—B. 3 hours and 25 minutes
C. 2 hours and 5 minutes
D. 4 hours and 10 minutes
E. 3 hours and 45 minutes
(3:432)

2. A G cylinder of oxygen has 1600 lbs. pressure in it and is running at a rate of 5 L/min. At this flow rate, how long will it take for the cylinder to run completely dry?

A. 11 hours and 49 minutes
B. 11 hours and 30 minutes
C. 12 hours and 5 minutes
—D. 12 hours and 50 minutes
E. 12 hours and 15 minutes
(3:432)

3. At a flow rate of 4 L/min, how long will it take for a full H cylinder to run completely dry?

A. 19 hours and 55 minutes
B. 29 hours and 15 minutes
C. 47 hours and 20 minutes
D. 30 hours and 10 minutes
— E. 28 hours and 45 minutes
(3:432)

4. An H cylinder of oxygen has 700 lbs. pressure and is delivering a flow of 7 L/min. Approximately how long will it take before it runs completely dry?

A. 6 hours and 45 minutes
B. 5 hours and 30 minutes
C. 6 hours and 15 minutes
D. 5 hours and 45 minutes
—E. 5 hours and 15 minutes
(3:432)

C. General FI_{O_2} Formula Pretest

Even when an oxygen analyzer is not available, the respiratory therapy practitioner can determine a patient's fractional inspired oxygen concentration (FI_{O_2}). This may be crucial in an emergency situation. This formula is as follows:

$$FI_{O_2} = \frac{[(0.21)(\text{No. Liters Air})] + [(1.00)(\text{No. Liters Oxygen})]}{\text{Total System Liter Flow}}$$

because O_2 occupies 20.95% of atmosphere — combined compressed Air + O_2

The following pretest was developed to help the candidate become proficient in this area.

1. The respiratory therapy practitioner is blending 6 L/min of oxygen and 9 L/min of air together into an oxygen hood. Approximately what concentration of oxygen will be administered under these circumstances?
   A. 25%
   B. 30%
   C. 35%
   D. 45%
   E. 50%
   (4:148)

2. The respiratory therapy practitioner is blending 5 L/min oxygen with 15 L/min air. What concentration of oxygen will be administered under these circumstances?
   A. 30%
   B. 55%
   C. 45%
   D. 40%
   E. 50%
   (4:148)

D. PIo₂ Formula Pretest

Because it is part of the alveolar air equation, the PI_{O_2} formula has many important laboratory and clinical applications. The formula is as follows:

$$PI_{O_2} = (FI_{O_2})\,(P_B - P_{H_2O})$$

The following pretest was developed to help the candidate become proficient in this area.

1. The respiratory therapy practitioner is asked to calculate a patient's PI_{O_2} given the following clinical conditions:

P_B	760 mm Hg
FI_{O_2}	0.21
P_{H_2O}	47 mm Hg

   Which of the following most accurately represents this value?
   A. 160 mm Hg
   B. 150 mm Hg
   C. 140 mm Hg
   D. 185 mm Hg
   E. 137 mm Hg
   (5:214) (2:235)

2. Calculate a patient's PI_{O_2} given the following clinical data:

FI_{O_2}	0.40
P_B	727 mm Hg
P_{H_2O}	47 mm Hg

Which of the following represents the value most accurately?
A.   250 mm Hg
B.   240 mm Hg
C.   270 mm Hg
D.   243 mm Hg
E.   120 mm Hg
(5:214) (2:235)

3.   Calculate the PI_{O_2} given the following clinical conditions:

FI_{O_2} 0.70
P_B 420 mm Hg
P_{H_2O} 47 mm Hg

Which of the following represents this value most accurately?
A.   480 mm Hg
B.   235 mm Hg
C.   260 mm Hg
D.   295 mm Hg
E.   280 mm Hg
(5:214) (2:235)

E. Alveolar Air Equation Pretest   P. 22 notes

Because the alveolar oxygen tension must be known to calculate the $P(A-a)_{O_2}$ and the intrapulmonary shunt fraction (when using the modified clinical shunt equation), the alveolar air equation is used very frequently by the respiratory therapy practitioner. Unfortunately, there are multiple versions of this equation. Thus, confusion sometimes exists concerning which equation is most appropriate. *Although this is certainly not the case in all laboratory and clinical situations on NBRC examinations, any one of the alveolar air equations is sufficiently accurate enough for the candidate to determine the correct answer.* I recommend that the candidate learn one of the simpler versions when preparing for these examinations. The suggested alveolar air equations appear below:

$$P_{AO_2} = [FI_{O_2}(P_B - P_{H_2O})] - \left[\frac{P_{aCO_2}}{R}\right]$$

or

$$P_{AO_2} = [FI_{O_2}(P_B - P_{H_2O})] - [(P_{aCO_2}) \times (1.25)]$$

These equations are suggested because they are highly accurate and relatively easy to remember. In an emergency or critical care setting, however, the busy practitioner might find it convenient to use a more simplified version that I call the *Emergency Alveolar Air Equation.* This appears below:

$$P_{AO_2} = (\text{Oxygen Percentage} \times 7) - (P_{aCO_2})$$

Surprisingly enough, this formula is accurate to within ±10 mm Hg throughout the entire range of FI_{O_2}'s.

The following pretest was developed to help the candidate to become proficient in this area.

1. Calculate the P_{AO_2} given the following clinical information:

P_B	760 mm Hg
FI_{O_2}	0.21
Pa_{CO_2}	40 mm Hg
Respiratory exchange ratio (R)	0.8

    Which of the following most accurately represents this value?
    A. 100 mm Hg
    B. 120 mm Hg
    C. 108 mm Hg
    D. 95 mm Hg
    E. 90 mm Hg
      (5:214) (2:235)

2. Calculate the P_{AO_2} given the following conditions:

P_B	640 mm Hg
FI_{O_2}	1.0
Pa_{CO_2}	30 mm Hg
Respiratory exchange ratio (R)	0.8

    Which of the following most accurately represents this value?
    A. 520 mm Hg
    B. 540 mm Hg
    C. 555 mm Hg
    D. 490 mm Hg
    E. 590 mm Hg
      (5:214) (2:235)

3. Given the following clinical data, which of the following choices most accurately represents a patient's P_{AO_2}?

P_B	730 mm Hg
FI_{O_2}	0.40
Pa_{CO_2}	55 mm Hg
Respiratory exchange ratio (R)	0.8

    A. 205 mm Hg
    B. 225 mm Hg
    C. 240 mm Hg
    D. 180 mm Hg
    E. 195 mm Hg
      (5:214) (2:235)

PART 1

F. Air Entrainment Formula Pretest

The air entrainment formula allows the respiratory therapy practitioner to determine how many liters of room air are entrained by a particular air entrainment valve per liter of source gas. It is assumed that this source gas is 100% oxygen. The formula is as follows:

$$\frac{\text{No. of Liters Air Entrained}}{\text{Liter Source Gas}} = \frac{1.0 - \text{FI}_{O_2}}{\text{FI}_{O_2} - 0.21}$$

To solve this equation, the practitioner must know the FI_{O_2} of the air entrainment valve being used. The most common practical application of this equation is the determination of total flow rate as delivered by a given air entrainment system. The formula for this is as follows:

$$\text{Total System Flow Rate} = \left(\frac{\text{No. of Liters}}{\text{Air Entrained}}\right) + \left(\frac{\text{Source Gas}}{\text{Liter Flow}}\right)$$

From this system it can be seen that in the case of a 3:1 ratio (such as exists with a 40% air entrainment system), a source gas flow of 10 L/min will yield a total flow of 40 L/min.

The following pretest was developed to help the candidate become proficient in this area.

1. The respiratory therapy practitioner is using an air entrainment valve that is designed to deliver an FI_{O_2} of 0.4. To do this it must entrain how many parts room air for each part source gas?
   A. 3
   B. 4
   C. 5
   D. 10
   E. 20
   (3:470–472)

2. An air entrainment valve is designed to deliver an FI_{O_2} of 0.6. To do this it must entrain how many parts room air for each part driving gas?
   A. 1.4
   B. 1.3
   C. 1.5
   D. 1.7
   E. 1.0
   (3:470–472)

3. According to the air entrainment formula, how many parts room air must be entrained for each part driving gas to obtain an FI_{O_2} of 0.24?
   A. 10
   B. 15
   C. 20
   D. 25
   E. 30
   (3:470–472)

4. An all-purpose pneumatic nebulizer is being driven by 8 L/min and the air entrainment valve is on the 40% setting. What is the total delivered flow rate?
    A. 37 L/min
    B. 40 L/min
    C. 32 L/min
    D. 27 L/min
    E. 45 L/min
    (3:470–472)

5. An all-purpose pneumatic nebulizer is being driven by 12 L/min and the air entrainment valve is set on 65%. What is the approximate total liter flow being delivered to the patient?
    A. 24 L/min
    B. 22 L/min
    C. 18 L/min
    D. 14 L/min
    E. 29 L/min
    (3:470–473)

6. A properly functioning 24% air entrainment mask is being driven by 4 L/min. What is the approximate total flow rate being delivered to the patient?
    A. 104 L/min
    B. 84 L/min
    C. 100 L/min
    D. 96 L/min
    E. 26 L/min
    (3:470–473)

G. Flowmeter Accuracy Calculations Pretest

Questions in this category are designed to assess the candidate's ability to determine the actual flow rate being administered by properly calibrated flowmeters being operated under unusual conditions.

The following self-study questions were developed to help the candidate become proficient in this area.

1. A properly calibrated backpressure-compensated oxygen flowmeter is being used to administer a mixture of 80% helium and 20% oxygen. The meter presently reads 10 L/min. Which of the following choices most accurately represents the flow rate in L/min that is actually being administered?
    A. 0
    B. 10
    C. 12
    D. 15
    E. 18
    (3:483) (4:78)

2. A properly calibrated backpressure-compensated oxygen flow-
    meter is being used to administer a mixture of 70% helium and
    30% oxygen. The flowmeter reads 10 L/min. Which of the fol-
    lowing choices represents the actual flow rate being admin-
    istered?
    A. 14 L/min
    B. 16 L/min
    C. 20 L/min
    D. 18 L/min
    E. 22 L/min
    (3:483) (4:78)

    70:30 = 1.6 times more diffusable

3. The respiratory therapy practitioner is administering oxygen
    through a properly calibrated backpressure-compensated Thorpe
    tube type flowmeter that reads 15 L/min. If the wall pressure is
    30 psig, what is the actual delivered flow rate?
    A. 6 L/min
    B. 12 L/min
    C. 9 L/min
    D. 8 L/min
    E. 10 L/min
    (69)

4. The respiratory therapy practitioner is administering oxygen
    through a properly calibrated backpressure-compensated flow-
    meter that reads 10 L/min. If the wall pressure is 65 psig, what is
    the actual delivered flow rate?
    A. 13 L/min
    B. 15 L/min
    C. 8 L/min
    D. 7 L/min
    E. 6 L/min
    (69)

H. Unusual Atmosphere Calculation Pretest

Questions in this category are designed to assess the candidate's ability
to apply his/her knowledge of medical gas therapy and respiratory physiology to patient care situations that involve unusual atmospheric conditions. The most common example of this occurs during the administration of hyperbaric medicine.

The following pretest was developed to help the candidate become
proficient in this area.

1. Which of the following choices most accurately represents the
    barometric pressure exerted on a diver who is submerged to a
    depth of 100 feet?
    A. One atmosphere
    B. Two atmospheres

    C.   Three atmospheres
    D.   Four atmospheres
    E.   Five atmospheres
      (3:706)

2.   Given a sample of gas under the following conditions, what is the partial pressure of oxygen (P sample O_2) of the gas?

P_B	2.0 atmospheres
FI_{O_2}	0.21
P_{H_2O}	47 mm Hg

    A.   340 mm Hg
    B.   310 mm Hg
    C.   280 mm Hg
    D.   420 mm Hg
    E.   330 mm Hg
      (3:706)

3.   A patient is in a hyperbaric chamber breathing 100% O_2 at 1.5 atmospheres. If his Pa_{CO_2} is 40 mm Hg and his respiratory exchange ratio is 0.8, which of the following most closely approximates this patient's P_{AO_2}?
    A.   1420 mm Hg
    B.   1660 mm Hg
    C.   1050 mm Hg
    D.   1010 mm Hg
    E.   1130 mm Hg
      (3:706) (2:235)

Part II
Humidity and Aerosol Therapy Calculations

Contents

A. Terminology Pretest

Questions in this category are designed to assess the practitioner's understanding of medical and scientific terms and symbols that are fundamental to the study of aerosol and humidity therapy.

The following pretest was developed to help the candidate become proficient in this area.

1. Which of the following sets of conditions are represented by the term STPD?
    I. $273°$ Absolute; one atmosphere; $P_{H_2O} = 0$ mm Hg
    II. $0°$ Centigrade; 1034 cm H_2O; $P_{H_2O} = 0$ mm Hg
    III. $459°$ Kelvin; 760 mm Hg; $P_{H_2O} = 0$ mm Hg
    IV. $0°$ Centigrade; 760 mm Hg; $P_{H_2O} = 0$ mm Hg
    V. $273°$ Kelvin; 760 mm Hg; $P_{H_2O} = 0$ mm Hg
        A. I, II, III, IV, and V
        B. II, III, IV, and V
        C. I, II, IV, and V
        D. I, II, III, and V
        E. I, II, III, and IV
    (9:14–19) (3:Chap 1)

37

2. Which of the following sets of conditions best represents the term *ATPD?*
    A. Ambient temperature; ambient pressure; $P_{H_2O} = 47$ mm Hg
    B. Ambient temperature; ambient pressure; $P_{H_2O} = 0$ mm Hg
    C. Ambient temperature; $P_B = 713$ mm Hg; $P_{H_2O} = 0$ mm Hg
    D. Body temperature; ambient pressure; $P_{H_2O} = 0$ mm Hg
    E. B and C are correct.
    (3:Chap 1)

3. Which of the following sets of conditions are represented by the term *ATPS?*
    A. Ambient temperature; ambient pressure; $P_{H_2O} = 47$ mm Hg
    B. Ambient temperature; ambient pressure; $P_{H_2O} = 0$ mm Hg
    C. Ambient temperature; ambient pressure; 100% relative humidity
    D. Ambient temperature; ambient pressure; $P_{H_2O} = 44$ mm Hg
    E. Ambient temperature; $P_B = 760$ mm Hg; $P_{H_2O} = 0$ mm Hg
    (3:Chap 1)

4. Which of the following sets of conditions are represented by the term *BTPD?*
    A. 310° Kelvin; ambient pressure; $P_{H_2O} = 47$ mm Hg
    B. 273° Centigrade; ambient pressure; $P_{H_2O} = 0$ mm Hg
    C. 37° Centigrade; ambient pressure; $P_{H_2O} = 0$ mm Hg
    D. Ambient temperature; ambient pressure; $P_{H_2O} = 0$ mm Hg
    E. A and C are correct.
    (3:Chap 1)

5. Which of the following sets of conditions are represented by the term *BTPS?*
    A. 37° Centigrade; ambient pressure; $P_{H_2O} = 47$ mm Hg
    B. 273° Kelvin; 760 mm Hg; $P_{H_2O} = 47$ mm Hg
    C. 273° Kelvin; ambient pressure; 100% body humidity
    D. All of the above
    E. A and C are correct.
    (3:Chap 1)

6. What is the water vapor tension of a sample of alveolar gas at BTPS?
    A. 44 mm Hg
    B. 47 mm Hg
    C. 37 mm Hg
    D. 101 mm Hg
    E. 52 mm Hg
    (1:165) (2:Chap 17)

7. Under the following conditions, what is the water vapor tension of a normothermic patient's alveolar gas?

P_B	390 mm Hg
FI_{O_2}	0.90
Pa_{CO_2}	65 mm Hg

PART II

A.   47 mm Hg
B.   44 mm Hg
C.   37 mm Hg
D.   100 mm Hg
E.   12 mm Hg
   (1:165) (2:Chap 17)

8. Which of the following accurately describe alveolar gas?
   I. P_{H_2O} = 44 mm Hg
   II.   Absolute humidity = 44 mg/L
   III. Relative humidity = 100%
   IV.   Percent body humidity = 100%
   V.   Water vapor density = 47 mg/L
   VI.   Exists at BTPS
     A.   I, II, III, IV, and V
     B.   II, III, IV, V, and VI
     C.   I, II, IV, V, and VI
     D.   II, III, IV, and VI
     E.   I, II, III, IV, V, and VI
  (1:165)

B. Absolute Humidity Pretest

Questions in this category are designed to assess the candidate's understanding of the concepts of absolute humidity. Absolute humidity is defined as the quantity of water vapor actually present in a gas sample. In human physiology this content is usually expressed in milligrams per liter (mg/L).

The following pretest was developed to help the candidate become proficient in this area.

1. Which of the following values represents the absolute humidity of a liter of gas at BTPS?
  A.   44 mg/L
  B.   47 mg/L
  C.   100 mg/L
  D.   37 g/L
  E.   310 g/L
   (2:Chap 17) (1:164–166)

2. A normothermic 100-kg patient is on a volume ventilator with a V_T of 850 mL. The FI_{O_2} is 45% and the P_B is 660 mm Hg. For this patient the absolute humidity of a liter of alveolar gas is represented most accurately by which of the following choices?
  A.   24 mg/L
  B.   44 mg/L
  C.   12 mg/L
  D.   38 mg/L
  E.   47 mg/L
   (2:Chap 17) (1:164–166)

Part II

3. What is the absolute humidity of a liter of gas that exists at condition of STPD? @ 0°C
   A. 37 mg/L
   B. 47 mg/L
   C. 44 mg/L
   D. 0.0 mg/L
   E. 97.5 mg/L
   (1:164–166) (2:Chap 17)

C. Percent Relative Humidity Pretest

Questions in this category are designed to assess the candidate's understanding of the concept of relative humidity. Relative humidity is defined as the degree to which a sample of gas is saturated with water expressed as a percent. This definition can be written algebraically as follows:

$$\text{Relative Humidity} = \frac{\text{Sample Absolute Humidity in mg/L}}{\text{Sample Water Vapor Capacity in mg/L}} \times 100$$

It is also helpful for the candidate to remember that a liter of alveolar gas is capable of holding 44 mg of water vapor when 100% saturated. at 37°C

The following pretest was developed to help the candidate become proficient in this area.

1. Calculate the relative humidity of a liter of gas under the following conditions:

Absolute humidity	31 mg/L
Temperature	37°C

   Which of the following choices most accurately represents this value?
   A. 30%
   B. 40%
   C. 50%
   D. 70%
   E. 100%
   (2:Chap 17) (1:164–166)

2. Calculate the relative humidity of a liter of sample gas under the following conditions:

Absolute humidity	9 mg/L
Temperature	310°K

   Which of the following choices most accurately represents this value?
   A. 15%
   B. 20%
   C. 28%
   D. 33%
   E. 50%
   (2:Chap 17) (1:164–166)

3. If a gas is capable of holding 28 mg H_2O/L when it is fully satu-
   rated, calculate the relative humidity if the absolute humidity is 4
   mg/L.
   A.   23%
   B.   10%
   C.   29%
   D.   15%
   E.   17%
   (2:Chap 17) (1:164–166)

   $\frac{4}{28} = 14\%$
   .14285 ≈ 15%

D. Percent Body Humidity Pretest

Questions in this category are designed to assess the candidate's
understanding of the concept of percent body humidity. The term *percent
body humidity* is used to describe gases being delivered during aerosol and
humidity therapy. The water vapor content of these gases is expressed as
a percentage of the water vapor content of gases at BTPS, such as alveolar gas. This definition can be written algebraically as follows:

$$\text{Percent Body Humidity} = \frac{\text{Sample Gas Absolute Humidity in mg/L}}{44 \text{ mg/L}} \times 100$$

Forty-four milligrams per liter, of course, is the absolute humidity of a
gas at BTPS.
The following pretest was developed to help the candidate become
proficient in this area.

1. Which of the following most accurately represents the percent
   body humidity of a sample of gas with an absolute humidity of 14
   mg/L?
   A.   25%
   B.   32%
   C.   40%
   D.   14%
   E.   30%
   (2:Chap 17) (1:164–166)

2. Which of the following choices represents the percent body
   humidity of a sample of gas at body temperature (37°C) with a
   relative humidity of 50%?
   A.   50%
   B.   45%
   C.   30%
   D.   20%
   E.   44%
   (2:Chap 17) (1:164–166)

E. Humidity Deficit Pretest

Questions in this category are designed to assess the candidate's understanding of the concept of humidity deficit. The term *humidity deficit* is defined as the absolute humidity of alveolar gas (44 mg/L) minus the absolute humidity of the inspired gases. This can be written algebraically as follows:

$$\text{Humidity Deficit in mg/L} = \left(\begin{array}{c} \text{Absolute Humidity} \\ \text{of Alveolar Gas} \\ \text{(44 mg/L)} \end{array} \right) - \left(\begin{array}{c} \text{Absolute Humidity} \\ \text{of Inspired Gas} \end{array} \right)$$

The following pretest was developed to help the candidate become proficient in this area.

1. Which of the following most accurately represents the humidity deficit if the patient is breathing gas with an H_2O content of 23 mg/L?
    A.   19 mg/L
    B.   24 mg/L
    C.   17 mg/L
    D.   26 mg/L
    E.   21 mg/L
    (2:Chap 17) (1:164–166)

2. Which of the following most accurately represents the humidity deficit of a patient who is breathing medical gas with a percent body humidity of 65%?
    A.   30 mg/L
    B.   19 mg/L
    C.   25 mg/L
    D.   15 mg/L
    E.   6 mg/L
    (2:Chap 17) (1:164–166)

Part III
Calculations Used in Continuous Ventilatory Support

Contents

A. The Flow Rate Formula Pretest

Few equations or calculations are as fundamental to the practice of respiratory therapy as the flow rate formula. Continuous ventilatory support cannot be administered intelligently without a thorough understanding of the concepts embodied in this formula:

$$\text{Flow Rate (L/sec)} = \frac{\text{Tidal Volume (L)}}{\text{Inspiratory Time (sec)}}$$

This formula will yield a flow rate in liters per second (L/sec). Should the practitioner desire this value in the more commonly used units of liters per minute, the original value must be multiplied by the factor 60 sec/min. As an example, a flow rate of 1 L/sec when multiplied by this factor yields the value 60 L/min.

The above formula, when manipulated algebraically to solve for the other two variables, yields the following forms:

$$\text{Tidal Volume} = (\text{Flow Rate})(\text{Inspiratory Time})$$

and

43

$$\text{Inspiratory Time} = \frac{\text{Tidal Volume}}{\text{Flow Rate}}$$

The following pretest was developed to help the candidate become proficient at the above calculations and techniques.

1. The respiratory therapy practitioner is using a volume-cycled constant flow generator in the intensive care unit. If the ventilator routinely delivers 850 cc of gas in 0.65 seconds, which of the following most accurately represents the average inspiratory flow rate?
   A.   1.3 L/sec
   B.   60 L/min
   C.   78 L/min
   D.   54 L/min
   E.   A and C are correct.
   (39:16–21) (81:Chap 1) (4:230)

2. A volume-cycled ventilator is delivering a tidal volume of 500 cc with an inspiratory time of 1.1 seconds. Based on this information, which of the following most accurately represents the ventilator's average inspiratory flow rate?
   A.   20 L/min
   B.   25 L/min
   C.   42 L/min
   D.   27 L/min
   E.   35 L/min
   (39:16–21) (81:Chap 1) (4:230)

3. A tidal volume of 75 cc is delivered over a 0.6-second inspiratory time. Which of the following is the average inspiratory flow rate?
   A.   75 mL/sec
   B.   7.5 L/min
   C.   150 mL/sec
   D.   750 mL/sec
   E.   75 L/min
   (39:16–21) (4:230) (81:Chap 1)

4. The inspiratory time for a volume-cycled ventilator with a flow rate of 500 mL/sec and a tidal volume of 650 cc is represented by which of the following choices?
   A.   1.3 seconds
   B.   1.2 seconds
   C.   3.2 seconds
   D.   1.0 seconds
   E.   1.1 seconds
   (4:230) (81:Chap 1)

5. Given a tidal volume of 950 cc and a flow rate of 35 L/min, the inspiratory time will be approximately:
   A.   2.1 seconds
   B.   1.8 seconds
   C.   3.1 seconds

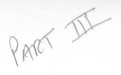

D.   1.7 seconds
E.   1.6 seconds
   (4:230) (81:Chap 1)

6.   Given a mean flow rate of 50 L/min and an inspiratory time of 1.2 seconds, the approximate tidal volume is represented by which of the following choices?
A.   1.0 liter
B.   1.1 liters
C.   830 cc
D.   1.2 liters
E.   900 cc
   (81:Chap 1) (4:230)

B. I:E Ratio Pretest

Questions in this category are designed to assess the candidate's ability to calculate the I:E ratio of a patient receiving continuous ventilatory support. Probably the simplest and most versatile formula for determining this is as follows:

$$(I + E) = \frac{\text{Inspiratory Flow Rate (L/min)}}{\text{Minute Ventilation (L/min)}}$$

What this formula states is that the numerical total of the inspiratory and expiratory ratio numbers is equal to the patient's minute ventilation divided by the average inspiratory flow rate. This is noted in the example below:

$$\frac{\text{Flow Rate} = 60 \text{ L/min}}{\text{Minute Ventilation} = 20 \text{ L/min}} = 3 = \text{I:E Ratio of 1:2}$$

Since only an I:E ratio of 1:2 has a numerical sum of 3, the correct answer can easily be determined. *From this equation, it can be seen that to obtain an I:E of 1:2, the patient's average inspiratory flow rate must be three times his mechanical minute volume.* By the same token, a flow rate four times the minute volume will yield a 1:3 ratio.

It is often useful to manipulate this formula to solve for other unknowns. These formulas are as follows:

$$\text{Flow Rate} = (\text{Minute Ventilation}) (I + E)$$
and
$$\text{Minute Ventilation} = \frac{\text{Flow Rate}}{(I + E)}$$

The following pretest was developed to help the candidate become proficient in the above calculations and techniques.

1.   What is the I:E ratio if the flow rate is 60 L/min and the minute ventilation is 20 L/min?
A.   1:1
B.   1:3
C.   1:2

    D. 1:4
    E. 2:1
      (4:230) (81:Chap 1) (72)

2. Which of the following most accurately represents the I:E ratio given a tidal volume of 1100 cc, a respiratory rate of 13/min, and an inspiratory flow rate of 40 L/min?
    A. 1:2.6
    B. 1:3.2   min. Vent $= RR \times V_T$
    C. 1:2.3
    D. 1:2.1
    E. 1:1.8
      (4:230) (81:Chap 1) (72)

3. What is the I:E ratio if the V_T is 25 mL, the respiratory rate is 42/min, and the flow rate is 75 mL/sec?   .025 ℓ
    A. 1:2.8 $75 \times 60 =$ ml/min $\to .075 \times 60 = 4.5$
    B. 1:2.6   ℓ/m
    C. 1:2.4
    D. 1:3.3
    E. 1:2.9
      (4:230) (81:Chap 1) (72)

4. What is the mean inspiratory flow rate necessary to maintain an I:E ratio of 1:2 if the tidal volume is 800 mL and the respiratory rate is 23/min?
    A. 50 L/min
    B. 55 L/min
    C. 32 L/min
    D. 60 L/min
    E. 80 L/min
      (39:16–21) (4:230) (81:Chap 1) (72)

5. What is the mean inspiratory flow rate necessary to maintain an I:E ratio of 1:3 if the ventilator's tidal volume is 300 cc and the respiratory rate is 33/min?
    A. 15 L/min
    B. 25 L/min
    C. 40 L/min
    D. 55 L/min
    E. 79 L/min
      (72) (81:Chap 1) (39:16–21)

6. The neonatologist asks the respiratory therapy practitioner to set up high-frequency ventilation on a 1100-g infant with severe infant respiratory distress syndrome. He wants a respiratory rate of 150/min and an inspiratory time of 0.20 second. What will the I:E ratio be under those circumstances?
    A. 1:1
    B. 1:0.5
    C. 1:1.5
    D. 1:1.2
    E. 1:1.3
      (4:230) (81:Chap 1) (72)

C. Corrected Tidal Volume and System Compliance Pretest

Questions in this category are designed to assess the candidate's ability to determine the actual or corrected tidal volume being delivered to the patient during the administration of continuous ventilatory support. The formula for corrected tidal volume is as follows:

$$\text{Patient's Corrected Tidal Volume} = \left(\begin{array}{c}\text{Ventilator}\\\text{Exhaled}\\\text{Tidal Volume}\end{array}\right) - \left(\begin{array}{c}\text{Compressed}\\\text{Volume}\end{array}\right)$$

Thus, the actual tidal volume received by the patient is equal to that volume delivered by the ventilator (preferably measured at the exhalation port) minus the volume compressed in the ventilator external tubing and humidifier system. To determine the compressed volume, the following formula must be used:

$$\overset{E\,\dot{V}_T}{\text{Compressed Volume (cc)}} = \left(\begin{array}{c}\text{Corrected Peak}\\\text{Pressure (cm } H_2O)\end{array}\right)\left(\begin{array}{c}\text{System Compliance}\\\text{Factor (cc/cm } H_2O)\end{array}\right)$$

There is a variation to this formula that is used whenever the practitioner is calculating the patient's effective static compliance (ESC). In this case, since pressure is measured during intervals of no gas flow, the patient's plateau pressure is substituted for the peak pressure as follows:

$$\overset{E\,\dot{V}_T}{\text{Compressed Volume (cc)}} = \left(\begin{array}{c}\text{Corrected Plateau}\\\text{Pressure (cm } H_2O)\end{array}\right)\left(\begin{array}{c}\overset{\text{TUBING}}{\text{System Compliance}}\\\text{Factor (cc/cm } H_2O)\end{array}\right)$$

It must be emphasized that for these and all other ventilator calculations, peak and plateau pressure measurements must be PEEP corrected if they are to be 100% accurate. Subtract

The system compliance noted above is frequently assumed to be 3.0 cc/cm H_2O and 1.0 cc/cm H_2O for adult and neonatal systems, respectively. This value can and, particularly for neonatal circuits, should be calculated. This formula is as follows:

$$\underset{\text{TUBING}\quad\text{"}}{\text{System Compliance (cc/cm } H_2O)} = \frac{\text{Test Volume (cc)}}{\text{Plateau Pressure (cm } H_2O)}$$

These values are obtained by delivering a small test volume (usually about 200 cc for adult and 50 cc for neonatal circuits) into the ventilator system and then noting the plateau pressure obtained at this time.

The following pretest was developed to help the candidate become proficient in these calculations and techniques.

1. The respiratory therapy practitioner is asked to calculate the system compliance for a Bennett MA-I ventilator. In so doing, he obtains an inspiratory plateau pressure of 61 cm H_2O with a test volume of 200 cc. Based on this information, which of the following choices most accurately represents this ventilator's system compliance factor?

A.   2.8 cc/cm H_2O
B.   4.4 cc/cm H_2O
C.   2.3 cc/cm H_2O
D.   3.0 cc/cm H_2O
E.   3.3 cc/cm H_2O
   (50) (70)

2. Which of the following most accurately represents the system compliance factor of a Sechrist ventilator if a plateau pressure of 56 cm H_2O is reached after delivering a flow rate of 3.0 L/min for 1 second into the ventilator system?
A.   1.25 cc/cm H_2O
B.   0.75 cc/cm H_2O
C.   0.50 cc/cm H_2O
D.   0.90 cc/cm H_2O
E.   3.0 cc/cm H_2O
   (50) (70)

50 cc/sec
56

3. What is the corrected (delivered) tidal volume if the set V_T is 890 mL, the peak pressure is 52 cm H_2O, and the tubing compliance factor is 2.1 cc/cm H_2O?
A.   900 cc
B.   830 cc
C.   740 cc
D.   780 cc
E.   760 cc
   (50) (70)

Compr. Vol = 52 × 2.1 = 109.2
890 − 109.2 = 780.8

4. Which of the following most accurately represents the corrected (delivered) tidal volume given the following conditions?

Set V_T	1100 cc
Peak pressure	73 cm H_2O
Compliance factor	3.8 cc/cm H_2O
PEEP	18 cm H_2O

A.   1030 cc
B.   890 cc
C.   930 cc
D.   845 cc
E.   742 cc
   (50) (70)

(73−18)(3.8)= 209
1100 − 209 = 891

5. Which of the following most accurately represents the corrected (delivered) tidal volume if the set V_T is 45 cc, the peak pressure is 58 cm H_2O, and the tubing compliance factor is 0.6 cc/cm H_2O?
A.   5 cc
B.   10 cc
C.   15 cc
D.   30 cc
E.   25 cc
   (50)

58 × .6 = 34.8
45 − 34.8 = 10.2

Part III

D. Effective Compliance and Resistance Pretest

Questions in this category are designed to evaluate the candidate's ability to assess pulmonary mechanics by calculating effective compliance and resistance values. The formulas for effective dynamic and static compliance are as follows:

$$\text{Effective Dynamic Compliance (EDC)} = \frac{\text{Corrected Tidal Volume (cc)}}{\text{Corrected Peak Pressure (cm } H_2O)}$$

$$\frac{EVt}{PIP} \, ?$$

and

$$\text{Effective Static Compliance (ESC)} = \frac{\text{Corrected Tidal Volume (cc)}}{\text{Corrected Plateau Pressure}}$$

$$\frac{EVt}{PLAT (PEEP)}$$

In order for these calculations to be accurate, all peak and plateau pressure measurements must be PEEP corrected. Additionally, when calculating ESC, compressed volume determinations should be performed using plateau, not peak, pressure measurements. (Please see the previous section, C, for further explanation.)

Using readily available data, the patient's effective airway resistance can be determined. The formula is as follows:

$$\text{Effective Airway Resistance (cm } H_2O/L/sec) = \frac{\text{(Proximal Airway Pressure)} - \text{(Plateau Pressure)}}{\text{Inspiratory Flow Rate (L/sec)}}$$

$$\frac{PIP - PLAT}{V}$$

This formula recognizes that the gradient between proximal and plateau pressures is due to nonelastic or "airway" resistance to gas flow. Widening of this gradient most typically occurs during episodes of bronchospasm or when excessive secretions accumulate in the airways.

The following pretest was developed to help the candidate become proficient in these calculations and techniques.

1. Which of the following choices most accurately represents a patient's effective dynamic compliance if the corrected tidal volume is 730 cc, the peak pressure is 38 cm H_2O, and the ventilator plateau pressure is 23 cm H_2O?
    A.   19 cc/cm H_2O
    B.   45 cc/cm H_2O
    C.   12 cc/cm H_2O
    D.   74 cc/cm H_2O
    E.   32 cc/cm H_2O
    (50) (2:222–226)

2. What is the effective static compliance if the corrected tidal volume is 620 mL, the ventilator plateau pressure is 42 cm H_2O, and the peak pressure is 59 cm H_2O?
    A.   28 cc/cm H_2O
    B.   39 cc/cm H_2O
    C.   10 cc/cm H_2O

    D.   22 cc/cm H_2O
    E.   15 cc/cm H_2O
    (50) (2:222–226)

3.   What is the effective static compliance if the corrected tidal volume is 880 mL, the ventilator plateau pressure is 53 cm H_2O, the peak pressure is 62 cm H_2O, and the patient is on 14 cm H_2O of PEEP?
    A.   47 cc/cm H_2O
    B.   17 cc/cm H_2O
    C.   23 cc/cm H_2O
    D.   12 cc/cm H_2O
    E.   29 cc/cm H_2O
    (50) (2:222–226)

4.   What is the effective static compliance if the plateau pressure is 56 cm H_2O, the system compliance factor is 4.2 cc/cm H_2O, and the uncorrected tidal volume is 1200 cc?
    A.   32 cc/cm H_2O
    B.   17 cc/cm H_2O
    C.   21 cc/cm H_2O
    D.   48 cc/cm H_2O
    E.   11 cc/cm H_2O
    (50) (2:222–226)

5.   Which of the following choices most accurately represents a patient's effective static compliance under the following clinical conditions?

Uncorrected tidal volume	920 cc
System compliance factor	2.4 cc/cm H_2O
Plateau pressure	44 cm H_2O
PEEP	16 cm H_2O

    A.   20 cc/cm H_2O
    B.   25 cc/cm H_2O
    C.   30 cc/cm H_2O
    D.   42 cc/cm H_2O
    E.   35 cc/cm H_2O
    (50) (2:222–226)

6.   Which of the following choices most accurately represents a patient's effective airway resistance under the following clinical conditions?

Corrected tidal volume	1.0 L
Proximal airway (peak) pressure	45 cm H_2O
Plateau pressure	33 cm H_2O
Mean inspiratory flow rate	60 L/min

A. 4 cm $H_2O/L/sec$
B. 8 cm $H_2O/L/sec$
C. 12 cm $H_2O/L/sec$
D. 14 cm $H_2O/L/sec$
E. 18 cm $H_2O/L/sec$
    (70)

7. Which of the following choices most accurately represents a patient's effective airway resistance under the following conditions?

Corrected tidal volume	700 cc
Proximal airway (peak) pressure	58 cm H_2O
Plateau pressure	47 cm H_2O
Mean inspiratory flow rate	35 L/min
PEEP	12 cm H_2O

not PEEP compensate ?!

A. 19 cm $H_2O/L/sec$
B. 12 cm $H_2O/L/sec$
C. 24 cm $H_2O/L/sec$
D. 6 cm $H_2O/L/sec$
E. 34 cm $H_2O/L/sec$
    (70)

PART III

E. PEEP Compliance Study Pretest

In the absence of cardiac output and other determinations only possible in patients whose pulmonary arteries have been catheterized, serial measurement of effective static compliance at different levels of PEEP is thought to be an effective method for determining the most appropriate dosage of this modality. The preferred level of PEEP is that which yields the highest effective static compliance.

The following pretest was developed to help the candidate become proficient in this technique.

1. The respiratory therapy practitioner is asked to place a patient on the lowest level of PEEP that yields the highest effective static compliance. After calculating the corrected tidal volume, which was adjusted to remain constant during this study, the following data were collected:

Level of PEEP (cm H_2O)	Plateau Pressure (cm H_2O)
3	34 = 31
6	35 = 29
9	37 = 28
12	41 = 29
15	45 = 30
18	49 = 31

Based on the above data, the preferred level of PEEP is:
A.   6 cm H_2O
B.   9 cm H_2O
C.   12 cm H_2O
D.   15 cm H_2O
E.   18 cm H_2O
   (47)

2.   The respiratory therapy practitioner is monitoring a 45-kg patient in the intensive care unit who is receiving continuous ventilatory support by way of a Servo 900 C ventilator. The patient's pulmonary wedge pressure (PWP) has risen rapidly over the past hour and is now 34 mm Hg. At this time the following clinical data are collected:

Pa_{O_2}	45 mm Hg
$S\bar{v}_{O_2}$	50%
$C(a-\bar{v})_{O_2}$	6.8 vol%
Peak pressure	48 cm H_2O
Plateau pressure	42 cm H_2O
PEEP	0 cm H_2O

Based on this information, the practitioner is asked to place the patient on the lowest level of PEEP that corresponds to the patient's highest effective static compliance. In so doing, the following data are collected:

Corrected Tidal Volume (cc)	Level of PEEP (cm H_2O)	Plateau Pressure (cm H_2O)	
550	0	42	13.1
550	3	44	13.4
550	6	45	14.1
550	9	47	14.5
550	12	48	15.28
550	15	49	16.2
550	18	54	15.27
550	21	58	14.9

Based on the above information, at which of the following levels of PEEP is the patient's effective static compliance highest?
A.   9 cm H_2O
B.   12 cm H_2O
C.   15 cm H_2O
D.   18 cm H_2O
E.   21 cm H_2O
   (47)

$$\frac{550}{PLAT - PEEP}$$

Part IV
Calculations Used to Assess Cardiopulmonary Status

Contents

A. Alveolar Ventilation Pretest

Because ventilation and oxygenation are the two major functions of the body's pulmonary system, few concepts are more fundamental than those of tidal, alveolar, and deadspace ventilation. Their relationship is expressed in the following formula:

$$V_A = V_T - V_D$$

53

This equation can also be rearranged so the practitioner can solve for the other two variables, as follows:

$$V_T = V_A + V_D$$
$$V_D = V_T - V_A$$

By inserting the patient's respiratory rate into these formulas, the values for minute alveolar ($\dot{V}_A$), deadspace ($\dot{V}_D$), and total minute ventilation ($\dot{V}_E$) can be determined.

The following pretest was developed to help the candidate become proficient in these calculations.

1. What is the alveolar ventilation under the following conditions?

V_T	950 cc
V_D	180 cc

    A. 490 cc
    B. 770 cc
    C. 560 cc
    D. 680 cc
    E. 720 cc
    (18:16–17) (7:72) (2:217–218)

2. What is the minute alveolar ventilation ($\dot{V}_A$) given the following conditions?

V_T	820 cc
V_D	230 cc
Respiratory rate	17/min

    A. 13.5 L/min
    B. 12.6 L/min
    C. 9.3 L/min
    D. 10.0 L/min
    E. 14.2 L/min
    (18:16–17) (7:72) (2:217–218)

    $820-230 = 590 \times 17$
    $\overline{1000}$

3. What is the minute deadspace ventilation ($\dot{V}_D$) given the following conditions?

V_A	260 mL
V_T	420 mL
Respiratory rate	42/min

    A. 1.4 L
    B. 10.3 L
    C. 5.9 L
    D. 7.6 L
    E. 6.7 L
    (2:217–218) (18:16–17) (7:72)

B. V_D/V_T Calculation Pretest

Questions in this category are designed to assess the candidate's ability to calculate and use the deadspace to tidal volume ratio (V_D/V_T). This value is most frequently determined by using the Enghoff modification to the Bohr equation. This formula is as follows:

$$V_D/V_T = \frac{Pa_{CO_2} - P\bar{E}_{CO_2}}{Pa_{CO_2}}$$

This value is readily determined at the patient's bedside by simultaneously obtaining samples of arterial blood and mixed expired gas and measuring their carbon dioxide tensions.

An application of the V_D/V_T relationship is its use in determining alveolar and physiologic deadspace ventilation by use of the following formulas:

$$V_A = (V_T)(1 - V_D/V_T)$$

and

$$V_D = (V_T)(V_D/V_T)$$

The following pretest was developed to help the candidate become proficient in these calculations.

1. The respiratory therapy practitioner is asked to calculate the V_D/V_T of a patient whose Pa_{CO_2} is 53 mm Hg and whose mixed expired carbon dioxide tension ($P\bar{E}_{CO_2}$) is 31 mm Hg. Which of the following choices most accurately represents this value?
    A. 0.42
    B. 0.53
    C. 0.67
    D. 0.37
    E. 0.32
       (2:217–218) (18:19–21)

2. The respiratory therapy practitioner is asked to determine the V_D/V_T given the following clinical data:

Pa_{CO_2}	40 mm Hg
$P\bar{E}_{CO_2}$	28 mm Hg

    A. 0.75
    B. 0.67
    C. 0.30
    D. 0.25
    E. 0.39
       (2:217–218) (18:19–21)

3. What is the V_D/V_T given the following conditions?

Pa_{CO_2}	85 mm Hg
$P\bar{E}_{CO_2}$	33 mm Hg

A. 0.46
B. 0.61
C. 0.29
D. 0.73
E. 0.87
    (2:217–218) (18:19–21)

4. Given the following clinical conditions, calculate the minute alve-
    olar ventilation ($\dot{V}_A$) for a patient who is receiving 50% oxygen by
    way of a T tube setup.

V_T	830 cc	$(.830)(1-.45)(27)$
Respiratory rate	27/min	
V_D/V_T	0.45	

Which of the following is the correct choice?
A. 10.1 L/min
B. 14.6 L/min
C. 12.3 L/min
D. 14.3 L/min
E. 9.4 L/min
    (18:16–17) (5:74–75) (2:217–218)

5. What is the minute alveolar ventilation ($\dot{V}_A$) given the following
    conditions?

V_T	1130 cc	or $1.13\ \ell$
Respiratory rate	29/min	
V_D/V_T	0.74	

A. 8.5 L/min
B. 4.7 L/min
C. 9.3 L/min
D. 12.4 L/min
E. 5.1 L/min
    (18:16–17) (2:217–218) (3:119–120)

$$\dot{V}_A = (V_T)(1 - V_D/V_T)$$
$$(1130)(.26) = 0.29 \times 29 = 8.5$$

C. Oxygen Content Calculation Pretest

Questions in this category are designed to assess the candidate's ability
to calculate the content of oxygen in samples of arterial and/or venous
blood. To do this the practitioner must remember that the total amount
of oxygen in any given sample of blood is equal to the sum of the quantity of oxygen combined with hemoglobin and the quantity of oxygen
dissolved in the plasma. This concept is represented by the following
formula:

PART IV *(handwritten)*

DISSOLVED IN (handwritten)

$$\text{Content O}_2 \text{ in Blood (CO}_2) = \left(\begin{array}{c}\text{Hemoglobin}\\\text{Concentration}\end{array}\right)(1.34)\left(\begin{array}{c}\text{Hemoglobin}\\\text{Saturation}\end{array}\right) + \left(\begin{array}{c}\text{DISSOLVED IN}\\\text{PLASMA}\\(P_{O_2})(0.003)\end{array}\right)$$

Of course, an oxygen carrying factor of 1.39 mL O_2/g Hb may be used when appropriate.

The following pretest was developed to help the candidate become proficient in this calculation.

assume fully saturated? (handwritten)

1. Which of the following choices most accurately represents the content of oxygen dissolved in the plasma of a patient whose Pa_{O_2} is 570 mm Hg?

    (15%)(1.34)(1.0) + (570)(.003)) ⟹ 1.71 (handwritten)

    A. 1.7 vol%
    B. 2.4 vol%   *do we omit this part (handwritten)*
    C. 1.9 vol%   *of the equation? yes becuz (handwritten)*
    D. 7.1 vol%   *the question asked for content in plasma (handwritten)*
    E. 1.5 vol%   *P.168 - S table 11-3 (handwritten)*

    Sh.- (1:~~123-125~~) (5:82–83) (2:239–240)
    168 (handwritten)

2. The respiratory therapy practitioner is asked to calculate the oxygen content of the arterial blood (Ca_{O_2}) given the following clinical data:

Pa_{O_2}	61 mm Hg
Sa_{O_2}	89%
Hb concentration	13.9 g/dL
O_2 carrying capacity	1.34 mL O_2/g Hb *(1.39)*

    Which of the following most correctly represents this value?
    A. 16.8 vol%   *(13.9)(1.34)(.89) + (61 × .003) (handwritten)*
    B. 17.9 vol%   *= 16.58   +   .183 (handwritten)*
    C. 13.0 vol%
    D. 17.2 vol%
    E. 17.4 vol%
    (1:123–125) (5:82–85) (2:239–240)

3. The respiratory therapy practitioner is asked to calculate the arterial oxygen content of a patient given the following clinical conditions:

Sa_{O_2}	85%
Hb concentration	22.4 g/dL
O_2 carrying capacity	1.39 mL O_2/g Hb

    Which of the following most correctly represents this value?
    A. 25.2 vol%
    B. 20.9 vol%   *Pa_{O_2}? (handwritten)*
    C. 25.9 vol%
    D. 26.6 vol%
    E. 28.4 vol%
    (1:123–125) (5:82–85) (2:239–240)

4. A severely anemic patient is receiving hyperbaric oxygen therapy. The respiratory therapy practitioner is asked to calculate this

1 atm = 760 mm Hg

patient's arterial oxygen content. Given the following clinical data, which of the following most accurately represents this value?

P_B	2.5 atmospheres *$(2.5)(760)$ = 1900 mm Hg*
$Paco_2$	35 mm Hg
$P(A-a)o_2$	240 mm Hg
Sao_2	100%
Hb concentration	3.6 g/dL
O_2 carrying capacity	1.39 mL O_2/g Hb

A. 8.1 vol%
B. 4.9 vol%
C. 5.0 vol%
D. 9.9 vol%
E. 8.6 vol%

(1:123–125) (2:239–240) (5:82–83)

D. P(A-a)o₂ Calculation Pretest

Questions in this category are designed to assess the candidate's ability to calculate the $P(A-a)o_2$. This is done by determining the alveolar oxygen tension from any one of the alveolar air equations and subtracting that value from the patient's arterial oxygen tension. This value is used to assess patient oxygenation status. In general, values greater than 40 mm Hg in patients breathing room air are an indication for oxygen administration. Values greater than 350 mm Hg in patients receiving high concentrations of oxygen indicate the presence of refractory oxygenation failure and usually require continuous ventilatory support with PEEP.

The following pretest was designed to help the candidate become proficient at this calculation.

1. Which of the following most accurately represents the $P(A-a)o_2$ for a patient on whom the following clinical data were obtained?

Pao_2	88 mm Hg
P_B	760 mm Hg
FIo_2	0.40
$Paco_2$	40 mm Hg
Respiratory exchange ratio (R)	0.8

A. 150 mm Hg
B. 175 mm Hg
C. 216 mm Hg
D. 125 mm Hg
E. 235 mm Hg

(1:118–120) (5:214–215) (3:717)

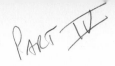

PART IV

2. Given the following clinical data, which of the following most accurately represents the $P(A-a)_{O_2}$?

Pa_{O_2}	148 mm Hg
P_B	710 mm Hg
FI_{O_2}	0.85
Pa_{CO_2}	73 mm Hg
Respiratory exchange ratio (R)	0.8

A. 285 mm Hg
B. 325 mm Hg
C. 345 mm Hg
D. 473 mm Hg
E. 360 mm Hg
   (1:118–120) (5:214–215) (3:717)

3. Given the following clinical data, which of the following most accurately represents this patient's Pa_{O_2}?

$P(A-a)_{O_2}$	486 mm Hg
FI_{O_2}	0.80
P_B	760 mm Hg
Pa_{CO_2}	40 mm Hg
Respiratory exchange ratio (R)	0.8

A. 80 mm Hg
B. 20 mm Hg
C. 35 mm Hg
D. 65 mm Hg
E. 192 mm Hg
   (1:118–120) (5:214–215) (3:717)

E. Right-to-Left Shunt (Q_S/Q_T) Equation Pretest (Advanced Level Only)

Questions in this category are designed to assess the candidate's ability to calculate Q_S/Q_T for patients receiving respiratory care. This calculation, like the alveolar air equation, may present some confusion because, as before, multiple equations exist. For an excellent discussion of the concept and clinical application of derived Q_S/Q_T values, the reader is referred to the following source:

Shapiro BA: *Clinical Application of Blood Gases,* 3rd ed, chap 18. Chicago, Year Book Medical Publishers, 1982.

In the interest of brevity and simplicity, only the two most common forms of these equations will be described here.

1. The Modified Clinical Shunt Equation
    This is probably the most familiar form of the shunt equation.
    This stems not from its clinical applicability (indeed, the reverse is
    true) but from the fact that it is the easiest to understand. This
    equation is as follows:

$$\dot{Q}_S/\dot{Q}_T = \frac{(P(A\text{-}a)o_2)\,(0.003)}{[C(a\text{-}\bar{v})o_2] + [(P(A\text{-}a)o_2)\,(.003)]}$$

For this equation to be accurate, the following limited clinical condition must be met. *The patient's hemoglobin must be 100% saturated
with oxygen.* This does not occur until the Pao_2 reaches 150 mm
Hg. It must be emphasized that this equation is accurate at *all*
FIo_2s as long as the Sao_2 is 100%. The actual clinical usefulness of
this equation is limited by the fact that the vast majority of
patients are managed at Pao_2s considerably less than 150 mm Hg.

For those clinical situations when this condition does not exist, the
practitioner will want to use the classic shunt equation described below.

2. The Classic Shunt Equation
    The advantage of this equation is considerable. *This is because it is
    accurate on all patients regardless of their FIo_2 or Pao_2.* The equation is
    also more concise as can be noted below:

$$\dot{Q}_S/\dot{Q}_T = \frac{Cc'o_2 - Cao_2}{Cc'o_2 - C\bar{v}o_2}$$

In this equation the content of oxygen in the end pulmonary capillaries ($Cc'\ o_2$) can be calculated most easily if the patient is
receiving an FIo_2 of 0.3 or greater. This oxygen concentration
should allow for a Pao_2 of greater than 150 mm Hg. The tension
of oxygen in end pulmonary capillary blood ($Pc'\ o_2$) is believed to
be equivalent to that of those ventilated alveoli they perfuse.
Thus, an $Sc'\ o_2$ of 100% can be assumed under these circumstances. When the Pao_2 is less than 150 mm Hg, the $Sc'\ o_2$ must
be determined by referring to the oxyhemoglobin dissociation
curve.

For either equation to be accurate, true mixed venous blood must be
available. Although the modified clinical shunt equation is perhaps more
frequently used, the classic version can be used on a larger patient popu-
lation. When used on identical sets of patient data, both yield the same
shunt fraction. This can be noted by solving pretest questions No. 2 and
No. 7 in this series.
The following pretest was developed to help the candidate become
proficient in these calculations and techniques.

1. The respiratory therapy practitioner is monitoring a 20-year-old
    patient in the intensive care unit who is receiving an FIo_2 of 1.0.
    A Pao_2 of 265 mm Hg and a $Paco_2$ of 40 mm Hg exist at a P_B of
    760 mm Hg. At the same time, a $C(a\text{-}\bar{v})o_2$ of 2.3 vol% is noted.

Based on this information, what is the patient's right-to-left shunt fraction (Q_S/Q_T)?

A. 39%
B. 23%
C. 30%
D. 43%
E. 34%

(5:210–224) (90:135–137)

2. Which of the following most accurately represents the percent right-to-left shunt (Q_S/Q_T) for a patient on whom the following clinical data were collected?

P_B	760 mm Hg
FI_{O_2}	1.0
Pa_{CO_2}	40 mm Hg
Pa_{O_2}	150 mm Hg — Hb sat ($S\bar{v}O_2$) 100%
Sa_{O_2}	100%
Hb concentration	15.0 g/dL
O_2 carrying capacity	1.34 mL O_2/g Hb
$C\bar{v}_{O_2}$	16.3 vol%
Respiratory exchange ratio (R)	0.8

A. 32%
B. 27%
C. 20%
D. 17%
E. 19%

(5:210–224) (90:135–137)

3. Which of the following choices most accurately represents the right-to-left shunt fraction (Q_S/Q_T) for a patient on whom the following data were collected?

Sa_{O_2}	100%
$P(A-a)_{O_2}$	500 mm Hg
$C(a-\bar{v})_{O_2}$	8.0 vol%

A. 12%
B. 19%
C. 32%
D. 47%
E. 16%

(5:210–224) (90:135–137)

4. Which of the following most accurately represents the right-to-left shunt fraction (Q_S/Q_T) for a patient on whom the following clinical data were collected?

Sa_{O_2}	100%
$P(A-a)_{O_2}$	500 mm Hg
$C(a-\bar{v})_{O_2}$	2.5 vol%

A. 34%
B. 38%
C. 29%
D. 21%
E. 46%
   (5:210–224) (90:135–137)

5. Which of the following choices most accurately represents the right-to-left shunt fraction (Q_S/Q_T) for a critically ill patient on whom the following data were collected?

Cc'_{O_2}	20.6 vol%
Ca_{O_2}	19.8 vol%
$C\bar{v}_{O_2}$	16.3 vol%

A. 10%
B. 24%
C. 38%
D. 19%
E. 14%
   (5:210–224) (90:135–137)

6. Which of the following choices most accurately represents the right-to-left shunt fraction (Q_S/Q_T) for a patient on whom the following clinical data were collected?

FI_{O_2}	0.4
P_B	760 mm Hg
P_{CO_2}	40 mm Hg
$P(A-a)_{O_2}$	175 mm Hg
Hb concentration	15.0 g/dL
Sa_{O_2}	91%
$P\bar{v}_{O_2}$	33 mm Hg
$S\bar{v}_{O_2}$	61%
O_2 carrying capacity	1.34 mL O_2/g Hb
Respiratory exchange ratio (R)	0.8

A. 27%
B. 35%
C. 21%
D. 8%
E. 44%
   (5:210–224) (90:135–137)

7. Which of the following most accurately represents the percent right-to-left shunt (Q_S/Q_T) for a patient on whom the following clinical data were collected?

P_B	760 mm Hg
Pa_{CO_2}	40 mm Hg

FI_{O_2}	1.0
Pa_{O_2}	150 mm Hg
Sa_{O_2}	100%
Hb concentration	15.0 g/dL
O_2 carrying capacity	1.34 ml O_2/g Hb
$C\bar{v}_{O_2}$	16.3 vol%
Respiratory exchange ratio (R)	0.8

A. 34%
B. 16%
C. 10%
D. 23%
E. 27%
   (5:210–214) (90:135–137)

F. a/A Ratio Pretest (Advanced Level Only)

Questions in this category are designed to assess the practitioner's ability to calculate and use the a/A ratio formula:

$$a/A \text{ Ratio} = \frac{Pa_{O_2}}{PA_{O_2}}$$

This value is used to assess patient oxygenation status. Clinically, values less than 0.60 are often believed to be an indication for oxygen administration. By the same token, values less than 0.15 are believed to indicate the presence of refractory oxygenation failure and usually the need for PEEP or CPAP therapy.

The following pretest was developed to help the candidate become proficient in the above calculations and techniques.

1. Which of the following most accurately represents a patient's a/A ratio, given the following clinical data?

P_B	760 mm Hg
P_{CO_2}	40 mm Hg
FI_{O_2}	1.0
$P(A\text{-}a)_{O_2}$	530 mm Hg
Respiratory exchange ratio (R)	0.8

A. 0.45
B. 0.20
C. 0.10
D. 0.15
E. 0.25
   (1:118–120) (5:214–215) (3:717)

2. Which of the following most accurately represents a patient's a/A ratio, given the following clinical data?

P_B	710 mm Hg
Pa_{O_2}	63 mm Hg
Pa_{CO_2}	47 mm Hg
FI_{O_2}	0.70
Respiratory exchange ratio (R)	0.8

A. 0.15
B. 0.30
C. 0.10
D. 0.25
E. 0.33
    (1:115–120) (5:214–215) (3:717)

G. Respiratory Index Pretest (Advanced Level Only)

Questions in this category are designed to assess the practitioner's ability to calculate the so-called respiratory index. The formula for this is as follows:

$$\text{Respiratory Index} = \frac{P(A\text{-}a)_{O_2}}{Pa_{O_2}}$$

This value is used to assess patient oxygenation status. Clinically, a value greater than 1.0 is often believed to be indicative for oxygen administration. By the same token, values greater than 6.0 are believed to indicate the presence of refractory hypoxemia and usually the need for PEEP or CPAP therapy.

The following pretest was developed to help the candidate become proficient in the above formulas and techniques.

1. Which of the following choices most accurately represents a patient's respiratory index, given the following clinical data?

Pa_{O_2}	85 mm Hg
Pa_{CO_2}	50 mm Hg
Respiratory exchange ratio (R)	0.8
FI_{O_2}	0.45
P_B	760 mm Hg

A. 1.8
B. 2.0
C. 2.2
D. 2.4
E. 3.1
    (102)

2. Which of the following choices most accurately represents a patient's respiratory index, given the following clinical data?

Pa_{O_2}	45 mm Hg
Pa_{CO_2}	65 mm Hg
Respiratory exchange ratio (R)	0.8
FI_{O_2}	0.8
P_B	760 mm Hg

A. 3.0
B. 4.2
C. 5.3
D. 7.8
E. 9.9
   (102)

H. $C(a-\bar{v})_{O_2}$ Pretest (Advanced Level Only)

Questions in this category are designed to assess the practitioner's ability to calculate the arterial minus venous oxygen content difference $(C(a-\bar{v})_{O_2})$. To determine this value, clinically the practitioner must have access to mixed venous blood from the pulmonary artery as well as an arterial sample. This value is used to assess cardiovascular reserves and, of course, is a necessary part of the shunt equations. Among critically ill patients whose oxygen consumption is within normal limits *and* who have minimal peripheral arteriovenous shunting, $C(a-\bar{v})_{O_2}$ values less than 4.0 vol% generally indicate the existence of good cardiovascular reserves whereas values greater than 6.0 vol% are believed to indicate poor cardiovascular reserves.

The following pretest was developed to help the candidate become proficient in calculating this value.

1. The respiratory therapy practitioner is monitoring a patient who is receiving continuous ventilatory support by way of a Servo 900 B ventilator. The following clinical data are obtained at this time from properly functioning central arterial and peripheral arterial lines:

Parameter	Arterial	Mixed Venous
P_{O_2}	53 mm Hg	29 mm Hg
S_{O_2}	85%	61%
Hb	9.7 g/dL	9.7 g/dL

Based on the above information, which of the following most accurately represents this patient's $C(a-\bar{v})_{O_2}$ (use an O_2 carrying capacity of 1.34 mL O_2/g Hb)?
A. 4.6 vol%
B. 1.9 vol%
C. 2.8 vol%
D. 3.6 vol%
E. 3.2 vol%
   (1:123–125) (5:82–85) (2:239–240)

2. Which of the following choices most accurately represents the $C(a-\bar{v})_{O_2}$ for a patient on whom the following clinical data are collected?

Pa_{O_2}	46 mm Hg
Sa_{O_2}	80%
Hb concentration	19.1 g/dL
$P\bar{v}_{O_2}$	26 mm Hg
$S\bar{v}_{O_2}$	49%
O_2 carrying capacity	1.34 mL O_2/g Hb

A. 4.7 vol%
B. 9.2 vol%
C. 1.6 vol%
D. 7.3 vol%
E. 8.0 vol%
   (1:123–125) (5:82–85) (2:239–240)

3. Which of the following choices most accurately represents the $C(a-\bar{v})_{O_2}$ for a patient on whom the following clinical data are collected?

Pa_{O_2}	235 mm Hg
Sa_{O_2}	100%
Hb concentration	22.3 g/dL
$P\bar{v}_{O_2}$	45 mm Hg
$S\bar{v}_{O_2}$	76%
Pa_{CO_2}	29 mm Hg
P_B	745 mm Hg
FI_{O_2}	0.8
O_2 carrying capacity	1.34 mL O_2/g Hb

A. 7.8 vol%
B. 6.7 vol%
C. 4.9 vol%
D. 5.2 vol%
E. 6.1 vol%
   (1:121–125) (5:82–85) (2:239–240)

I. Fick Equation Pretest (Advanced Level Only)

Questions in this category are designed to assess the practitioner's ability to perform hemodynamic calculations using the Fick equation. This equation is as follows:

$$\text{Oxygen Consumption} = (\text{Cardiac Output})\,(C(a\text{-}\bar{v})o_2)$$

The units for this equation are as follows:

$$\frac{\text{mL Oxygen}}{\text{min}} = \left(\frac{\text{mL Blood}}{\text{min}}\right)\left(\frac{\text{mL Oxygen}}{100\text{ mL Blood}}\right)$$

Thus, in a healthy, resting subject:

$$\frac{250\text{ mL Oxygen}}{\text{min}} = \left(\frac{5000\text{ mL Blood}}{\text{min}}\right)\left(\frac{5.0\text{ mL Oxygen}}{100\text{ mL Blood}}\right)$$

This equation can be rearranged to solve for cardiac output and $C(a\text{-}\bar{v})o_2$ as follows:

$$\text{Cardiac Output} = \frac{\text{Oxygen Consumption}}{C(a\text{-}\bar{v})o_2}$$

and

$$C(a\text{-}\bar{v})o_2 = \frac{\text{Oxygen Consumption}}{\text{Cardiac Output}}$$

The following pretest was developed to help the candidate become proficient in these calculations.

1. Given the following clinical data, which of the following represents the oxygen consumption ($\dot{V}o_2$) for a 50-kg patient?

    Cardiac output ($\dot{Q}_T$)   3.9 L/min
    $C(a\text{-}\bar{v})o_2$ 6.8 vol%

    A. 310 mL/min
    B. 265 mL/min
    C. 250 mL/min
    D. 422 mL/min
    E. 235 mL/min
    (5:51 and 211–213) (2:955)

2. Given the following clinical data, calculate the oxygen consumption ($\dot{V}o_2$) for the following patient:

    Cardiac output ($\dot{Q}_T$)   4.8 L/min
    $C(a\text{-}\bar{v})o_2$ 2.4 vol%

    Which of the following is the most correct choice?
    A. 115 mL/min
    B. 130 mL/min

C. 96 mL/min
D. 105 mL/min
E. 200 mL/min
    (5:51 and 211–213) (2:955)

3. The respiratory therapy practitioner is monitoring the cardiopulmonary status of a patient who is receiving continuous ventilatory support. The following clinical data are made available at this time:

Cardiac output	9.8 L/min
Pa_{O_2}	53 mm Hg
$P\bar{v}_{O_2}$	29 mm Hg
Sa_{O_2}	84%
$S\bar{v}_{O_2}$	55%
Hb concentration	16.8 g/dL
O_2 carrying capacity	1.39 mL O_2/g Hb

Based on the above information, which of the following most accurately represents this patient's oxygen consumption ($\dot{V}_{O_2}$)?
A. 560 mL/min
B. 575 mL/min
C. 610 mL/min
D. 720 mL/min
E. 670 mL/min
    (5:51 and 211–213) (2:955)

4. Given the following clinical information, calculate this patient's cardiac output ($\dot{Q}_T$):

Oxygen consumption ($\dot{V}_{O_2}$)	250 mL/min
$C(a-\bar{v})_{O_2}$	4.0 vol%

A. 6.7 L/min
B. 4.7 L/min
C. 6.3 L/min
D. 5.8 L/min
E   9.6 L/min
    (5:51 and 211–213) (2:955)

5. Given the following clinical information, calculate the $C(a-\bar{v})_{O_2}$ for this 70-kg patient:

Cardiac output ($\dot{Q}_T$)	8.3 L/min
Oxygen consumption ($\dot{V}_{O_2}$)	380 mL/min

Which is the single best choice?
A. 2.1 vol%
B. 3.9 vol%
C. 4.4 vol%
D. 8.9 vol%
E. 4.6 vol%
    (5:51, 52, and 211–213) (2:955)

J. Pulmonary Vascular Resistance Pretest (Advanced Level Only)

Questions in this category are designed to assess the practitioner's ability to calculate pulmonary vascular resistance. This formula like all resistance formulas is derived from the Poiseuille and Ohm formulas. Therefore, just as the airway resistance formula asks one to divide the pressure drop across the conducting airways by the inspiratory flow rate, the pulmonary vascular resistance formula asks that one divide the pressure drop across the pulmonary vascular circuit by the flow rate of blood through that circuit (i.e., the cardiac output). This formula is as follows:

$$\text{Pulmonary Vascular Resistance} \atop \text{(mm Hg/L/min)} = \frac{\text{PAM} - \text{LVEDP}}{Q_T}$$

In the above equation, PAM stands for the pulmonary arterial mean pressure and LVEDP is the left ventricular end diastolic pressure. Clinically, the pulmonary wedge pressure (PWP) is usually an accurate approximation of the LVEDP. Consequently, it may be substituted in the equation. The normal range for pulmonary vascular resistance (PVR) is 1.0 mm Hg to 3.0 mm Hg/L/min. For an individual with perfectly normal pulmonary arterial pressures, the calculation would be as follows:

$$\text{PAM} = 15 \text{ mm Hg}$$
$$\text{PWP} = 9 \text{ mm Hg}$$
$$Q_T = 6.0 \text{ L/min}$$

$$\frac{15 \text{ mm Hg} - 9 \text{ mm Hg}}{6.0 \text{ L/min}} = 1.0 \text{ mm Hg/L/min}$$

This equation clearly shows that the drop in pressure from the right to the left ventricle increases in direct proportion to the resistance to flow within that circuit.

Another variation in the above formula asks that the derived value be multiplied by a factor of 80 to yield a value in dyne·seconds·cm^{-5} (see reference 79:220). This method is primarily used in cardiologic studies, and NBRC candidates need not concern themselves with it.

Clinically, a reliable estimate of the pulmonary vascular resistance can be gathered by subtracting the pulmonary wedge pressure (PWP) from the pulmonary artery diastolic pressure (PAD). A PAD − PWP gradient greater than 5 mm Hg is believed to indicate abnormal resistance to right ventricular output (see reference 41).

The following pretest was developed to help the candidate become proficient in this area.

1. The respiratory therapy practitioner is monitoring a critically ill patient in the intensive care unit. The following clinical data are collected from the patient's balloon-tipped pulmonary artery catheter:

Pulmonary artery mean pressure	20 mm Hg
Cardiac output	6.0 L/min
Pulmonary wedge pressure	8 mm Hg

Which of the following choices most accurately represents this patient's pulmonary vascular resistance?
A.   4.5 mm Hg/L/min
B.   2.0 mm Hg/L/min
C.   1.3 mm Hg/L/min
D.   6.0 mm Hg/L/min
E.   12.2 mm Hg/L/min
   (79:220)

2.   Given the following information, calculate the pulmonary vascular resistance:

Pulmonary artery mean pressure	38 mm Hg
Cardiac output	3.9 L/min
Pulmonary wedge pressure	4 mm Hg

A.   4.0 mm Hg/L/min
B.   8.1 mm Hg/L/min
C.   9.7 mm Hg/L/min
D.   16.3 mm Hg/L/min
E.   8.7 mm Hg/L/min
   (79:220)

3.   Given the following information, calculate the pulmonary vascular resistance:

Pulmonary artery mean pressure	20 mm Hg
Cardiac output	3.0 L/min
Pulmonary wedge pressure	13 mm Hg

A.   1.7 mm Hg/L/min
B.   19.4 mm Hg/L/min
C.   2.3 mm Hg/L/min
D.   7.9 mm Hg/L/min
E.   5.2 mm Hg/L/min
   (79:220)

Part V
Calculations Used in Pulmonary Function Testing

Contents

A. Lung Volume and Capacity Pretest
B. Spirometry Pretest (Advanced Level Only)
C. Residual Volume Pretest (Advanced Level Only)

A. Lung Volume and Capacity Pretest

Questions in this category are designed to assess the practitioner's ability to calculate the various lung volumes and capacities given appropriate laboratory data. These calculations and their solutions are all derived from the familiar lung volume and capacity diagram for a 70-kg patient that appears below:

		I	IRV
T	V	C	3.1L
L	C	3.6L	
C			TV
	4.8L	F R C	ERV
6.0L		2.4L	1.2L
	RV 1.2L		RV
			1.2 L

The following pretest was developed to help the candidate become proficient in these techniques.

1. In response to a physician's order, the respiratory therapy practitioner gathers the following laboratory data:

IRV	2150 cc
TV	480 cc
ERV	2340 cc
RV	1470 cc

    Based on the above information, which of the following most accurately represents this patient's total lung capacity?
    A. 5830 cc
    B. 7220 cc
    C. 6260 cc
    D. 6440 cc
    E. 7000 cc
       (16:2)

2. Based on the following laboratory data, which of the choices most accurately represents the patient's vital capacity?

IRV	1725 cc
TV	355 cc
FRC	1630 cc
RV	920 cc

    A. 2790 cc
    B. 4230 cc
    C. 3660 cc
    D. 2940 cc
    E. 3920 cc
       (16:2)

3. Given the following information, calculate the ERV.

IRV	3940 cc
FRC	2680 cc
TV	555 cc
RV	1175 cc

    A. 2135 cc
    B. 1175 cc
    C. 1205 cc
    D. 1675 cc
    E. 1505 cc
       (16:2)

4. Given the following information, calculate the inspiratory reserve volume.

VC	1350 cc
FRC	1030 cc

RV	675 cc
TV	135 cc

A. 740 cc
B. 690 cc
C. 820 cc
D. 910 cc
E. 860 cc *850*
   (16:2)

5. Given the following information, calculate the RV/TLC ratio.

IRV	1050 cc
TV	330 cc
FRC	1905 cc
VC	2670 cc

A. 19%
B. 13%
C. 32%
D. 10%
E. 25%
   (16:2)

B. Spirometry Pretest (Advanced Level Only)

Clinical spirometry is an area from which many different types of questions may be drawn. Some of these are as follows:

1. Percent Predicted Question
   To determine the value, the following formula is used:

$$\% \text{ Predicted} = \frac{\text{Observed Value}}{\text{Predicted Value}}$$

2. Bell Factor Question
   A spirometer's "bell factor" is the number of cc's of gas that must be displaced in order to move the bell and pen assembly 1.0 mm. For instance, if a particular spirometer has a factor of 41.27 cc/mm, a 25-mm vertical excursion noted on the recording paper will be generated each time 1030 cc is moved in or out of the bell. This volume, like all recorded volumes, must be expanded from ATPS to BTPS.

3. Percent Improvement After Bronchodilation (BD) Question
   The formula for this is:

$$\% \text{ Improvement After BD} = \frac{\left(\begin{array}{c}\text{Value Observed}\\ \text{After BD}\end{array}\right) - \left(\begin{array}{c}\text{Value Observed}\\ \text{Before BD}\end{array}\right)}{\begin{array}{c}\text{Value Observed}\\ \text{Before BD}\end{array}}$$

The following pretest was developed to help the candidate become proficient in these calculations and techniques.

1. From the following information, calculate the $\dfrac{FEV_1}{FVC}\%$.

$$\begin{array}{ll} FVC & 4.12 \text{ L} \\ FEV_1 & 3.06 \text{ L} \\ FEF_{200-1200} & 6.53 \text{ L/sec} \\ FEF_{25-75} & 3.82 \text{ L/sec} \end{array}$$

    A. 83%
    B. 80%
    C. 74%
    D. 72%
    E. 68%
    (16:30)

2. From the following information, calculate the $\dfrac{FEV_3}{FVC}\%$.

Measured excursion of FVC	42 mm
Measured excursion of FEV_3	36 mm
Bell factor	41.27 cc/mm
ATPS to BTPS correction factor	1.096

    A. 74%
    B. 92%
    C. 53%
    D. 81%
    E. 86%
    (16:30)

3. The practitioner has just performed an FVC test on a patient with obstructive lung disease. In calculating the results of this effort, he/she makes hatch marks at points that are equal to 25% and 75% of the volume measured by the FVC tracing. The practitioner then draws a line through these two points, making sure the line crosses two vertical time lines representing 1 second. The tangent crosses the first time line at a volume of 11,300 cc and the second time line at 8250 cc. Subsequently, the following data are noted:

ATPS to BTPS correction factor	1.102
Predicted FEF_{25-75}	4.95 L/sec

    Based on the above data, what percent of predicted is this patient's observed FEF_{25-75}?
    A. 72%
    B. 68%
    C. 85%
    D. 60%
    E. 42%
    (16:32–33)

4. Following administration of 0.5 cc of 1:200 isoproterenol, a patient's FEF_{25-75} is noted to increase from 1.35 L/min to 1.90 L/min. Which of the following choices most accurately represents the percent improvement experienced by this patient?
    A. 40%
    B. 50%
    C. 25%
    D. 35%
    E. 15%
    (96)

C. Residual Volume Pretest (Advanced Level Only)

Questions in this category are designed to assess the practitioner's ability to calculate a patient's residual volume, functional residual capacity, or total lung capacity by open circuit nitrogen washout or closed circuit helium dilution methods. The formulas for these are as follows:

1. Open Circuit Nitrogen Washout Formula

$$FRC = \frac{\left(\begin{array}{c}\text{Final Nitrogen}\\\text{Percentage in}\\\text{Tissot Spirometer}\end{array}\right)\left(\begin{array}{c}\text{Volume of Gas in}\\\text{Tissot Spirometer}\end{array}\right)}{0.75}$$

2. Closed Circuit Helium Dilution Formula

$$FRC = \left(\frac{\begin{array}{c}\text{Initial}\quad\quad\text{Final}\\\text{Helium \% } - \text{ Helium \%}\end{array}}{\begin{array}{c}\text{Final}\\\text{Helium \%}\end{array}}\right)\left(\begin{array}{c}\text{Initial Volume}\\\text{in Spirometer}\end{array}\right)$$

As usual, these values must be expanded from ATPS to BTPS.

The following pretest was developed to help the candidate become proficient in these calculations.

1. The physician's order reads: "Patient to go to Pulmonary Function Lab for determination of all lung volumes and capacities." The following information is obtained by the respiratory therapy practitioner:

Spirometer Data	
VC at ATPS	5240 cc
TV at ATPS	950 cc
IRV at ATPS	3110 cc
Correction factor from ATPS to BTPS	1.102

Data from 7-Minute Nitrogen Washout

Volume in Douglas bag	38.5 L
Concentration of final N_2 in Douglas bag	8.2%
Alveolar N_2 concentration	75%

Based on the above information, which of the following choices most correctly represents this patient's residual volume?
A. 1.8 L
B. 2.4 L
C. 3.0 L
D. 1.6 L
E. 3.3 L
   (16:5)

2. A patient is seen in the pulmonary function laboratory for determination of his total lung capacity. From the following information, calculate its value.

Spirometric Data

IRV at ATPS	1.52 L
TV at ATPS	0.32 L
VC at ATPS	2.66 L
Correction factor from ATPS to BTPS	1.085

Data from 7-Minute Nitrogen Washout

Volume in Tissot spirometer	41.8 L
Concentration of N_2 in spirometer	6.7%
Alveolar N_2 concentration	75%

Based on the above data, which of the following most accurately represents this patient's TLC?
A. 6.05 L
B. 5.2 L
C. 4.8 L
D. 3.8 L
E. 5.6 L
   (16:5)

3. Data were obtained from a closed circuit helium dilution study. The subject was a 63-year-old woman with an 80 pack/year history:

Original volume in spirometer	2.8 L
Original concentration of helium	10.6%
Final concentration of helium	4.3%
Temperature correction factor	1.102

Based on the above information, which choice most accurately represents this patient's FRC?
A.   3.6 L
B.   4.1 L
C.   4.5 L
D.   2.7 L
E.   2.3 L
   (16:7)

Part VI
Calculations Used in Pharmacology

Contents

A. Units of Measurement Pretest

Questions in this category are designed to assess the practitioner's understanding of the various units of measurement commonly used in respiratory pharmacotherapeutics.

The following pretest was developed to help the candidate become proficient in these techniques.

1. Which of the following most accurately represents the weight of a volume of water 1 cc in size?
    A.   1.0 g
    B.   2.0 g
    C.   1000 mg
    D.   100 mg
    E.   A and C are correct.
       (3:679–703) (2:497) (53:Chap 2)

2. Which of the following most accurately represents the weight of a volume of water 1 mL in size?
    A.   1.0 g
    B.   1000 mg
    C.   10 g
    D.   1.0μg
    E.   A and B are correct.
       (2:497) (3:699–703) (53:Chap 2)

79

3. Approximately how many milliliters are contained in a sample of water that occupies 1000 cc?
   A.   1.0
   B.   1000
   C.   50
   D.   5000
   E.   500
      (2:497) (3:699–703) (53:Chap 2)

4. How many milligrams are there in 0.016 g?
   A.   160
   B.   16
   C.   1.6
   D.   320
   E.   640
      (2:497) (3:699–703) (53:Chap 2)

5. How many micrograms are there in 1.0 mg?
   A.   1000
   B.   10,000
   C.   100,000
   D.   10
   E.   100
      (3:699–703) (2:497) (53:Chap 2)

6. How many standard drops does it take to equal 1 mL of H_2O?
   A.   65
   B.   125
   C.   64
   D.   32
   E.   15
      (2:497) (53:Chap 2)

7. One standard household tablespoon is equal to approximately how many milliliters?
   A.   15
   B.   20
   C.   30
   D.   10
   E.   5
      (2:497) (53:Chap 2)

8. One standard household teaspoon is equal to approximately how many milliliters?
   A.   10
   B.   15
   C.   20
   D.   5
   E.   25
      (2:497) (53:Chap 2)

B. Percent and Ratio Solution Pretest

To understand these concepts, it is best to start by defining the following terms:

Solute—the solid drug that is dissolved in the solvent.

Solvent—the liquid media into which the drug (solute) is dissolved. Most drugs are dissolved in an aqueous solvent (H_2O). It is important to remember that 1.0 mL of H_2O weighs almost exactly 1 g. Thus, 100 mL of water will weigh 100 g.

Solution—the mixture of solid solute and aqueous solvent. Interestingly enough, when relatively small quantities of solute are dissolved in an aqueous medium, the total *volume* of the solution does not change appreciably. Thus, if 1000 mg of a drug is added to 100 mL of the H_2O, the resulting solution would weigh 101 g but still occupy 100 mL.

There are basically two types of solutions that the respiratory therapy practitioner will encounter:

1. Percent Solutions

$$\text{Solution Percentage} = \left(\frac{\text{Weight}}{\text{Solution}} \div \frac{\text{Volume}}{\text{Solvent}}\right) \times 100$$

Thus, in the previous example 1000 mg of a given drug added to 100 mL of H_2O will result in a 1.0% solution. Percent solutions are sometimes called weight-to-volume (W/V) solutions.

2. Ratio Solutions
    A ratio solution is defined by the following formula, which indicates the ratio of solute weight to solvent weight:

$$\text{Solution Ratio} = \text{Weight Solute} \div \text{Weight Solvent}$$

Thus, in the continuing example, 1000 mg of a given drug added to 100 mL of aqueous solution will result in a 1:100 solution. Ratio solutions are sometimes referred to as weight-to-weight (W/W) solutions.

Concentration—When applied to pharmacologic agents, this refers to the quantity of solute per unit of final solution. The most commonly used units for concentration are mg/mL. Thus, both a 1.0% (W/V) solution and a 1:100 (W/W) solution have a concentration of 10 mg/mL.

The following pretest was designed to test the candidate's understanding of these concepts and computations.

1. The respiratory therapy practitioner is asked to add 1.0 g of metaproterenol to 100 mL of aqueous solvent. This will result in which of the following concentrations?
    I.   1:1000
    II. 0.1%
    III. 1:100
    IV. 1.0%
    V.   0.01%

[handwritten notes: 1000 g = 1L, 1000 mL = 1L, 1g → 100 mL, 1:100 or 1%]

A.   I and II
B.   III only
C.   I and IV
D.   III and IV
E.   V only
(2:497) (53:Chap 2)

2. If 250 mg of solute is added to 100 mL aqueous solvent, the result
    will be which of the following solutions?
    I.   0.4%
    II.   1:400
    III. 0.25%
    IV.   1:200
    V.   1:250

    250 mgs = 250 mls
    250 :100 = 25:10
    5:2

         A.   II and III
         B.   III and IV
         C.   III only
         D.   I and II
         E.   I and V
    (2:497) (53:Chap 2)

    = 1/10 g/ml

3. If the practitioner adds 100 mg of a drug to 100 mL aqueous sol-
    vent, the result will be which of the following solutions?
    I.   0.1%
    II.   0.01%
    III. 1.0%
    IV.   1:1000
    V.   1:10,000

    100 mgs ≈ 1g ≈ 1 cc ml
    1000 cc = 1L
    1000 ml = 1L

         A.   II and IV
         B.   I and IV
         C.   II and V
         D.   III and IV
         E.   I and III
    (2:497) (53:Chap 2)

4. If the practitioner adds 2.0 g solute to 100 mL of aqueous solu-
    tion, the result will be which of the following solutions?
    I.   1:250
    II.   1:50
    III. 2%
    IV.   1:400
    V.   4%

    100 ml = 100 cc
    2g → 20 mg = 20 mg/cc
    100 cc   1000 mgs/cc

         A.   II and III
         B.   I and III
         C.   II and V
         D.   IV only
         E.   I and V
    (2:497) (53:Chap 2)

1000 mgs = 1 cc

PART II B . . .

1% sol = 10 mg/1 cc

5. The practitioner is asked to administer 1.0 mL of a 1.0% solution of isoetharine to an asthmatic patient. How many milligrams of drug does this represent?
    A. 10   *10 mg/1 cc = 1%*
    B. 20
    C. 100
    D. 1000
    E. 1.0
    (2:497) (53:Chap 2)

6. The respiratory therapy practitioner is asked to administer 0.5 mL of a 1:200 solution of isoetharine. How many milligrams of drug does this represent?   *1:200 = .5%*
    A. 5.0
    B. 2.5   *.5 ml*
    C. 10
    D. 4.0
    E. 1.0
    (2:497) (53:Chap 2)

7. The respiratory therapy practitioner is asked to administer 3.0 mL of a 0.17% solution of bronchodilator to an asthmatic patient. Approximately how many milligrams of drug does this represent?
    A. 1.0
    B. 2.5
    C. 5
    D. 10
    E. 24
    (2:497) (53:Chap 2)

8. The physician's order reads: "Administer 5 mg metaproterenol via hand-held nebulizer." How many milliliters of a 1:100 solution should be used?
    A. 0.5
    B. 1.0
    C. 1.5
    D. 2.0
    E. 2.5
    (2:497) (53:Chap 2)

9. The physician's order reads: "Administer 75 mg Decadron® via hand-held nebulizer." How many milliliters of a 2.5% solution should be used?
    A. 2.2
    B. 0.5
    C. 3.0
    D. 1.5
    E. 4.5
    (2:497) (53:Chap 2)

10. The physician's order reads: "Administer 15 mg metaproterenol via hand-held nebulizer." How many milliliters of a 2% solution

should be used?
A.   1.0
B.   1.5
C.   0.75
D.   1.75
E.   0.5
   (2:497) (53:Chap 2)

C. Drug Dilution Pretest

Questions in this category are designed to assess the candidate's ability to dilute various pharmacologic agents from an original concentration to a desired concentration in accordance with a physician's order. The formula for this is as follows:

$$\begin{array}{c} \text{Volume of Diluent} \\ \text{to be Added} \end{array} = \left(\begin{array}{c} \text{Total or} \\ \text{New Volume} \\ \text{of Drug} \end{array} \right) - \left(\begin{array}{c} \text{Original Volume} \\ \text{of Drug} \end{array} \right)$$

$$\text{Total (New) Volume} = \frac{\text{(Original Volume) (Original Concentration)}}{\text{New (Desired) Concentration}}$$

Thus, if the physician wants a 5% solution of acetylcysteine made up and 20 mL of a 20% solution is all there is, the calculation is as follows:

$$\frac{(20 \text{ mL}) (20\%)}{(5\%)} = 80 \text{ mL}$$

It is therefore known that the total volume of the new solution is 100 mL. Inserting this value into the original formula reveals the following:

$$\begin{array}{c} \text{Volume of Diluent} \\ \text{to be Added} \end{array} = (80 \text{ mL}) - (20 \text{ mL}) = 60 \text{ mL}$$

Thus, 80 mL of diluent (H_2O) must be added to 20 mL of a 20% solution to yield a 5% solution.

The following pretest was developed to help the candidate become proficient in these calculations and techniques.

1.   The respiratory therapy practitioner is asked to dilute 100 mL of a 2% solution of beclomethasone to a 1.0% concentration. How many milliliters of water must be added to the original mixture to obtain the desired concentration?
A.   100
B.   50
C.   200
D.   150
E.   10
   (2:497) (3:63–64)

2. How many milliliters of water must be added to 10 mL of a 20%
    solution of acetylcysteine to dilute it to a 5% concentration?
    A. 40
    B. 30
    C. 50
    D. 20
    E. 10
       (2:497) (3:63–64)

3. The physician's order reads: "Instill 5 mL 5% $NaHCO_3$ q. 4h
    and p.r.n." All that is on hand are 50-mL ampules of an 8.4%
    solution. How many milliliters of distilled water must be added to
    obtain a 5% solution?
    A. 10
    B. 21
    C. 34
    D. 42
    E. 84
       (2:497) (3:63–64)

4. The medical director requests that a large quantity of 35%
    ETOH be made up. Using 500 mL of a 95% solution, approxi-
    mately how much of the new solution can be made up?
    A. 1250 mL
    B. 1360 mL
    C. 1400 mL
    D. 1500 mL
    E. 1175 mL
       (2:497) (3:63–64)

Answer Key

Part I

A. 1. D
2. A
3. D
4. D

B. 1. B
2. D
3. E
4. E

C. 1. E
2. D

D. 1. B
2. C
3. C

E. 1. A
2. C
3. A

F. 1. A
2. E
3. D
4. C
5. B
6. A

G. 1. E
2. B
3. E
4. A

H. 1. D
2. B
3. C

Part II

A. 1. A

2. B
3. C
4. C
5. A
6. B
7. A
8. D

B. 1. A
2. B
3. D

C. 1. D
2. B
3. D

D. 1. B
2. A

E. 1. E
2. D

Part III

A. 1. E
2. D
3. B
4. A
5. E
6. A

B. 1. C
2. E
3. D
4. B
5. C
6. A

C. 1. E

2. D
3. D
4. B
5. B

D. 1. A
2. E
3. C
4. B
5. C
6. C
7. A

E. 1. B
2. C

Part IV

A. 1. B
2. D
3. E

B. 1. A
2. C
3. B
4. C
5. A

C. 1. A
2. A
3. D
4. D

D. 1. A
2. B
3. C

E. 1. E

2. B
3. E
4. B
5. D
6. C
7. E

F. 1. B
2. A

G. 1. B
2. E

H. 1. E
2. E
3. A

I. 1. B
2. A
3. E
4. C
5. E

J. 1. B
2. E
3. C

Part V

A. 1. D
2. A
3. E
4. E
5. A

B. 1. C
2. E
3. B

2. B
3. E
4. B
5. D
6. C
7. E

F. 1. B
2. A

Part VI

A. 1. E
2. E
3. B
4. B
5. A
6. E
7. A
8. D

B. 1. D
2. A
3. B
4. A
5. A
6. B
7. C
8. A
9. C
10. C

C. 1. A
2. B
3. C
4. B

4. A

C. 1. E
2. A
3. C

UNIT II

Situational Set Pretest (Entry Level Only)

Approximately 10% of the questions on the NBRC Entry Level Examination are presented in the situational set format. Similar to the more sophisticated latent image branching-logic problems presented on the NBRC Clinical Simulation Examination, these case presentations assess the candidate's ability to manage a patient and/or respiratory care equipment within the clinical setting. The situational set begins with a short scenario. This narrative typically contains appropriate clinical data such as blood gas results, cardiopulmonary vital signs, results of chest radiography, and so on. By analyzing this information carefully, the candidate will be able to solve the problem that is presented. The scenario is followed by three to five questions; these test the candidate's ability to assess the nature and extent of the clinical problem and to make appropriate decisions regarding respiratory care.

The following section contains 20 situational sets that are presented more or less in order of difficulty.

Set 1
Chronic Obstructive
Pulmonary Disease I

A 59-year-old patient with a history of COPD is brought to the emergency department after several days of increasing respiratory distress. Baseline blood gases are drawn and the patient is placed on 1 L oxygen via nasal cannula. Data from the original and a subsequent arterial sample appear below:

	Room Air Sample	1 Liter Nasal O_2
Pa_{O_2}	36 mm Hg	46 mm Hg
Pa_{CO_2}	84 mm Hg	80 mm Hg
pH	7.24	7.30
HCO_3^-	32 mEq/L	34 mEq/L

1. Based on the foregoing data, the most appropriate recommendation for the respiratory therapy practitioner to make at this time would be:
    A. Increase oxygen flow to 2 L/min
    B. Make no change in therapy
    C. Intubate and place patient on continuous ventilatory support
    D. Place patient on 35% air entrainment mask
    E. Decrease oxygen to 0.5 L/min
    (1:479–483) (5:179–183)

2. Conservative and supportive therapy is the general rule in managing acute respiratory insufficiency superimposed on COPD. Which of the following is *not* a reason for this?
    A. Poor tolerance of continuous mechanical ventilation
    B. General success of respiratory therapy
    C. Favorable response to oxygen therapy in this group
    D. Reversible nature of bronchospasm
    E. Rarity of severe and life-threatening distress in these patients
    (32:93–95) (7:83–85) (1:479–483) (49)

3. Physical examination of the patient reveals a loose cough productive of moderate quantities of rusty-colored secretions. Which of the following is likely to be responsible for this finding?
    A. Bronchial asthma
    B. Pseudohemoptysis

C. Pneumococcal pneumonia
D. *Pseudomonas* pneumonia
E. Anaerobic lung abscess
(2:263)

4. Which of the following is not considered part of the conservative supportive approach to the management of the COPD patient who requires hospitalization?
A. IPPB
B. Antibiotic therapy
C. Continuous ventilatory support
D. Chest physical therapy
E. Oxygen therapy
(7:83–84) (32:93–95) (38:64–66) (49)

5. The decision to intubate and initiate continuous ventilatory support in patients with severe chronic obstructive pulmonary disease is made on demonstration of all of the following *except:*
A. $Paco_2$ greater than 70 mm Hg
B. Inability to protect the airway
C. Sudden onset of severe cardiovascular symptomatology
D. Progressive acidosis despite controlled oxygen administration
E. Worsening fatigue and sensorium
(49) (32:93–95) (38:64–65)

Set 2
Epiglottitis

A severely distressed 3-year-old girl is brought to the emergency department by her parents. Physical signs include a loud barking cough and high-pitched inspiratory stridor. She is unable to swallow and is noted to be drooling profusely. Her mother says that she did not become ill until approximately 4 hours prior to admission. Arterial blood gas analysis on 3 L oxygen via cannula reveals the following data:

Pao_2	53 mm Hg
$Paco_2$	27 mm Hg
pH	7.40
HCO_3^-	14.8 mEq/L
Base excess	−4.5 mEq/L

1. Which of the following is the correct interpretation of this
    patient's arterial blood gas data?
    A. Fully compensated respiratory acidosis
    B. Partially compensated respiratory alkalosis
    C. Metabolic acidosis with respiratory alkalosis
    D. Fully compensated metabolic alkalosis
    E. Partially compensated metabolic acidosis
        (5:Chaps 12 and 13)

2. The clinical presentation of epiglottitis differs from that of croup
    in which of the following respects?
    I.   The onset of symptoms is more rapid.
    II.   It usually affects a neonatal population.
    III. It is a more common presentation.
    IV.   Distress is generally more severe.
        A. I, III, and IV
        B. II, III, and IV
        C. I, II, III, and IV
        D. I and IV
        E. I and III
    (32:133–135) (13:104–108)

3. Which of the following pathogens is most frequently associated
    with epiglottitis?
    A. Viral agents
    B. *Escherichia coli*
    C. *Pseudomonas*
    D. *Hemophilus influenzae*
    E. *Bacillus fragilis*
        (13:105)

4. Examination of the pharynx in patients with epiglottitis:
    I.   May result in complete upper airway obstruction
    II.   Will typically reveal a cherry-red epiglottis
    III. Should only be performed by a nurse practitioner
        A. I and III
        B. I, II, and III
        C. II and III
        D. I and II
        E. I only
    (13:105–106) (32:130–134)

Set 3
Chronic Obstructive Pulmonary Disease II

A 44-year-old woman with advanced cystic fibrosis is admitted to the emergency department. The patient is cyanotic, febrile, and confused. Arterial blood is drawn just prior to and 20 minutes after she is placed on 3 L oxygen via nasal cannula. These data are reported below:

	Room Air Sample	3 L Nasal Oxygen
Pa_{O_2}	35 mm Hg	46 mm Hg
Pa_{CO_2}	73 mm Hg	97 mm Hg
pH	7.31	7.17
HCO_3^-	37 mEq/L	32 mEq/L

1. Based on the foregoing information, which of the following recommendations should the respiratory therapy practitioner make at this time?
   A. Increase oxygen to 4 L/min
   B. Decrease oxygen to 1 L/min
   C. Intubate and place on a ventilator with an FI_{O_2} of 0.35
   D. Intubate and place on an FI_{O_2} of 0.35 via T tube
   E. Make no change in therapy
   (32:95)

2. In most patients suffering from chronic hypercapnia who require oxygen therapy, the hazard of CO_2 retention can usually be minimized by keeping the Pa_{O_2} between _____ mm Hg.
   A. 30–40
   B. 40–50
   C. 50–70 — hypercapnic ?
   D. 60–80
   E. 70–90
   (32:95) (1:483)

3. Which of the following statements regarding the use of the continuous ventilatory support in the management of COPD is *not* true?
   A. Barotrauma is a known complication.
   B. Worsening of V/Q relationships is common.
   C. The patient's work of breathing frequently increases following placement on continuous ventilatory support.
   D. Ventilator dependence may occur.
   E. Nosocomial infections may prolong course.
   (49) (38:64–66) (32:93–95) (1:483) 1979 ed.

Set 4
Pulmonary Function Testing

A 71-year-old patient is admitted to the hospital for a cholecystectomy. Preoperative lung function tests are performed on this 65-kg patient with the following results:

	Observed	% Predicted
FVC	1.74 L	39
FEV_1	0.82 L	30
$\dfrac{FEV_1}{FVC}\%$	31%	—
$FEF_{200\text{-}1200}$	1.89 L/sec	31
$FEF_{25\text{-}75}$	0.34 L/sec	12
FRC	3.52 L	140

1. On the basis of the foregoing data, which of the following pulmonary mechanical defects is most likely present?
   A. Restrictive lung disease
   B. Normal study
   C. Upper airway obstruction only
   D. Mild obstructive pulmonary disease
   E. Severe obstructive pulmonary disease
   (2:210–212)

2. Which of the following best describes this patient's risk of developing postoperative pulmonary complications?
   A. No risk
   B. Low risk
   C. Moderate risk
   D. High risk
   E. Not enough information available
   (1:464–467)

3. Which of the following is considered the best test for detecting early obstructive changes in the smaller airways?
   A. $FEF_{200\text{-}1200}$
   B. MVV
   C. $FEF_{25\text{-}75}\%$
   D. FEV_1
   E. $\dfrac{FEV_1}{FVC}\%$
   (2:208–211)

4. In this patient, the elevated FRC is *least* suggestive of which of the following abnormalities?
   A. Loss of pulmonary elastic recoil
   B. Emphysema
   C. Air trapping
   D. Diffuse parenchymal consolidation
   E. Obstruction to expiratory airflow
   (11:Chap 7)

Set 5
Flail Chest

A 16-year-old, 60-kg automobile accident victim is rushed to the emergency department by ambulance. The victim is unconscious, deeply cyanotic, and in life-threatening distress. Respirations are extremely labored and his right anterior chest wall is noted to move inward on inspiration. Multiple lacerations and contusions are present from which the patient is bleeding profusely. As paramedics bring him into the trauma room he is noted to be receiving 10 L oxygen via simple oxygen mask.

1. Which of the following actions should the respiratory therapy practitioner take at this time?
   A. Palpate the carotid pulse
   B. Assist in hemostasis
   C. Establish an airway
   D. Assess level of consciousness
   E. Begin external cardiac compressions
   (37:12–15)

2. Which of the following statements is (are) true regarding flail chest?
   I. Double fractures of several adjacent ribs may be etiologic.
   II. Lung contusion is a rare accompanying pathology.
   III. Continuous ventilatory support is always indicated.
       A. II and III
       B. I and II
       C. I only
       D. I, II, and III
       E. I and III
   (1:503–505) (7:344)

3. Following successful intubation, the physician asks the respiratory therapy practitioner to place the patient on a volume ventilator.

Which of the following modes of continuous mechanical ventilation is (are) believed to aid in stabilization of the chest wall?
  I. Pharmacologic paralysis in conjunction with large tidal volumes
  II. Pharmacologic paralysis in conjunction with positive end-expiratory pressure (PEEP) therapy
  III. Pharmacologic paralysis in conjunction with negative end-expiratory pressure (NEEP) therapy
  A. I and III
  B. II and III
  C. III only
  D. I and II
  E. I only
  (1:503–505) (64)

4. Continuous ventilatory support in the patient with flail chest:
  I. May be necessary for 1 or more weeks
  II. May be helpful in preventing hypoxia
  III. May be complicated by pulmonary barotrauma
  A. I, II, and III
  B. II and III
  C. I and II
  D. I only
  E. I and III
  (1:503–505) (7:344–349) (46)

Set 6
Bronchiectasis

A 45-year-old patient was admitted to the respiratory service 2 weeks ago. His relevant history began in childhood with a pneumonia that did not receive adequate medical attention. Since that time his pulmonary symptomatology has become increasingly pronounced. This is his sixth hospitalization, but it is the first time he has been examined by a pulmonary specialist.

1. The chief complaint of the patient with bronchiectasis is:
  A. Orthopnea
  B. Easy fatigability
  C. Dyspnea
  D. Sleep apnea
  E. Cough and sputum production
  (11:114)

2. In general, sputum produced by the patient with bronchiectasis is:
    I.   Mucoid
    II. Copious
    III. Purulent
    IV. Scanty
        A. II and IV
        B. I and III
        C. I and IV
       —D. II and III
        E. I and II
    (11:115)

3. Definitive diagnosis of bronchiectasis is made on the basis of which of the following?
    A. History and physical examination
    B. Sputum culture and sensitivity
   —C. Bronchography
    D. Angiography
    E. Pulmonary tomography
    (14:115)

4. Pulmonary function and arterial blood studies on a bronchiectasis patient typically reveal:
    I.   Decreased expiratory flow rates
    II. Increased inspiratory capacity
    III. Hypoxemia
    IV. Massive intrapulmonary shunting
        A. II and III
        B. I and II
        C. III and IV
       —D. I and III
        E. I, II, III, and IV
    (11:115)

5. All of the following have a place in this patient's home care program. Which is believed to be the most indispensable aid to maintaining bronchial hygiene?
    A. Aerosol therapy
    B. Hyperinflation therapy
   —C. Pulmonary drainage techniques
    D. Antibiotic therapy
    E. Breathing exercises
    (11:115–118)

Set 7
Ventilator Emergency
I

The respiratory therapy practitioner is assigned to a ventilator patient in the cardiac care unit. While making rounds the therapist hears the ventilator's high pressure alarm sounding. Although unconscious, the patient is diaphoretic, cyanotic, and in respiratory distress.

1. What is the first thing that must be done to alleviate this patient's distress?
   A. Check the ventilator to see if it is malfunctioning
   B. Take the patient off the ventilator and ventilate manually
   C. Go to the nurses' station and get help
   D. Have a physician paged
   E. Measure the patient's blood pressure
   (32:209)

2. Following the action outlined in the previous question, which *two* of the following actions must be taken simultaneously?
   I.   Call for a stat chest roentgenogram
   II. Check the ventilator for malfunction
   III. Have a partner bag the patient with 100% O_2
   IV. Examine the patient's chest to determine the cause of distress
   V.   Check the patient's blood pressure
      A. I and III
      B. IV and V
      C. III and IV
      D. III and V
      E. II and III
   (32:209)

3. Percussion at this time reveals sharply diminished aeration on the left side and a hyperresonant percussion note on the right side. Which of the following disorders is (are) most likely to be responsible for this finding?
   I.   Intubation of the right mainstem bronchus
   II. Right-sided pneumothorax
   III. Right-sided hemothorax
   IV. Acute pulmonary edema
      A. I and II
      B. II and IV
      C. I and III

    D. II and III
    E. I, II, and IV
  (32:210 and 212)

4. While waiting for the physician to arrive, the practitioner notes that the patient is becoming increasingly cyanotic. Soon, the carotid pulse is not palpable. Over the past 2 minutes the cardiac rate has dropped from 200 to approximately 20. Based on this information, the therapist should:
    A. Draw a stat arterial blood gas sample
    B. Insert a 16-gauge needle in the second or third interspace of the affected side
    C. Advance the airway slightly
    D. Auscultate the chest
    E. Begin external cardiac compressions
  (37:19) (25:Chap 6, p 9)

Set 8
Cardiogenic
Pulmonary Edema

A severely distressed 45-year-old man is brought to the emergency department by paramedics who were called when an anginal episode did not respond to administration of several nitroglycerin tablets. The patient is suffering from tachycardia, hypertension, and tachypnea. Auscultation of the chest reveals wet inspiratory rales and scattered wheezes.

1. The physician wants the respiratory therapy practitioner to administer IPPB via a Bird Mark 7® ventilator. Which of the following is most appropriate at this time?
    A. Air dilution in system with Q.S. 60% to 80% ethyl alcohol
    B. Air dilution out of system with Q.S. 10% to 20% ethyl alcohol
    C. Air dilution out of system with Q.S. 20% to 50% ethyl alcohol
    D. Air dilution in system with Q.S. 50% to 70% ethyl alcohol
    E. Air dilution out of system with Q.S. 60% to 80% ethyl alcohol
  (1:435–436) (3:434–437)

quantity required?

2. This patient's wheezes:
    A. Are most likely the result of bronchial asthma
    B. Are a characteristic finding in left ventricular failure
    C. May be termed cardiac asthma
    D. B and C are correct.
    E. All of the above are correct.
      (11:177) (1:432)

3. Venous return may be reduced by which of the following therapeutic modalities?
      I.   Use of positive pressure ventilation
      II.   Use of diuretics
      III. Morphine administration
      IV.   Bronchodilator therapy
        A. I and II
        B. I, II, and IV
        C. III and IV
        D. II, III, and IV
        E. I, II, and III
      (1:434–435) (3:435–436)

4. Which of the following are reasons why IPPB may prove useful in the emergency treatment of acute cardiogenic pulmonary edema?
      I.   100% O_2 may be administered.
      II.   Positive pressure may improve cardiac performance.
      III. Antifoaming agents may be administered.
      IV.   Dyspnea may be relieved.
        A. II, III, and IV
        B. I, II, and IV
        C. I, II, III, and IV
        D. I and IV
        E. I, III, and IV
      (1:435–436) (3:434–437)

Set 9
Guillain-Barré
Syndrome

A 52-year-old man is brought to the emergency department. For the past 2 days he has been experiencing progressive numbness and weakening of the extremities. When several hours ago he found he could not catch his breath after walking across the room, he had a neighbor drive him to the hospital. Physical findings include tachypnea, dysphagia, and slurred speech. Antecedent history was unremarkable except for an upper respiratory tract infection in the past 2 weeks. Arterial blood gases drawn on room air just prior to direct admission to the intensive care unit were:

Pa_{O_2}	81 mm Hg
Pa_{CO_2}	52 mm Hg
pH	7.30
Base excess	-3.9 mEq/L
HCO_3^-	20 mEq/L

1. True statements regarding the patient's blood gas and acid-base status include:
    I.   Respiratory acidosis exists.
    II. A widened $P(A-a)_{O_2}$ exists.
    III. Physiologic shunting is evident.
    IV. Metabolic acidosis is present.
        A. I and IV
        B. II and III
        C. I, II, and IV
        D. I, III, and IV
        E. II and IV
    (2:Chap 18)

2. Which of the following statements regarding the Guillain-Barré syndrome is (are) true?
    I.   It may lead to respiratory muscle paralysis.
    II. It is considered an obstructive disorder. *RESTRICTIVE*
    III. Its primary pathology involves neuromuscular blockade. *MY. GRAVIS*
    IV. It is a common cause of adult respiratory distress syndrome.
        A. I, II, and IV
        B. III and IV
        C. I only
        D. I, II, III, and IV
        E. I, III, and IV
    (11:205–206) (5:188)

3. Which of the following statements regarding the clinical picture of patients with Guillain-Barré syndrome is (are) true?
    I.   Loss of vital capacity is a consistent finding.
    II. Pulmonary edema is frequently severe.
    III. Increased anteroposterior diameter is a common radiologic finding.
    IV. Cough with sputum is the chief complaint.
        A. I and III
        B. II, III, and IV
        C. I, III, and IV

D.   I only
E.   II and III
(11:205–206)

4.   True statements regarding the use of mechanical ventilation in patients with Guillain-Barré syndrome include:
   I.   PEEP therapy is usually required.
  II.   It is indicated when the vital capacity is less than 20% of predicted.
 III.   Mechanical hyperventilation is indicated to reduce intracranial pressure.
  IV.   It may be required for several weeks or longer.
       A.   I and IV
       B.   II, III, and IV
       C.   III and IV
       D.   II and IV
       E.   I, II, III, and IV
   (7:359–360)

Set 10
Croup

A 13-month-old, well-nourished infant is brought to the emergency department in respiratory distress. His mother says that he has had a cold for the past 2 days. About 18 hours ago he developed a loud barking cough and began making "crowing" sounds on inspiration. Symptoms slowly continued to deteriorate, necessitating his admission.

1.   All of the following physical findings were seen in this patient. Which is the most characteristic of the pediatric croup syndrome?
   A.   Tachycardia
   B.   Fever
   C.   Inspiratory stridor
   D.   Tachypnea
   E.   Productive cough
      (32:131)

2.   Which of the following is the most common causative agent in episodes of croup?
   A.   *Hemophilus influenzae*
   B.   *Bacillus pneumoniae*
   C.   Viral organisms

     D.   *Escherichia coli*
     E.   *Bordetella pertussis*
      (32:131)

3. Which of the following statements regarding croup is (are) true?
     I.   It is also known as laryngotracheobronchitis.
    II.   The underlying pathology involves pharyngeal edema.
   III.   It is known to respond to aerosol therapy.
      A.   I and II
      B.   II and III
      C.   I and III
      D.   II only
      E.   III only
      (32:133–135) (13:104–108)

4. Which of the following statements regarding croup as compared with epiglottitis is (are) true?
     I.   Symptoms are generally more severe.
    II.   Onset of symptoms is more rapid.
   III.   An emergency airway is required less frequently.
      A.   I and III
      B.   II and III
      C.   I and II
      D.   I only
      E.   III only
      (32:133–135) (1:512–513) (13:104–108)

Set 11
Pediatric Cardiopulmonary Resuscitation

A 6-year-old boy is brought to the emergency department after being struck by an automobile while riding his bicycle. On admission he is comatose and cyanotic. As he is rushed in by paramedics, it is noted that he is receiving 8 L oxygen via mask and that an overly large oropharyngeal airway has been taped in place. Gross inspection at this time also reveals multiple lacerations and contusions over his thorax, abdomen, and legs. Rapid assessment of this patient reveals the absence of air movement and ventilatory efforts.

1. Based on the above information, the practitioner would now:
   A. Check the carotid pulse
   B. Assess pupillary response
   C. Give four quick breaths
   D. Administer a precordial thump
   E. Give four back blows
   (37:16)

2. Use of an improperly sized oropharyngeal airway in conjunction with an oxygen mask is particularly hazardous for which of the following reasons?
   A. It can lead to an increased mechanical deadspace.
   B. It will lower the effective FIo_2.
   C. It can lead to vomiting.
   D. It may cause reflex tachycardia.
   E. It may impinge on the soft palate.
   (25:Chap IV, p 2) (1:237)

3. True statements about rescue breathing in the child include:
   I. The side effect of gastric distention is more common than it is in the adult.
   II. When accompanying external cardiac compressions, the rate should be 25/min.
   III. Mouth-to-nose ventilation is generally preferred.
   IV. It should be administered during the downstroke of every fifth compression.
   A. II, III, and IV
   B. I, III, and IV
   C. II and III
   D. I only
   E. I, II, and IV
   (37:20 and 31–33)

4. Which of the following statements regarding airway obstruction in children is (are) true?
   I. It is more common than in adults.
   II. It is commonly caused by toys and peanuts.
   III. The emergency procedure does not include back blows.
   A. I and II
   B. I, II, and III
   C. III only
   D. II and III
   E. I and III
   (37:31–32) (32:133–134)

5. Emergency cardiac compressions in the child:
   I. Should be administered at a rate of 80/min
   II. Should compress the sternum ½ to 2 inches
   III. Can frequently be performed with the heel of one hand

A. I and III
B. II and III
C. I, II, and III
D. II only
E. I and II
(37:33)

Set 12
Ventilator Emergency II

The respiratory therapy practitioner is treating a patient who has become acutely dyspneic while being ventilated by a Siemens Servo ventilator. Chest physical assessment at this time reveals a dull percussion note on the right side and a hyperresonant percussion note on the left. At the same time, the patient's trachea is noted to be deviated to the right side.

1. Based on the above data, which of the following is most likely responsible for the above abnormality?
   A. Left-sided pneumothorax
   B. Right mainstem intubation
   C. Right-sided pleural effusion
   D. Massive left-sided atelectasis
   E. Herniation of the endotracheal tube cuff
   (11:190–192)

2. Which of the following will usually lead to decreases in effective static compliance?
   I. Bronchospasm
   II. Cardiogenic pulmonary edema
   III. Endotracheal tube cuff herniation
   IV. Tension pneumothorax
   A. I and III
   B. II and III
   C. I and IV
   D. III and IV
   E. II and IV
   (34:122–126) (32:Chap 12)

3. Which of the following groups of patients is *least* likely to develop a pneumothorax while receiving continuous ventilatory support?
    A. Those with lung abscess
    B. Those with chest trauma
    C. Those with neuromuscular disease
    D. Those with pulmonary emphysema
    E. Those who require PEEP
    (46) (11:190–192)

4. The respiratory therapy practitioner should recommend which of the following to establish a definitive diagnosis in this case?
    A. Obtain a chest roentgenogram
    B. Advance the endotracheal tube a few centimeters
    C. Perform a thoracotomy
    D. Check the ventilator circuit for leaks
    E. Perform arterial blood gas analysis
    (11:191)

Set 13
Upper Airway Emergency

The respiratory therapy practitioner is paged to the cardiac care unit to check the equipment storeroom. As he walks by the adjacent visitors' waiting room, he notices an elderly woman slump over in her chair and fall to the floor.

1. All of the following are steps that are followed in performing basic cardiopulmonary resuscitation. Please place them in correct order.
    I.   Check for pulse.
    II.   Give four quick breaths.
    III. Establish unconsciousness.
    IV.   Hyperextend neck and check breathing.
    V.   Begin external cardiac compressions.
    VI.   Call for help.
        A. III, VI, IV, I, II, and V
        B. III, VI, IV, II, I, and V
        C. III, VI, II, I, IV, and V
        D. VI, IV, III, I, V, and II
        E. VI, II, I, III, IV, and V
    (37:11)

2. Single-rescuer cardiopulmonary resuscitation of the adult victim consists of:
    A. 15 compressions followed by two ventilations
    B. 10 compressions followed by two ventilations
    C. 5 compressions followed by one ventilation
    D. 15 compressions followed by two back blows
    E. 15 compressions followed by four ventilations
        (37:23–25)

3. The therapist attempts to deliver four quick breaths to this victim but is unable to move air into the lungs. All of the following are steps in the procedure to relieve complete airway obstruction in the unconscious adult victim. Please place them in proper order.
    I.   Give four stomach or chest thrusts.
    II. Give four back blows.
    III. Sweep the mouth with your fingers.
    IV. Reposition the head and neck and try to ventilate.
        A. I, II, IV, and III
        B. II, I, IV, and III
        C. II, I, III, and IV
        D. I, III, II, and IV
        E. I, II, III, and IV
    (37:47)

4. According to the American Heart Association, the chest thrust may be preferable to the abdominal thrust in which of the following cases?
    I.   Comatose victims
    II. Pregnant victims
    III. Very obese victims
    IV. Infants
    V.   Children
        A. I, III, IV, and V
        B. II, III, and IV
        C. II, III, and V
        D. I, II, III, IV, and V
        E. II, III, IV, and V
    (37:28–31)

5. After several repetitions of the above procedure, the therapist is able to dislodge a large piece of food from the victim's airway. By this time help has arrived. Place the following lifesaving steps in their proper order.
    I.   Give four quick breaths.
    II. Check for pulse.
    III. Begin two-rescuer cardiopulmonary resuscitation.
        A. III, II, and I
        B. II, III, and I
        C. I, III, and II
        D. I, II, and III
        E. III, I, and II
    (37:25)

Set 14
Cystic Fibrosis

An infant is admitted to the seventh floor pediatric ward with a tentative diagnosis of "failure to thrive." Four months ago this patient was sent home with her mother following an uneventful delivery. Since then she has had several upper respiratory tract infections and a persistent cough. Her main problem at this time has been an inability to gain weight despite apparently normal feeding habits. Abdominal distention and bulky, foul-smelling stools are pertinent features of this infant's clinical picture.

1. True statements regarding cystic fibrosis include:
   I. It is a chronic, restrictive pediatric pulmonary disorder.
   II. It may also be called mucoviscidosis.
   III. It is a hereditary disorder of the body's endocrine system.
   IV. It is rarely fatal.
   V. Primary pulmonary pathology involves hypersecretion of mucus.
   A. I, II, IV, and V
   B. I, III, IV, and V
   C. II and V
   D. III and V
   E. I, II, III, and V
   (11:119–212)

2. Which of the following is most helpful in establishing the diagnosis of cystic fibrosis?
   A. Pulmonary tomography
   B. Measurement of sweat electrolytes
   C. Angiograms
   D. Lung biopsy
   E. Sputum culture and sensitivity
   (11:119)

3. Retained pulmonary secretions in the patient with cystic fibrosis *least* frequently leads to:
   A. Atelectasis
   B. Pneumonia
   C. Left ventricular failure
   D. Increased work of breathing
   E. Blood gas abnormalities
   (11:120–121)

4. Pulmonary function testing in the patient with cystic fibrosis usually shows evidence of:
   I. Decreased FEF_{25-75}

II. Increased $\dfrac{FEV_1}{FVC}\%$

III. Increased residual volume
IV. Decreased inspiratory flow rates
    A. I and III
    B. I, III, and IV
    C. I only
    D. I, II, and IV
    E. III and IV
  (11:121)

5. Oxygen administration to the patient with cystic fibrosis:
  I. May cause respiratory acidosis
  II. Will have no effect on arterial hypoxemia
  III. Is rarely necessary
    A. I and III
    B. I, II, and III
    C. II and III
    D. I only
    E. II only
  (13:121) (2:394–395)

Set 15
Drug Overdose

A 15-year-old is brought by paramedics to the emergency department with an esophageal obturator airway in place. She is being ventilated by a manual resuscitator that is connected to supplemental oxygen. Her height is average and her weight is well in excess of 100 kg. Spontaneous respirations are 6/min and shallow. Skin color is ashen but not cyanotic. Pulse is 130, the blood pressure is 70/40, and the patient does not respond to painful stimuli.

1. Which of the following should the respiratory therapy practitioner recommend at this time?
  A. Pass a nasogastric tube
  B. Intubate and support ventilation
  C. Obtain stat arterial blood gas analysis
  D. Begin hemodialysis
  E. Remove the esophageal obturator airway
  (1:499–500) (7:370)

2. Which of the following best describes this patient's sensorium?
    A.   Alert and oriented
    B.   Restless and agitated
    C.   Lethargic and confused
    D.   Light coma
    E.   Deep coma
       (33:400 and 452)

3. An arterial blood sample is drawn while the patient is breathing
    room air. The results appear below:

Pa_{O_2}	35 mm Hg
Pa_{CO_2}	65 mm Hg
pH	7.20
HCO_3^-	26 mEq/L
Base excess	−4.0 mEq/L

    Based on the above information, the patient's hypoxemia is most
    likely due to:
    A.   Hypoventilation
    B.   Shunting
    C.   Low V/Q
    D.   High V/Q
    E.   A and C are correct.
       (2:243) (32:63–66)

4. Regarding this patient's acid-base status:
    A.   A mixed respiratory and metabolic acidosis exists.
    B.   A mixed respiratory and metabolic alkalosis exists.
    C.   Respiratory acidosis alone exists.
    D.   Partially compensated metabolic alkalosis exists.
    E.   A partially compensated respiratory acidosis exists.
       (5:Chap 12)

Set 16
Adult Respiratory
Distress Syndrome I

The respiratory therapy practitioner is monitoring a 25-year-old man
who was admitted after an industrial accident involving inhalation of
chlorine gas. Eight hours post admission the patient has tachycardia,

tachypnea, and hypertension. Auscultation of the chest reveals diminished breath sounds bibasally and scattered inspiratory rales. Arterial blood sampled with the patient breathing 8 L oxygen via simple oxygen mask yields the following data:

Pa_{O_2}	34 mm Hg
Pa_{CO_2}	23 mm Hg
pH	7.50
HCO_3^-	18 mEq/L

1. Which of the following is most likely to be responsible for this patient's arterial hypoxemia?
   A. Low V/Q
   B. High V/Q
   C. Diffusion defect
   D. Intrapulmonary shunting
   E. Hypoventilation
   (46) (2:394–395) (38:62–65)

2. Administration of 100% oxygen to this patient at this time would most likely have which of the following effects?
   I. Widening of the $P(A-a)_{O_2}$
   II. Dramatic increase in the Pa_{O_2}
   III. Narrowing of the $P(A-a)_{O_2}$
      A. III only
      B. I only
      C. II and III
      D. II only
      E. I and II
   (2:394–395) (46) (47)

3. The physician wants to place the patient on the level of PEEP that will yield the highest systemic oxygen transport. Which of the following is believed to be the best indicator of this?
   A. Pa_{O_2}
   B. Cardiac output
   C. $P(A-a)_{O_2}$
   D. $S\bar{v}_{O_2}$
   E. Effective static compliance
   (46) (47)

4. In an attempt to determine the optimal therapeutic level of PEEP, the following information is gathered:

Level of PEEP (cm H_2O)	Sa_{O_2} (%)	$S\bar{v}_{O_2}$ (%)
0	74	40
3	74	47
6	76	53
9	78	58
12	80	53
15	76	50

Based on the above information, the best level of PEEP for the patient is:
A.   3 cm H_2O
B.   6 cm H_2O
C.   9 cm H_2O
D.   12 cm H_2O
E.   15 cm H_2O
   (46) (47)

5.   Four days later, the patient is on an FI_{O_2} of 0.6 with 10 cm H_2O PEEP. Arterial blood gas data obtained at this time with the patient in the assist/control mode are as follows:

Pa_{O_2}	151 mm Hg
Pa_{CO_2}	32 mm Hg
pH	7.46
HCO_3^-	22 mEq/L

Based on the above information, which of the following setting changes should the respiratory therapy practitioner recommend at this time?
A.   Decrease the PEEP to 5 cm H_2O and add 100 cc mechanical deadspace
B.   Decrease the FI_{O_2} to 0.5
C.   Decrease the FI_{O_2} to 0.5 and add 500 cc mechanical deadspace
D.   Decrease the PEEP to 8 cm H_2O and place patient on intermittent mandatory ventilation
E.   Decrease the FI_{O_2} to 0.3 and raise the PEEP to 12 cm H_2O
   (46) (1:351–352)

Set 17
Status Asthmaticus

A 50-year-old man is brought to the emergency department in severe respiratory distress. The patient is dusky but not cyanotic, and his wheezing can be heard across the room. This admission was preceded by an upper respiratory infection that had increased in severity over the past week. The patient is immediately placed on 3 L nasal oxygen and an arterial blood sample is drawn. The following arterial gas and acid-base data are obtained at this time:

Pao_2	68 mm Hg
Paco_2	29 mm Hg
pH	7.50
HCO$_3^-$	22 mEq/L
Base excess	+1.0 mEq/L

1. Which of the following is the correct interpretation of the above acid-base status?
   A. Partially compensated respiratory alkalosis
   B. Partially compensated metabolic acidosis
   C. Uncompensated respiratory alkalosis and uncompensated metabolic acidosis
   D. Uncompensated metabolic acidosis and partially compensated respiratory alkalosis
   E. Uncompensated respiratory alkalosis
      (5:137–139, 198, and 201)

2. Which of the following statements regarding the use of continuous ventilatory support in the management of the status asthmaticus patient is *not* true?
   A. The majority should be managed without it.
   B. Patient ventilator tolerance is a common problem.
   C. It often results in cardiogenic pulmonary edema.
   D. Tension pneumothorax is a known complication.
   E. It may allow decreasing of bronchodilator dosage.
      (1:506) (32:161)

3. Two hours later, the patient has become severely obtunded. Sinus tachycardia with frequent premature ventricular contractions is noted on the monitor. Auscultation reveals sharply diminished air entry bilaterally. All of the following actions are believed to be indicated at this time. Which is the number one priority?
   A. Drawing an arterial blood sample
   B. Initiation of continuous ventilatory support
   C. Insertion of a Swan-Ganz catheter
   D. Obtaining a chest roentgenogram
   E. Monitoring blood pressure
      (32:161)

Set 18
Aspiration Pneumonia

A 19-year-old woman is intubated and placed on a Bennett MA-I ventilator subsequent to having aspirated gastric contents during obstetric surgery. She is receiving an FIo_2 of 1.0 with no PEEP and a V_T of 10 cc/kg. Arterial blood gas and acid-base data obtained with the ventilator in the control mode are as follows:

Pao_2	56 mm Hg
$Paco_2$	47 mm Hg
pH	7.47
HCO_3^-	17 mEq/L
Base excess	-4.9 mEq/L

1. Which of the following is the most correct interpretation of this patient's acid-base status?
    A. Metabolic acidosis with respiratory alkalosis
    B. Mixed respiratory and metabolic acidosis
    C. Fully compensated respiratory acidosis
    D. A laboratory error exists.
    E. Metabolic acidosis alone exists.
    (5:Chap 12)

2. Episodes of aspiration that occur while the patient is in a supine position are known to most frequently involve which of the following areas of the lung?
    A. Right lower lobe, superior segment
    B. Right lower lobe, medial support
    C. Right lower lobe, anterior segment
    D. Right lower lobe, lateral segment
    E. Right lower lobe, posterior segment
    (32:13)

3. Which of the following is *not* a method of reducing the *severity* of episodes of gastric aspiration?
    A. Keeping patient N.P.O.
    B. Administering narcotic agents
    C. Applying nasogastric suction
    D. Administering antacids
    E. Administering cimetidine
    (31:346-347)

4. Four days later, the patient is alert and is receiving an FIo_2 of 0.6 with 10 cm H_2O PEEP and a V_T of 12 cc/kg in the assist/control mode. At that time the following blood gas data are reported:

Pao_2	183 mm Hg
$Paco_2$	27 mm Hg
pH	7.44
HCO_3^-	20 mEq/L

Based on the above information, which of the following would be the most appropriate recommendation for the respiratory therapy practitioner to make at this time?
    A. Lower the PEEP and add mechanical deadspace

B.   Lower the FI_{O_2} and place the patient on intermittent manda-
     tory ventilation
C.   Increase the tidal volume and lower the FI_{O_2}
D.   Increase the tidal volume and lower the PEEP
E.   Place the patient on intermittent mandatory ventilation with
     other settings unchanged
   (46) (49)

Set 19
Tension
Pneumothorax

A 19-year-old man is brought to the emergency department after
experiencing sharp chest pain while playing basketball. Gross observation reveals a tall, thin man in severe distress. Despite receiving 10 L
oxygen via simple oxygen mask, the patient is deeply cyanotic. Percussion of the chest yields a dull note on the right side and a hyperresonant
note on the left. Additionally, a distinct shift in the trachea toward the
right side is noted. Cardiac leads are attached and the monitor shows
multifocal premature ventricular contractions and sinus tachycardia.
The blood pressure is measured at this time to be 40/0.

1.   Which of the following should the respiratory therapy practitioner
     recommend at this time?
     A.   Obtaining stat arterial blood sample
     B.   Obtaining stat chest roentgenogram
     C.   Inserting a needle in the eighth interspace of the left chest
          wall
     D.   Administration of intermittent positive pressure breathing
     E.   Inserting a needle in the third interspace of the left chest wall
        (25:Chap 14, p 18)
2.   Which of the following is the most correct diagnosis?
     A.   Open pneumothorax
     B.   Traumatic tension pneumothorax
     C.   Bronchopulmonary dysplasia
     D.   Spontaneous tension pneumothorax
     E.   Open tension pneumothorax
        (11:190–191) (7:344–350)

3. Which of the following is the most probable cause of this patient's cyanosis?
   A. Decreased cardiac output
   B. Right-to-left physiologic shunting
   C. Anemia
   D. Ventilation in excess of perfusion
   E. A and B are correct.
   (11:191)

Set 20
Adult Respiratory Distress Syndrome II

A 23-year-old man is brought to the emergency department following a hiking accident. The patient is severely distressed, is comatose, and is noted to have multiple facial, head, and chest trauma. Closer evaluation of this patient reveals considerable bleeding from pharyngeal tissues.

1. Considering the foregoing information, the respiratory therapy practitioner would now recommend which of the following?
   A. Intubate and place on an FI_{O_2} of 0.6
   B. Perform emergency tracheotomy and place on 30% oxygen via heated aerosol system
   C. Obtain an arterial sample and a chest roentgenogram stat
   D. Place on nonrebreathing type mask at 12 L/min O_2 flow
   E. C and D are correct.
   (1:499)

2. Twelve hours later the patient is in the intensive care unit and is receiving 70% oxygen via T tube setup. Arterial blood gases drawn at this time reveal:

Pa_{O_2}	40 mm Hg
Pa_{CO_2}	35 mm Hg
pH	7.43
HCO_3^-	26 mEq/L

   Based on the above information, which of the following is the most correct recommendation?
   A. Place on 5 cm H_2O PEEP with an FI_{O_2} of 0.4

B. Place on continuous ventilatory support with an FI_{O_2} of 0.9
C. Place on 5 cm H_2O CPAP with an FI_{O_2} of 0.8
D. Increase FI_{O_2} to 1.0 on T tube
E. Place on continuous ventilatory support with a tidal volume of 18 cc/kg and an FI_{O_2} of 1.0
    (46) (38:63–65)

3. Three days later, with the patient on 40% oxygen and 15 cm H_2O PEEP, the following arterial blood gas data were obtained:

Pa_{O_2}	132 mm Hg
Pa_{CO_2}	32 mm Hg
pH	7.53
HCO_3^-	29.3 mEq/L

Based on the foregoing information, which of the following modifications should the respiratory therapy practitioner recommend?
A. Lower PEEP to 12 cm H_2O
B. Add 150 cc mechanical deadspace and lower the PEEP to 10 cm H_2O
C. Lower the FI_{O_2} to 0.3
D. Place on 15 cm H_2O CPAP with an FI_{O_2} of 0.6
E. Lower the PEEP to 10 cm H_2O and the FI_{O_2} to 0.3
    (46)

4. Two days later, the patient is on an FI_{O_2} of 0.4 with no PEEP. Because of substantial improvement in the patient's clinical picture, the physician asks the respiratory practitioner to collect appropriate weaning criteria. The following data are charted at this time:

Pa_{O_2}	117 mm Hg
Pa_{CO_2}	37 mm Hg
pH	7.42
HCO_3^-	23 mEq/L
Negative inspiratory force	88 cm H_2O
Vital capacity	49 cc/kg
Resting spontaneous minute volume	8.1 L/min

Based on this information, the respiratory therapy practitioner should now recommend:
A. Place patient on T tube with an FI_{O_2} of 0.4
B. Place on intermittent mandatory ventilation with an FI_{O_2} of 0.4
C. Place on intermittent mandatory ventilation with an FI_{O_2} of 0.5
D. Place on T tube with an FI_{O_2} of 0.5
E. Place on T tube with an FI_{O_2} of 0.7
    (2:668–670) (1:324–348)

Answer Key

Set 1
1. A
2. E
3. C
4. C
5. A

Set 2
1. C
2. D
3. D
4. D

Set 3
1. C
2. C
3. C

Set 4
1. E
2. D
3. C
4. D

Set 5
1. C

2. C
3. D
4. A

Set 6
1. E
2. D
3. C
4. D
5. C

Set 7
1. B
2. C
3. A
4. E

Set 8
1. C
2. D
3. E
4. C

Set 9
1. A
2. C

3. D
4. D

Set 10
1. C
2. C
3. C
4. E

Set 11
1. C
2. C
3. D
4. A
5. A

Set 12
1. A
2. E
3. C
4. A

Set 13
1. B
2. A
3. C

4. E
5. D

Set 14
1. C
2. B
3. C
4. B
5. D

Set 15
1. B
2. E
3. E
4. A

Set 16
1. D
2. B
3. B
4. C
5. B

Set 17
1. E
2. C

3. B

Set 18
1. D
2. A
3. B
4. B

Set 19
1. E
2. D
3. E

Set 20
1. A
2. C
3. A
4. D

UNIT III

Hemodynamics Review and Pretest (Advanced Level Only)

Part I
Hemodynamics
Review

It has been well documented (see references 45 and 80) that the respiratory care practitioner plays an important role in the management of patients with cardiovascular disorders. These individuals frequently require procedures such as continuous ventilatory support and arterial blood gas analysis. Increasingly, the management of these patients is being guided by valuable information obtained from flow-directed, balloon-tipped pulmonary artery catheters. Information from these devices is extremely important to the respiratory therapy practitioner since it allows therapeutic modalities such as positive end-expiratory pressure (PEEP) and oxygen to be administered in precise dosages. A common clinical problem is the management of those patients with large physiologic shunts complicated by marginal cardiovascular reserves. These patients often would benefit from PEEP therapy. Unfortunately, cardiovascular depression seen with this modality may be pronounced. Cardiovascular support with fluids and inotropic agents is frequently indicated to minimize these side effects. However, these support agents have their unwanted actions as well. In particular, excessive fluid administration may increase intrapulmonary shunting, and sympathomimetics can precipitate cardiovascular failure.

Unfortunately, when one system is treated, another often gets worse. This pathophysiologic standoff has stumped clinicians since Hippocrates' day and continues to do so. Consequently, it is not difficult to see how the ability to monitor cardiac output, pulmonary wedge pressure, and Q_S/Q_T can simplify matters greatly.

This part reviews the important concepts necessary in understanding the clinical assessment of central and peripheral vascular hemodynamics. To help make this material more accessible, this outline is followed:

 I. General Principles
 II. The Central Circulation
     A. Pulmonary wedge pressure (PWP)
        1. Physiology
        2. Increased PWP
           a. Left ventricular failure
           b. Left ventricular failure vs. hypervolemia

        3.   Decreased PWP
        4.   Effect of PEEP on PWP measurements
   B.   Pulmonary arterial pressures
        1.   Pulmonary hypertension
        2.   Pulmonary vascular resistance
        3.   Pulmonary hypotension
   C.   Other measurements available with pulmonary artery catheterization
        1. $C(a\text{-}\bar{v})o_2$ measurement
        2. $S\bar{v}o_2$ and $P\bar{v}o_2$ measurements
        3.   Central venous pressure
III.   Peripheral Circulation
   A.   Hypertension
        1.   Chronic hypertension
        2.   Acute hypertension
   B.   Hypotension
        1.   Decreased cardiac output
        2.   Decreased peripheral vascular resistance

Obviously, this is a broad subject. An in-depth discussion of all of these topics is beyond the scope of one examination review text. It is also unnecessary since these topics are comprehensively covered in many fine standard textbooks. The following selected readings are recommended to supplement the following discussion:

Reference 1: Chaps 2, 26, and 27
Reference 5: Chap 18
Reference 11: Chap 20
Reference 25
Reference 31: Chap 9
Reference 41
Reference 46
Reference 61
Reference 100: Chap 20
Reference 101: Chaps 2 and 6

General Principles

It is the function of the powerful left ventricle to perfuse the high pressure, high resistance peripheral circulation. Concurrently, the considerably less muscled right ventricle pumps an identical output through the low pressure, low resistance central vasculature.

A healthy 70-kg subject has a circulating blood volume of approximately 6 L. At rest, roughly two thirds of this volume is in the venous system and another fourth is in the arterial system. The remaining 10% is in the pulmonary vasculature (see reference 1:Chap 2).

In conceptualizing the body's circulatory system, it is important to remember that (under normal circumstances) the right and left sides of the heart are parallel circuits with *exactly* the same output. Should these outputs not match one another down to the smallest fraction of a milliliter, right- or left-sided congestive heart failure is inevitable. The following scenario illustrates this fact (see reference 100: Chap 20).

Consider a 70-kg patient with a cardiac rate of 100 beats/min. If the stroke volume of this patient's right and left ventricles is 70 mL, then both sides of the heart will have an identical output of 7 L/min. What would happen if the left ventricle suffered an ischemic episode and its stroke volume decreased 0.1 mL to 69.9 mL? *Within 1 hour the volume of blood within the pulmonary vasculature would have doubled (to 1200 mL) and the patient would be in left-sided congestive heart failure.*

Clinically, this patient would display signs of increased cardiorespiratory workloads, and should a pulmonary artery catheter be in place, a substantial increase in the pulmonary wedge pressure (PWP) would be noted. Oxygen administration, inotropic stimulation, diuresis, and pharmacologic reduction of venous return all have their place in correcting myocardial workload/demand imbalances such as this and would undoubtedly be of great benefit to this patient (see reference 100:Chap 20).

The Central Circulation

The central or pulmonary circulation begins with the right atrium and ends at the aortic valve. It is characterized as a low pressure, low resistance system. This is due to the copiousness of this vascular bed. It is perhaps best thought of as an enormous sheet of blood with a surface area roughly two thirds of the alveolar septum (45 m^2). This is the reason postpneumonectomy patients may not develop pulmonary hypertension. This, unfortunately, is not the case with many critically ill patients. Hypoxemia, hypercarbia, and acidosis are all potent constrictors of pulmonary arterioles. It is this fact that is responsible for the widespread use of Swan-Ganz catheters. Thus, the following concept must be understood from the outset if one is to grasp the clinical significance of pulmonary artery catheterization:

> In a patient with normal pulmonary vascular resistance and a healthy right ventricle, the central venous pressure (CVP), usually measured at the mouth of the right atrium, will accurately represent left ventricular filling (preload) pressures. However, if the pulmonary vascular resistance is increased, the CVP may be falsely elevated and thus cannot be relied on to assess left ventricular status (see reference 101:Chap 2).

Therein lies the problem with CVP measurement. The patients on whom it is accurate frequently do not need it. The clinical importance of pulmonary artery catheterization then can be summed up as follows: *it allows for measurement of the PWP. This value is not affected by changes in pulmonary vascular resistance. Thus, under most clinical circumstances it accurately reflects left ventricular filling pressures* (see reference 101:Chap 2).

Pulmonary Wedge Pressure (PWP)

Physiology

The normal range of values for the PWP is generally stated to be 5 mm Hg to 12 mm Hg, with an average value of 9 mm Hg. When a pulmonary artery catheter is in the "wedge" position, the pressure transducer measures vascular system backpressure under <u>conditions of no blood flow</u>. By inflating the catheter's balloon and stopping blood flow through that particular pulmonary artery branch, the clinician eliminates the component of pulmonary vascular resistance: <u>no flow</u>, <u>no resistance</u>—it is as simple as that (see reference 100:Chap 20).

The respiratory therapy practitioner employs this principle every time he or she occludes a ventilator's exhalation valve to obtain a plateau pressure. By stopping flow at end inspiration, the component of airway resistance is eliminated. The resulting static pressure is believed to approximate alveolar pressure and thus not be influenced by changes in airway caliber or flow characteristics. This plateau pressure can, therefore, only be affected by changes in the relationship between lung volume and lung thorax elastance: that is, static lung-thorax compliance (C_{LT}).

By the same token, when the clinician inflates a pulmonary artery catheter's balloon and measures the PWP, he or she is actually getting a reflection of the hydrostatic pressures within the left ventricle. In the absence of blood flow, the catheter's transducer "reads" the pressure of a static column of blood extending from the pulmonary capillaries into the pulmonary vein and finally into the left atrium. The mean left atrial pressure represents the filling pressure of the left ventricle at end-diastole. This left ventricular end diastolic pressure (LVEDP) is a major determinant of stroke volume and therefore cardiac output. Like ventilator plateau pressure, the LVEDP is a reflection of the relationship between the volume within the left ventricle and the elastic forces of the myocardium itself (see reference 101:Chap 2). This, the Frank-Starling relationship, is expressed most clearly by constructing a myocardial compliance/performance curve such as that which appears below.

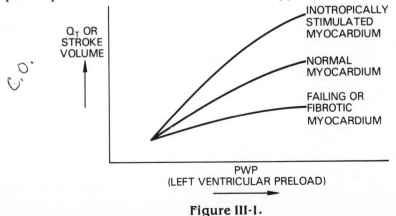

Figure III-1.

From this illustration it is not hard to see that both a low PWP (hypovolemia) and a loss of myocardial muscle tone (such as occurs following infarction) will both lead to a decrease in outflow. Again, one can draw a parallel between cardiovascular and pulmonary systems since both are affected adversely by poor volume/pressure relationships (see reference 101:Chap 6).

Increased PWP

The most important clinical problem associated with increases in the PWP is the development of pulmonary edema. This is believed to be inevitable whenever the pressure rises above 25 mm Hg (see references 42 and 99). Among critically ill patients, especially those with poor nutritional status, clinically significant edema often develops at considerably lower pressures (see reference 99). Lacking an adequate protein source, the serum albumin levels of these patients may drop to dangerously low levels. This and other serum proteins are responsible for maintaining intravascular volume because of the colloidal osmotic pressure they exert.

Also at risk of developing pulmonary edema at relatively low PWPs are those patients with adult respiratory distress syndrome (ARDS). These patients have experienced alveolar capillary damage through one mechanism or another (e.g., liquid aspiration or Gram-negative sepsis). The inflamed parenchyma is known to become extremely edematous even in the presence of normal serum protein and PWP levels (see reference 32:Chap 12).

Many clinical conditions have been associated with increases in the PWP. Fortunately, most of these are rare. Thus, NBRC candidates need concern themselves with only the following two disorders as illustrated by the preceding Frank-Starling curve. Left ventricular dysfunction and hypervolemia are, by far, the most common and clinically significant of these disorders (see references 41 and 101:Chap 2). Consider the following self-study question:

Question:
Which of the following disorders are known to cause the PWP to become elevated?
  I.   Adult respiratory distress syndrome
 II.   Left ventricular failure
III.   Right ventricular failure
IV.   Hypervolemia
  V.   Increased pulmonary vascular resistance
        A.   I, III, and IV
        B.   II, III, and IV
        C.   I and V
        D.   II and V
        E.   II and IV
Answer: E

Only choices II and IV will lead to this. Increases in pulmonary vascular resistance, as described earlier, is what the PWP was designed *not* to reflect. Right ventricular failure will not increase the PWP and neither will adult respiratory distress syndrome.[1] Patients with right ventricular failure or adult respiratory distress syndrome often have increased PWPs, but it is almost invariably due to concurrent left ventricular dysfunction or hypervolemia. Indeed, left ventricular failure is the most common clinical cause of right ventricular failure.

Left Ventricular Failure

The left ventricle is a pump. Failure of this pump will result in blood backing up and engorging the pulmonary vasculature. One of the major indications for PWP measurement is the early detection of left ventricular dysfunction. Because it directly reflects left-sided heart activity, the PWP is generally considered the most sensitive indicator of impending left ventricular failure (see reference 101:Chap 2).

Left ventricular failure may be caused by an acute ischemic episode such as a myocardial infarction. It may also result from increased myocardial workloads such as may result from mitral and aortic valvular disease or more commonly from arterial hypertension.

Therapy for left ventricular failure includes increasing myocardial contractile force and decreasing venous return. The former may be accomplished by using pharmacologic agents such as dopamine, dobutamine, and digitalis, all of which have a positive inotropic effect. Venous return (the PWP or preload) is usually reduced pharmacologically by administering diuretics and/or morphine. The latter has a potent dilatory effect on the venules. Other methods, such as positive pressure ventilation and rotating tourniquets, may also be of value.

The following self-study question illustrates these points.

Question:
The following data were collected on a 70-kg patient in the cardiac care unit:

Pulmonary artery systolic	53 mm Hg
Pulmonary artery diastolic	39 mm Hg
PWP	32 mm Hg
Cardiac output	3.4 L/min
$C(a-\bar{v})o_2$	7.3 vol%
Temperature	36.8°C

---

[1]One possible exception to this is so-called neurovasogenic ARDS. Here, acute and massive increases in intracranial pressure cause profound increases in systemic vascular resistance (Cushing effect). This can lead to large (but transient) increases in the PWP. Most observers, however, prefer to think of the phenomenon as transient left ventricular failure secondary to an acutely increased afterload (see reference 2:754).

Which of the following pharmacologic agents would the respiratory therapy practitioner be *least* likely to recommend for this patient?

A. Dopamine
B. Morphine
C. Oxygen
D. Propranolol
E. Furosemide

Answer: D

Propranolol is known to inhibit the action of B_1-receptors in the myocardium. Thus, its negative inotropic actions would make its administration unadvisable. All the other values listed in the question are typical for a patient with left ventricular failure. Note the severely decreased cardiac output and widened $C(a-\bar{v})_{O_2}$. Clinically, a cardiac index of less than 2.2 $L/min/m^2$ or a $C(a-\bar{v})_{O_2}$ of greater than 6.0 vol% in the absence of hypermetabolism or peripheral arteriovenous shunting is believed to indicate the presence of poor cardiovascular reserves (see reference 5:Chap 18).

Left Ventricular Failure vs. Hypervolemia

An increased PWP due to left ventricular failure can frequently be differentiated from that caused by hypervolemia if the cardiac output or a good indicator such as the $C(a-\bar{v})_{O_2}$ is known. The following self-study question should be helpful in illustrating this fact.

Question:
The following data were collected on a 70-kg patient in the cardiac care unit:

Pulmonary artery systolic	53 mm Hg
Pulmonary artery diastolic	34 mm Hg
PWP	28 mm Hg
Cardiac output	10.6 L/min
$C(a-\bar{v})_{O_2}$	2.7 vol%
Oxygen consumption ($\dot{V}_{O_2}$)	285 mL/min

$$C.O. \times c(a-\bar{v})_{O_2}$$

Based on the above information, which of the following is most likely to be responsible for this patient's elevated PWP?

A. Hypervolemia
B. Hypovolemia
C. Left ventricular failure
D. Adult respiratory distress syndrome
E. Right ventricular failure

Answer: A

The reasoning for this becomes clear if one remembers that it is impossible for a patient in left ventricular failure to have a cardiac output nearly twice the normal. Left ventricular failure leads to a *decreased* cardiac output. In examining the Frank-Starling curve (Figure III-1), the reader will notice that as the PWP goes up, the cardiac output increases. Eventually, a point is reached at which output falls precipitously, but initially output increases. Again note the relationship between the cardiac output and the $C(a-\bar{v})o_2$. Because of the very large Q_T and narrow $C(a-\bar{v})o_2$, this patient's cardiovascular reserves would have to be considered excellent (see reference 5:Chap 18).

Decreased PWP

The PWP is considered decreased whenever it falls below 5 mm Hg. By far, the most common clinical cause of this is hypovolemia. The case history presented below represents a typical patient.

Question:
The following data were collected on a 70-kg patient seen in the intensive care unit:

Pulmonary artery systolic	22 mm Hg
Pulmonary artery diastolic	6 mm Hg
PWP	2 mm Hg
$C(a-\bar{v})o_2$	7.9 vol%
Temperature	37°C

Which of the following assessments regarding the above patient are most likely to be true?
  I.   The patient is hypovolemic.
 II.   Left ventricular failure exists.
III.   The cardiac output is probably decreased.
IV.   Pulmonary edema is inevitable.
    A.   I and III
    B.   II and IV
    C.   I and II
    D.   I, II, and III
    E.   I, III, and IV

Answer: A

The patient's PWP indicates the probable presence of hypovolemia. Regarding the patient's cardiovascular reserves, they are apparently anything but excellent. With few exceptions (massive catabolism and hyperthyroidism among them) a $C(a-\bar{v})o_2$ of 7.9 vol% in a normothermic patient would indicate the existence of a severely decreased cardiac output (see reference 5:Chap 18).

Effect of PEEP on PWP Measurements

If the catheter tip is properly placed in a zone III artery, the effect of mild to moderate doses of PEEP on PWP measurements is usually minimal. It has been suggested that on an average the PWP will increase approximately 1 mm Hg for each 5 cm H_2O of PEEP (see reference 46). Ways of reducing PEEP-induced artifact include the use of strip rather than digital recorders, as well as taking measurements at end expiration (see reference 100:Chap 20).

Pulmonary Arterial Pressures

The following table lists the normal values for the pressures within the pulmonary artery (P.A.):

Pressure	Range of Clinical Normals	Laboratory Normals
P.A. systolic	20–35	25
P.A. diastolic	5–15	8
P.A. mean	10–20	15

When the pulmonary artery catheter balloon is deflated, the transducer will record the pulmonary arterial systolic and diastolic pressures. Electronic instrumentation will derive the pulmonary arterial mean pressure from this information. The NBRC may use a question such as the one that follows to assess the candidate's understanding of the pulmonary arterial pressures.

Question:
The respiratory therapy practitioner is monitoring a patient in the intensive care unit. The following clinical data are gathered at this time:

P.A. systolic	26 mm Hg
P.A. diastolic	8 mm Hg
P.A. mean	15 mm Hg
PWP	28 mm Hg
Cardiac output	6.0 L/min

Which of the following is the most appropriate assessment regarding the above information?
A.   The data are in error.
B.   Left ventricular dysfunction exists.
C.   The pulmonary vascular resistance is elevated.
D.   The patient is hypervolemic.
E.   The above represents a normal study.
Answer: A

Since it is the function of the right ventricle to deliver blood to the left ventricle and not the other way around, it is impossible for the PWP to exceed the P.A. systolic pressure. It would be equally impossible for peripheral venous pressures to exceed peripheral arterial pressure. Blood flows forward, not backward. The PWP is usually slightly lower than the P.A. diastolic pressure unless the pulmonary vascular resistance is increased; then it is *considerably* lower (see reference 41).

Pulmonary Hypertension

Pulmonary hypertension is said to exist whenever the pressures in the pulmonary arterial circuit are greater than 35/15 (see reference 11:Chap 20). This is known to occur most commonly as the result of one of three disorders:

1. Left ventricular dysfunction
2. Hypervolemia
3. Increased pulmonary vascular resistance (PVR)

Since left ventricular failure and hypervolemia were discussed in the section on increased PWP, only PVR will be discussed here.

Pulmonary Vascular Resistance

Clinically, the PVR is considered elevated whenever the gradient between P.A. diastolic and the PWP (PAD−PWP) is greater than 5 mm Hg (see reference 41). This may be calculated more accurately by dividing the difference between the P.A. mean and the PWP (PAM−PWP) by the cardiac output. This calculation is discussed in more detail in the mathematics review section of this book (see page 69). PAP

The PVR may be increased either by factors that constrict the pulmonary arterioles or by factors that destroy or obstruct the pulmonary vascular bed (see reference 11:Chap 20). Acidosis, hypercarbia, and particularly hypoxemia all have a profound effect on pulmonary arteriolar smooth muscle tone. Thus, these are the most common causes of increased PVR seen clinically. Pulmonary embolization, alveolar septal destruction, and surgical removal of lung tissue, although less common and usually less severe, will also increase the PVR. One of the major values of PWP measurement is that pulmonary hypertension due to increased PVR may be differentiated from that caused by left ventricular problems and hypervolemia (see reference 41). The following case history illustrates this.

Question:
The following data were collected on a 50-kg patient seen in the intensive care unit:

P. A. systolic	43 mm Hg
P. A. diastolic	21 mm Hg
CVP	12 mm Hg
PWP	3 mm Hg
$\dot{Q}_T$	3.9 L/min
$C(a-\bar{v})_{O_2}$	7.2 vol%
Oxygen consumption ($\dot{V}_{O_2}$)	280 mL/min

Which of the following statements regarding the patient is (are) most likely to be true?
I. Left ventricular failure exists.
II. The patient is probably hypovolemic.

III.   Cardiovascular reserves are excellent.
IV.   The pulmonary vascular resistance is increased.
    A.   I, II, and III
    B.   II and IV
    C.   I and III
    D.   II and III
    E.   I only
Answer: B

Since the PAD−PWP gradient is 18 mm Hg, the PVR is considerably elevated. By looking at the CVP or the pulmonary artery pressures, the clinician would have had little idea that hypovolemia existed. In fact, just the opposite might have occurred. The clinician, faced with elevated pressures and signs of diminished perfusion, might have believed left ventricular dysfunction to be the chief problem. Had this erroneous assessment 'ed to the decision to administer a diuretic, the result could conceivably have been catastrophic.

Pulmonary Hypotension

For all practical intents and purposes, there is only one cause of decreased central vascular pressures and that is hypovolemia (see reference 101:Chap 2). This holds true for all the pulmonary arterial pressures as well as the PWP and the CVP.

Other Measurements Available with Pulmonary Artery Catheterization

$C(a\text{-}\bar{v})o_2$ Measurement

The $C(a\text{-}\bar{v})o_2$ is believed to be a reliable indicator of cardiac output whenever the oxygen consumption is relatively normal and constant. Fortunately, this is frequently the case (see reference 5:Chap 18).

The following table relates cardiac output and $C(a\text{-}\bar{v})o_2$ to the cardiovascular reserves of a 70-kg critically ill patient with normal oxygen consumption:

Cardiovascular Reserves	Excellent	Good	Marginal	Poor
Cardiac output	10 L/min	7.5 L/min	5.0 L/min	↓ 4.0 L/min
$C(a\text{-}\bar{v})o_2$	2.5 vol%	3.5 vol%	5.0 vol%	↑ 6.0 vol%

It must be emphasized that the above values are for a critically ill patient. Among the critically ill, an average $C(a\text{-}\bar{v})o_2$ is 3.5 vol%. This is in contrast to the laboratory normal of 5.0 vol%, which is measured on a healthy subject at rest (see reference 5:Chap 18).

$S\bar{v}o_2$ and $P\bar{v}o_2$ Measurements

These are believed to be the most reliable indicators of tissue oxygenation status (see references 46 and 100:Chap 20). The following table illustrates this:

Tissue Oxygenation Status	$P\bar{v}o_2$	$S\bar{v}o_2$
Normal	35–45 mm Hg	65–75%
Mild to moderate hypoxia	30–35 mm Hg	55–65%
Severe hypoxia	↓ 30 mm Hg	↓ 55%

From the above table it can be appreciated that because of the steepness of the oxyhemoglobin dissociation curve in this range, a drop in $P\bar{v}o_2$ of several millimeters of mercury may be of great significance. The $S\bar{v}o_2$ is perhaps the more reliable of the two because it is not affected by changes in the positioning of the oxyhemoglobin dissociation curve. The addition of an oximeter to the standard four-channel pulmonary artery catheter allows for continuous readout of $S\bar{v}o_2$ at the patient's bedside. This is becoming an increasingly valuable tool to guide the administration of cardiorespiratory therapy.

Central Venous Pressure

The central venous pressure (CVP) is usually measured at the mouth of the right atrium. It can be measured with a CVP catheter (designed to measure only the CVP) or with three- and four-channel pulmonary artery catheters. The normal range for the CVP is usually between 5 mm Hg and 15 mm Hg (see reference 101:Chap 2). The CVP usually is equal to the pulmonary arterial diastolic pressure or is slightly higher, since some blood flow exists at its site of measurement. Clinically, the CVP may be decreased if the patient becomes hypovolemic. Increases in CVP most frequently result from the increased work of having to pump blood through a hypertensive pulmonary vascular system.

As has been noted previously, the fact that the CVP can be elevated by an increased PVR means that it frequently does not accurately reflect left ventricular filling pressures (preload). The very real need for a means of assessing the left ventricle in these patients led, ultimately, to the development of the balloon-tipped, flow-directed pulmonary artery catheter (see reference 101:Chap 2).

Peripheral Circulation

The peripheral circulation begins with the aortic valve and ends at the mouth of the right atrium. It is characterized as a high pressure, high resistance circulation. This is because its pressures and resistance to blood flow represent a fivefold to tenfold increase over those in the central circuit (see reference 101:Chap 2).

The normal arterial blood pressure is generally stated to be 120/80, but patients are generally not considered hypertensive or hypotensive until a wider range of 90/60 through 140/90 is exceeded. As is so often the case, what is normal for one patient may not be for another.

Hypertension

In general, hypertension is not believed to exist until the peripheral arterial diastolic pressure exceeds 90 mm Hg. Mild to moderate elevations in this value (90 mm Hg to 100 mm Hg) are often unaccompanied by overt symptomatology but nonetheless viewed with concern. Severe elevations (greater than 110 mm Hg) are usually the result of significant organic pathology and generally necessitate prompt intervention (see reference 94:Chap 6).

Chronic Hypertension

Unfortunately, chronic hypertension is a very common problem, but it can be managed adequately in the majority of cases. Mild to moderate elevations in the diastolic blood pressure (90 mm Hg to 110 mm Hg) may be caused by nothing more than an overly stressful life-style. Severe hypertension (↑ 110 mm Hg) usually indicates some degree of irreversible sclerotic changes in the arterial wall. For the sake of completeness, it should be mentioned that peripheral arterial hypertension will increase left ventricular workloads. Thus, hypertension is one of the risk factors associated with the development of congestive heart failure. Accordingly, peripheral arterial vasodilators such as nitroprusside (Nipride®) are frequently used in the management of chronic hypertension patients who develop congestive heart failure. Their use to decrease left ventricular afterload is frequently rewarded with an increase in cardiac output (see reference 101:Chap 2).

Acute Hypertension

Acute elevations in systemic blood pressure are part of the body's generalized response to stress of any source. Physiologically, these elevations represent an attempt to shunt blood away from the tissue beds to the central organs and skeletal muscles where it can be used for the fight or flight response. This response is mediated in large part by the release of norepinephrine from sympathetic fibers located in arteriolar smooth muscle fibers. In general, elevations of greater than 30/15 from baseline are considered medically significant. Severe stress or illness may result in elevations of 60/30 from baseline. In many of these instances, failure to intervene immediately may result in a life-threatening emergency (see reference 94:Chap 6).

For the sake of completeness, the so-called Cushing effect should be mentioned here. Cushing was the first to describe the sudden and often massive increases in arterial blood pressure that occur following acute increases in intracranial pressure associated with neuropathology. This represents an autoregulatory mechanism designed to maintain cerebral perfusion pressure within its normal range of 60 mm Hg to 100 mm Hg (see reference 100:Chap 18). This relationship is shown as follows:

$$\text{Cerebral Perfusion Pressure} = (\text{Mean Arterial Pressure}) - (\text{Intracranial Pressure})$$

$$60\text{–}100 \text{ mm Hg} = (70\text{–}110 \text{ mm Hg}) - (10\text{–}20 \text{ mm Hg})$$

It is not uncommon for patients suffering from acute neurologic emergencies (e.g., cerebrovascular accident, neurotrauma) to present with blood pressures in excess of 200/150.

Hypotension

A patient is not generally considered hypotensive until the arterial blood pressure falls below 90/60. When these episodes are prolonged or severe enough, circulatory failure or shock is said to exist. A good definition of shock is as follows: *a state of circulatory failure characterized by peripheral arterial hypotension and tissue hypoxia* (see reference 94).

From a pathophysiologic standpoint, there are two causes of hypotension:

1. Decreased cardiac output
2. Decreased peripheral vascular resistance

Decreased Cardiac Output

This is most commonly caused by left ventricular failure and hypovolemia (see reference 101:Chap 2). Differential diagnosis is accomplished most easily by measuring PWP. The following two self-study questions illustrate this clearly.

1. The following clinical data were gathered on a 70-kg adult patient in an intensive care unit:

Cardiac output	3.1 L/min
PWP	36 mm Hg
$C(a\text{-}\bar{v})_{O_2}$	7.9 vol%
Oxygen consumption ($\dot{V}_{O_2}$)	245 mL/min

    Which of the following mechanisms is most likely responsible for this patient's low cardiac output?
    A. Right ventricular failure
    B. Left ventricular failure
    C. Hypovolemia
    D. Increased PVR

E.   Adult respiratory distress syndrome
Answer: B

2.   The following clinical data were gathered on a 70-kg adult patient in an intensive care unit:

Cardiac output	3.1 L/min
PWP	3 mm Hg
$C(a\text{-}\bar{v})_{O_2}$	7.9 vol%
Oxygen consumption ($\dot{V}_{O_2}$)	245 mL/min

Which of the following mechanisms is most likely responsible for this patient's low cardiac output?
A.   Right ventricular failure
B.   Left ventricular failure
C.   Hypovolemia
D.   Adult respiratory distress syndrome
E.   Increased PVR
Answer: C

The PWP is used clinically to approximate left ventricular filling pressures. It is well known medically that the cardiac output is largely dependent on the filling pressure of the left ventricle. This is, of course, the Frank-Starling relationship, and it is illustrated once again below:

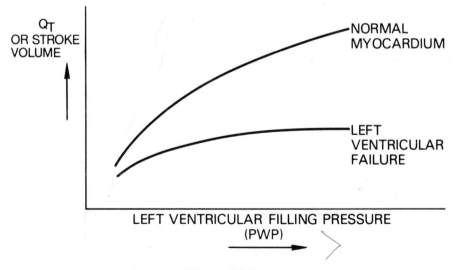

Figure III-2.

The graph clearly shows that the cardiac output is low at low pressures. Clinically, a low PWP in conjunction with a low cardiac output usually indicates hypovolemia. It is also noted above that the failing ventricle possesses a low output.

Decreased Peripheral Vascular Resistance

Septic, anaphylactic, and neurogenic shock all lead to circulatory failure via the same pathway: generalized peripheral vasodilation. This increase in the vascular space without an increase in vascular volume will lead to arterial hypotension (see reference 1). When arterial hypotension is widespread, the heart becomes unable to mobilize the blood trapped in peripheral vessels. This stagnant blood becomes increasingly acidotic and in severe cases may begin to clot. When clotting is extensive, disseminated intravascular coagulation (DIC) is said to exist (see reference 33).

Sepsis and anaphylaxis are known to cause vasodilation through release of large quantities of the vasoactive chemicals histamine, serotonin, and bradykinin. These inflammatory mediators are not only powerful vasodilators but also play important roles in activating complement and clotting mechanisms (see reference 12). Neurogenic shock is the result of the loss of sympathetic (alpha) innervation to the periphery. Sympathectomy may be traumatic or anoxic in origin. Cervical spine transection and low brain (hypothalamic) death are good representative examples. It must be pointed out, however, that hypotension is an uncommon manifestation of neuropathology. Hypertension is, in fact, seen much more frequently. The increase in arterial blood pressure that accompanies increased intracranial pressure is called the Cushing effect and is designed to maintain adequate cerebral perfusion pressure (see reference 100:Chap 18).

Part II
Hemodynamics
Pretest

The following four case studies are designed to assess the candidate's understanding of the hemodynamic concepts just discussed. Each case is followed by a brief discussion designed to reinforce these concepts. As the candidate reads through these, should he or she have additional questions, the appropriate section on the previous pages should be referred to.

Hemodynamics Case I

An unconscious 70-kg patient is brought to the emergency department by paramedics. Barbiturate intoxication is suspected. The patient is immediately intubated and placed on continuous ventilatory support. Because profound hypotension exists, a large quantity of crystalloid is administered. The patient is then transferred to the intensive care unit where she is placed on a Bourns Bear ventilator with an FI_{O_2} of 0.4.

Eight hours later the patient's chest roentgenogram shows evidence of alveolar and interstitial edema. The following data are gathered at this time, with the patient on an FI_{O_2} of 0.6 in the assist/control mode:

Pa_{O_2}	34 mm Hg
Pa_{CO_2}	34 mm Hg
pH	7.28
HCO_3^-	14 mEq/L
Base excess	−7.8 mEq/L
Oxygen consumption ($\dot{V}_{O_2}$)	250 mL/min
$C(a\text{-}\bar{v})_{O_2}$	2.9 vol%
PWP	27 mm Hg
$P\bar{v}_{O_2}$	24 mm Hg
$S\bar{v}_{O_2}$	46%

(handwritten annotations:) Combo acidosis; C.O. ↑; ↑ LVF R/O due to ↓ Ca₂-v̄p₂ ↑↑ C.O.

135

1. Which of the following is most likely to be responsible for this patient's base deficit?
   A. Renal insufficiency
   B. Gastric hyperactivity
   C. Anaerobic metabolism
   D. Metabolic compensation
   E. Normocarbia
   Answer: C

2. Assessment of which one of the above parameters would lead the practitioner to rule out left ventricular failure as the cause of this patient's acute pulmonary edema?
   A. $C(a\text{-}\bar{v})_{O_2}$
   B. PWP
   C. Pa_{O_2}
   D. Arterial pH
   E. Base deficit
   Answer: A

3. Which of the following should the respiratory therapist recommend at this time?
   I. Increase FI_{O_2} to 1.0
   II. Administer diuretics
   III. Begin PEEP therapy
   IV. Administer ¼ normal saline intravenously
   A. II and IV
   B. I, III, and IV
   C. II and III
   D. III only
   E. I only
   Answer: C

4. If the patient's effective static compliance had been monitored over the past few hours, which of the following would most likely have been noted?
   A. Widening of the gradient between peak and plateau pressures
   B. Increase in plateau pressure and increase in peak pressure
   C. Decrease in plateau pressure
   D. No change in peak pressure and increase in plateau pressure
   E. Decrease in pulmonary elastance
   Answer: B

Case I Discussion

Question 1

The tip-off in this question is the critically low $P\bar{v}_{O_2}$. This indicates the presence of severe tissue hypoxia. The resultant production of lactic acid is most likely responsible for this patient's metabolic acidosis.

Question 2

The very low $C(a-\bar{v})o_2$ coupled with the normal oxygen consumption ($\dot{V}o_2$) indicates a high cardiac output, thus ruling out left ventricular failure. An elevated PWP without a diminished cardiac output is associated with uncomplicated hypervolemia.

Question 3

The presence of refractory hypoxemia in the presence of an increased cardiac output is a reasonably clear indication for PEEP therapy. Diuretics are needed to lower the PWP and reduce pulmonary edema. Increasing the FIo_2 to 1.0 would probably not be of significant benefit since the hypoxemia is due to physiologic shunting (see reference 47).

Question 4

Peak and plateau pressure monitoring is often an effective method of anticipating the need for therapeutic intervention. In this case, gradual increases in both peak and plateau pressures would have alerted the practitioner that pulmonary pathology was worsening.

Hemodynamics Case II

A 53-year-old man with a long history of drug abuse is brought to the emergency department following aspiration of gastric contents. After successful resuscitation he is transferred to the intensive care unit where he is placed on a Bourns Bear I ventilator with an FIo_2 of 0.6 and 10 cm H_2O PEEP. Arterial blood gas analysis at this time reveals the following information:

Pao_2	41 mm Hg
$Paco_2$	43 mm Hg
pH	7.26
HCO_3	13.6 mEq/L
Base excess	−9.7 mEq/L

Par. comp. resp. acid

1. The physician believes that the patient's hypoxia would be easier to manage if a Swan-Ganz catheter were present. The respiratory therapy practitioner is asked to assist in its placement. During the procedure, the therapist notes the following waveform on the monitor:

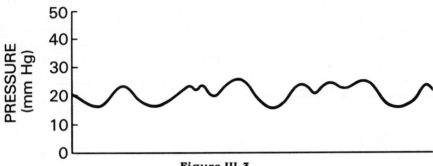

Figure III-3.

Which of the following statements about the above is (are) true?
I.   A pulmonary arterial tracing is noted.
II. The catheter should be retracted.
III. The catheter is in the wedge position.
IV. The catheter should be flushed with a heparin solution.
    A. I and IV
    B. I only
    C. III and IV
    D. II and III
    E. III only
Answer: E

2. Following successful placement and calibration, the following values were obtained:

P.A. systolic	56 mm Hg
P.A. diastolic	41 mm Hg
PWP	30 mm Hg
CVP	14 mm Hg
$C(a-\bar{v})o_2$	7.2 vol%
Oxygen consumption ($\dot{V}o_2$)	280 mL/min

Based on the above information, the most likely cause for the above data is which of the following?
    A. Right ventricular failure
    B. Left ventricular failure
    C. Adult respiratory distress syndrome
    D. Hypervolemia
    E. Hypovolemia
Answer: B

3. Based on the foregoing information, which of the following should the respiratory therapist recommend at this time?
    A. Increase the level of PEEP
    B. Administer inotropic agents
    C. Administer dromotropic agents
    D. Increase venous return
    E. Increase FIo_2
Answer: B

4. Which of the following statements regarding this patient's pulmo-
    nary arterial pressures is (are) true?
    I.   They are normal.
    II. Pulmonary hypertension exists.
    III. They are affected by the PVR.
        A. I only
        B. II and III
        C. III only
        D. I and III
        E. II only
    Answer: B

Case II Discussion

Question 1

Based on the information presented, the catheter is in the wedge
position.

Question 2

The presence of an elevated PWP with a severely widened $C(a\text{-}\bar{v})_{O_2}$ is
most suggestive of left ventricular failure. A $C(a\text{-}\bar{v})_{O_2}$ greater than 6.0
vol% frequently indicates the presence of poor cardiovascular reserves.

Question 3

Of the choices presented, increasing administration of inotropics is by
far the best choice. Additionally, the medical staff would probably be
attempting to decrease venous return and be considering a lower level of
PEEP.

Question 4

Pulmonary arterial pressures greater than 35/15 are believed to indicate pulmonary hypertension. Pulmonary arterial pressures are affected
by changes in PVR. Because the patient's PAD−PWP gradient is
greater than 5 mm Hg, the PVR must be considered elevated.

Hemodynamics Case III

A 38-year-old patient was admitted to the emergency department in
hemorrhagic shock following a motorcycle accident. Because of profound
hypotension and arrhythmias, basic and advanced cardiac life support

measures were used. Following stabilization the patient was transferred to the intensive care unit and placed on a Bennett MA-II ventilator with an FIO_2 of 0.6 in the control mode without PEEP. Blood gas data obtained at that time were as follows:

$$Pao_2 \qquad 41 \text{ mm Hg}$$
$$Paco_2 \qquad 45 \text{ mm Hg}$$
$$pH \qquad 7.28$$
$$HCO_3^- \qquad 18.2 \text{ mEq/L}$$

1. Based on the above information, which of the following modifications should the respiratory therapy practitioner make at this time?
    A. Increase the FIO_2 to 0.9
    B. Decrease the respiratory rate and increase the FIO_2
    C. Increase the tidal volume and the FIO_2
    D. Place on 10 cm H_2O PEEP with an FIO_2 of 0.6
    E. Place on 10 cm H_2O CPAP with an FIO_2 of 0.6
    Answer: D

2. The physician believes that this patient's management should be guided by serial PWP measurements. After cutting down to the subclavian vein, a balloon-tipped catheter is inserted. During the procedure the following tracing was noted:

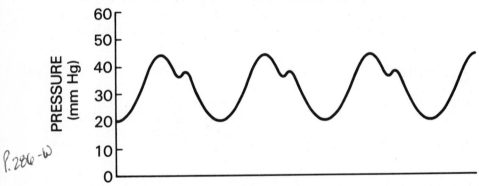

P. 286 -w

Figure III-4.

Which of the following statements regarding the above waveform is (are) true?
I.   The catheter is in the pulmonary artery.
II.   The catheter may be advanced.
III. The catheter is in the wedge position.
IV.   The catheter is in the left ventricle.
    A. I only
    B. I and II
    C. III only
    D. II only
    E. IV only
Answer: B

3. Following successful placement the following data were obtained:

P.A. systolic	48 mm Hg
P.A. diastolic	32 mm Hg
PWP	22 mm Hg
CVP	15 mm Hg
$C(a\text{-}\bar{v})_{O_2}$	2.6 vol%

Based on the above information, the most likely assessment is which of the following?
A. Hypovolemia
B. Hypervolemia
C. Left ventricular failure
D. Acute pulmonary embolus
E. Tension pneumothorax
Answer: B

4. Based on the foregoing information, which of the following should the therapist recommend?
A. Increase venous return
B. Administer diuretics
C. Administer fluids
D. Administer norepinephrine
E. Wean from the ventilator
Answer: B

Case III Discussion

Question 1

Because refractory hypoxemia exists, the patient needs a trial of PEEP. CPAP is usually not appropriate during the acute phase of respiratory failure because of increases in work of breathing that may result from its application.

Question 2

The pulmonary arterial waveform can be recognized by the wide swings in pressure and by the presence of the dicrotic notch. This latter represents closure of the pulmonic valve.

Question 3

The presence of an increased PWP and an increased cardiac output is most suggestive of hypervolemia. A $C(a\text{-}\bar{v})_{O_2}$ of less than approximately 4.0 vol% generally indicates the presence of good cardiovascular reserves.

Question 4

Diuresis is indicated to lower the PWP and treat pulmonary edema. The patient is not able to be weaned from the ventilator at this time.

Hemodynamics Case IV

A 68-year-old man is admitted to the intensive care unit after falling at a local nursing home. He is comatose and febrile and has a blood pressure of 40/0. The patient's appearance suggests protracted poor oral intake. The admission workup also shows a fractured right femur and swelling in the pelvic region that is suggestive of hemorrhage. Because of this he is scheduled for emergency surgery. In the operating room profound hypotension continues despite administration of two units of blood and 3 L crystalloid. After successful control of all bleeding, he is returned to the intensive care unit. Data obtained at that time include:

FIo_2	0.40 (via T tube system)
Pao_2	83 mm Hg
$Paco_2$	65 mm Hg
pH	7.20
Base excess	-5.1 mEq/L
Pulse	130
BP	70/40
CVP	20 mm Hg

1. True statements regarding the above information include which of the following?
    I.   Refractory hypoxemia exists.
    II. Ventilatory support is indicated.
    III. Systemic hypotension exists.
    IV. The CVP is elevated.
        A. II, III, and IV
        B. I and II
        C. I, II, and III
        D. I, III, and IV
        E. I, II, and IV
    Answer: A

2. The elevated CVP indicates right ventricular insufficiency. This would most likely have been precipitated by which of the following?
    I.   Left ventricular failure
    II. Hypervolemia
    III. Increased PVR
        A. II only
        B. I, II, and III

C.   II and III
D.   I and III
E.   I only
Answer: B

3.   The physician believes the CVP line is inadequate. To help guide
this patient's volume replacement, he decides to place a pulmonary artery catheter. Subsequently, a 7 French catheter is inserted
percutaneously into the subclavian vein. During the procedure,
the following waveform is seen:

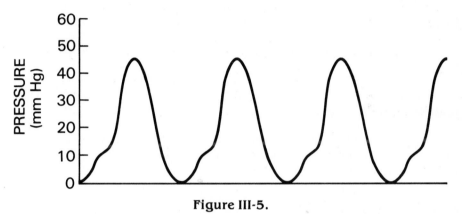

Figure III-5.

Which of the following is the true statement regarding the previ-
ous tracing?
A.   The catheter tip is in the right ventricle.
B.   The catheter tip is in the wedge position.
C.   The catheter tip should be retracted.
D.   The catheter tip is in the pulmonary artery.
E.   Artifact is present.
Answer: A

4.   Following placement of the pulmonary artery catheter, the following data were obtained:

P.A. systolic	43 mm Hg
P.A. diastolic	26 mm Hg
PWP	3 mm Hg
CVP	20 mm Hg

Based on the above information, which of the following is the
most likely cause of the above results?
A.   Left ventricular failure
B.   Hypervolemia
C.   Hypovolemia with increased PVR
D.   Adult respiratory distress syndrome
E.   Aortic stenosis
Answer: C

Case IV Discussion

Question 1

The Pa_{CO_2} of 65 mm Hg in the presence of a severely acidotic pH is a clear indication for ventilatory support. Surprisingly, even with the systemic hypotension and the mixed acidosis, the patient is not severely hypoxemic. The normal CVP is 5 mm Hg to 15 mm Hg.

Question 2

All of these may contribute to the increased CVP. Please see text for further discussion.

Question 3

A right ventricular waveform can be identified by wide swings in pressure and a diastolic pressure that falls to approximately 0 mm Hg. Also note the absence of the dicrotic notch.

Question 4

The PWP of 3 mm Hg most likely indicates the presence of hypovolemia. The PAD−PWP gradient is 23 mm Hg. Because this is considerably greater than the normal of less than 5 mm Hg, this patient's PVR must definitely be considered elevated.

UNIT IV

Examination Category Review and Pretest

NBRC examinations have been carefully designed to determine whether candidates possess a level of competence that would allow them to practice respiratory therapy on an entry or an advanced practitioner level. The 1981 NBRC Job Survey painstakingly identified 398 separate tasks that comprise the profession of respiratory therapy (see references 45 and 80). The survey further delineated which of these tasks were performed by individuals just entering the field (entry level) and those by individuals who are recognized experts (advanced practitioners). The NBRC has designed examinations to assess the candidate's ability to perform these entry and advanced level tasks in a patient care setting.

For all its exhaustive specificity and detail, the 1981 NBRC Job Survey is built on the simple fact that much of the practice of respiratory care starts with a physician's written instructions. Once the order is transcribed, an appropriate health care practitioner is assigned to carry out its letter and intent. For the individual respiratory therapy practitioner, the NBRC indicates that this consists of three phases. These are listed below.

1. *Gather and analyze pertinent clinical data.* The respiratory therapy practitioner, once assigned to a particular patient, goes first to the ward station and reviews the patient's chart and other pertinent records. He or she then collects and evaluates additional data at the patient's bedside. After analyzing the foregoing information, the practitioner may deem it appropriate to recommend that additional data be obtained. The therapist may be required to obtain or perform these additional studies himself/herself. Finally, the practitioner must assess the overall appropriateness of the therapeutic plan and, whenever necessary, participate in its development.

2. *Bring all appropriate respiratory care equipment to the patient's bedside.* After all appropriate clinical information has been gathered, the practitioner must then select the appropriate equipment for safe and proper performance of the diagnostic and therapeutic procedures ordered by the physician. Accordingly, the therapist must be able to assemble and check this equipment for proper function. Of course, should the equipment not operate properly, the practitioner must be able to correct any malfunctions. This latter statement is meant to include those actions necessary to ensure cleanliness and calibration of all equipment.

3. *Perform prescribed respiratory therapeutic procedures.* Finally, the practitioner must perform the therapeutic procedures that have been ordered by the physician. It is in the performance of these procedures that the analytical and judgmental skills of the practitioner are perhaps most considerable. For not only must the therapist be well versed in initiating and performing these procedures, but he or she must also be capable of assessing the patient's response to therapy. Should the patient experience an adverse reaction or if in the therapist's judgment optimal therapeutic benefit is not being derived, the therapist must appropriately modify therapy. In the event that this modification requires a change in the physician's order, the practitioner must then communicate his or her recommendations promptly and along established lines of communication.

The specifications of both the Entry Level and Advanced Practitioner Examinations were written around the above job description. Thus, each examination is divided into the above *three* major content categories. These three are divided into 21 subcategories, which on the 1981 Job Survey were broken down into the 398 tasks mentioned previously. The questions in this book and on the NBRC examinations are written specifically to assess the candidate's ability to understand the significance of and to perform each one of these 398 tasks. Therefore, in order to evaluate his or her proficiency in each one of these areas, the reader is asked to look up each of these 21[1] exam content categories in the Table of Contents and review the self-study examination questions contained therein. For now, however, please note that the examination specification table (see Table 1 below) contains the percentage of questions appropriated to each content category. These percentages reflect the number of tasks involved in each, respectively, and further establish the validity of the NBRC examination process in assessing clinical competency.

---

[1]We will use 26 exam content categories in this book. See page 201 for further explanation.

Table 1. Entry Level and Advanced Practitioner Examination Content Matrix.

		Entry Level		Advanced Level	
	Content Category	Percentage Breakdown	Numerical Breakdown (200 total)	Percentage Breakdown	Numerical Breakdown (100 total)
I.	Clinical Data	30	60	25	25
A.	Review patient records	4.5	9	10	10
B.	Collect and evaluate clinical information	10.5	21	5	5
C.	Recommend and obtain diagnostic procedures	3	6	0	0
D.	Perform and evaluate laboratory procedures	6	12	10	10
E.	Assess therapeutic plan	6	12	0	0
II.	Equipment	25	50	10	10
A.	Select equipment	6	12	2	2
B.	Assemble, note operation, and correct equipment malfunctions	15	30	4	4
C.	Ensure cleanliness of equipment	4	8	1	1
D.	Perform quality control and calibration procedures	0	0	3	3
III.	Therapeutic Procedures	45	90	65	65
A.	Educate patients	1.5	3	0	0
B.	Control infection	2	4	0	0
C.	Maintain airway	4	8	3	3
D.	Mobilize and remove secretions	4.5	9	0	0
E.	Ensure ventilation	5.5	11	7	7
F.	Ensure oxygenation	5.5	11	3	3
G.	Assess patient response to therapy	5.5	11	20	20
H.	Modify therapy	5	10	7	7
I.	Recommend modifications in therapy	4	8	22	22
J.	Initiate cardiopulmonary resuscitation	5.5	11	0	0

Table 1. Entry Level and Advanced Practitioner Examination Content Matrix.

Content Category	Entry Level		Advanced Level	
	Percentage Breakdown	Numerical Breakdown (200 total)	Percentage Breakdown	Numerical Breakdown (100 total)
K. Maintain records and communication	1.5	3	0	0
L. Assist physician with special procedures	0	0	3	3

As the candidate will note, each of the three major sections and 21 sub-sections is described and discussed on the following pages.

Part I
Clinical Data

Thirty percent of the questions on the Entry Level Examination and 25% of the questions on the Advanced Practitioner Examination are taken from this content category. These questions assess the candidate's ability to gather and analyze appropriate clinical information prior to selecting equipment or performing therapy. The NBRC 1981 Job Survey identifies five major competencies in this category:

1. Review patient records
2. Collect and evaluate clinical information
3. Recommend and obtain diagnostic procedures (entry level only)
4. Perform and evaluate laboratory procedures
5. Assess therapeutic plan (entry level only)

Each one of these areas will be discussed in further detail in the following pages.

A. Review Patient Records

Questions in this category are designed to assess the candidate's ability to evaluate information found in the patient's chart prior to performing therapy. This information can often alert the practitioner to potential hazards. For instance, if in reading the patient's chart the practitioner notes that the patient has severe coronary artery disease and that this patient is also to receive a sympathomimetic aerosol, the practitioner would want to monitor this patient's cardiovascular status very carefully during therapy. Questions in this category will also test the candidate's knowledge of medical terminology and of laboratory values.

Entry Level Pretest

According to the NBRC, 4.5% of the questions on the Entry Level Examination are from the review patient records category. In addition, the Composite Examination Matrix (see reference 80) states that questions in this category will test the candidate's ability to assess the following pertinent data:

1. Patient history, physical examination, and current vital signs
2. Admission and current respiratory care orders
3. Patient progress notes
4. Results of electrolytes, hemoglobin, white blood cell count analyses and/or chemistries
5. Pulmonary function values and blood gas results
6. Chest roentgenography results
7. Sputum culture and/or Gram's stain results
8. Results of ventilatory monitoring (including tidal volume, minute volume, respiratory rate, I:E ratio, negative inspiratory force, maximum expiratory force, and vital capacity)
9. Results of blood pressure and heart rate monitoring

The following self-study questions were developed from the NBRC Composite Examination Matrix:

1. In reviewing the chart of a patient with cystic fibrosis, the respiratory therapy practitioner would most likely note that the patient's chief complaint is which of the following?
    A. Cough with copious sputum production
    B. Sleep apnea
    C. Nocturnal dyspnea
    D. Chest pain on exertion
    E. Orthopnea
        (11:124)

2. In reviewing a patient's chart prior to therapy, the respiratory therapy practitioner notes that a 30-year-old patient's peak expiratory flow rate is 10.2 L/sec. This value is most consistent with which of the following?
    A. Obstructive defect
    B. Restrictive defect
    C. Small airways disease
    D. Normal study
    E. Oxygenation failure
        (16:36)

3. In reviewing a patient's chart prior to therapy, the respiratory therapy practitioner notes that the 40-year-old patient's arterial blood pressure is 160/120. This value is most consistent with:
    A. Myocardial infarction
    B. Arterial hypertension
    C. Normotension
    D. Arterial hypotension
    E. Shock
        (94:147)

4. Which of the following most closely approximates the content of oxygen in the arterial blood of a healthy young adult breathing ambient gas at sea level?
    A. 12 vol%
    B. 15 vol%

C. 18 vol%
D. 20 vol%
E. 25 vol%
   (3:106)

5. Which of the following represents the normal percent to which the arterial blood of a healthy young adult is saturated?
   A. 90
   B. 97
   C. 80
   D. 75
   E. 100
   (3:106)

6. The expected inspiratory capacity for a young, healthy, 70-kg individual would be approximately:
   A. 4.2 L
   B. 3.6 L
   C. 4.8 L
   D. 2.8 L
   E. 2.1 L
   (16:3)

7. Which of the following is the normal arterial oxygen tension for a healthy 60-year-old individual?
   A. 50 mm Hg
   B. 60 mm Hg
   C. 70 mm Hg
   D. 80 mm Hg
   E. 90 mm Hg
   (32:62)

8. The normal value for whole blood buffer base is approximately:
   A. 22–26 mEq/L
   B. 34–38 mEq/L
   C. 46–50 mEq/L
   D. 60–64 mEq/L
   E. 280–290 mEq/L
   (2:245)

9. In reviewing a patient's orders prior to performing therapy, the respiratory therapy practitioner notes that the physician wants a sputum sample sent to the oncology laboratory for cytologic studies. From this information the therapist may safely assume that:
   A. The patient is in strict isolation.
   B. The patient may have tuberculosis.
   C. An anaerobic pneumonitis is suspected.
   D. The physician suspects a pulmonary neoplasm.
   E. The patient is terminally ill.
   (3:226)

Answer Key

1. A	3. B	5. B	7. D	9. D
2. D	4. D	6. B	8. C	

Advanced Practitioner Pretest

According to the NBRC, 10% of the questions on the Advanced Practitioner Examination are from the review patient records category. In addition, the Composite Examination Matrix (see reference 80) states that questions in this category will assess the candidate's ability to assess the following pertinent data:

1. Pulmonary function values and blood gas results
2. Results of ventilatory monitoring (including tidal volume, minute volume, respiratory rate, I:E ratio, negative inspiratory force, maximum expiratory force, and vital capacity)
3. Results of hemodynamic monitoring
   a. Central venous pressure, pulmonary capillary wedge pressure, pulmonary artery pressures, and cardiac output
   b. The electrocardiogram
   c. Fluid intake and output
   d. The amount and character of pleural drainage

The following self-study questions were developed from the NBRC Composite Examination Matrix:

1. In reading a patient's chart prior to administering ultrasonic therapy, the respiratory therapy practitioner notes a history of paralysis involving the recurrent laryngeal nerve. This patient would *most* likely:
   A. Be comatose
   B. Be unable to cough effectively
   C. Have a vital capacity below 5 mL/kg
   D. Be combative
   E. Have diplopia
   (1:162)

2. Which of the following statements is (are) true regarding pleural transudates?
   I. They may be caused by left ventricular failure.
   II. They are a clear, straw-colored liquid.
   III. They are associated with lung abscess.
   IV. They have a very high protein content.
   A. II and III
   B. I and II
   C. I and IV
   D. III and IV
   E. III only
   (11:187–189) (94:179–181) (12:317)

3. On reading a patient's chart prior to administering IPPB therapy, the respiratory therapy practitioner notes that the patient's FEF_{25-75} was 0.22 L/sec. On the basis of this information, the therapist can safely assume that:
   A. A severe restrictive disorder exists.
   B. The patient would most likely benefit from incentive spirometry.
   C. A mild obstructive disorder exists.
   D. The patient has no demonstrable pulmonary problems.
   E. A severe obstructive disorder exists.
   (16:33)

4. Which of the following should the respiratory therapy practitioner consider the upper limit of normal for intracranial pressure among adult patients?
   A. 10 mm Hg
   B. 20 mm Hg
   C. 30 mm Hg
   D. 40 mm Hg
   E. 50 mm Hg
   (23) (25:Chap 15, p 13)

5. In reading a patient's chart prior to performing postural drainage and percussion techniques, the respiratory therapy practitioner notices in the admission notes that the patient is suffering from senile emphysema. True statements regarding this include:
   I. It is a congenital disorder of the mucociliary blanket.
   II. It is considered a restrictive disorder.
   III. It is a viral disorder affecting primarily the elderly.
   IV. It is believed to be responsible for the "normal" hypoxemia of old age.
   A. I and III
   B. IV only
   C. III and IV
   D. I and IV
   E. I and II
   (38:10–12) (24:220)

6. In reading a patient's chart prior to performing IPPB, the respiratory therapy practitioner notes an electrophoresis study that indicates a very low serum concentration of the enzyme α-1-antitrypsin. The practitioner would expect the patient to have which of the following pulmonary disorders?
   A. Centrolobular emphysema
   B. Panlobular emphysema
   C. Collagen vascular disease
   D. Pancoast superior sulcus syndrome
   E. Idiopathic pulmonary hemosiderosis
   (24:220)

7. The normal value for D_{LCO} when performed by the single breath method is:
    A. 12 mm Hg/mL/sec
    B. 15 mL/min/mm Hg
    C. 25 mL/min/mm Hg
    D. 8 mL/mm Hg/min
    E. 45 mL/mm Hg/min
       (15:71)

8. A 22-year-old man is admitted to the emergency department in a coma. A deep and slow ventilatory pattern as well as pinpointed pupils are noted by the respiratory therapy practitioner. Which of the following is most likely to be responsible for the above presentation?
    A. Oxygen induced hypoventilation
    B. Barbiturate overdose
    C. Diabetic acidosis
    D. Narcotic overdose
    E. Hypothyroidism
       (5:187) (31:336–337)

9. Which of the following most accurately represents an average $C(a\text{-}\bar{v})o_2$ for a critically ill patient with good cardiovascular reserves?
    A. 11.0 vol%
    B. 3.5 vol%
    C. 5.5 vol%
    D. 7.5 vol%
    E. 10.0 vol%
       (5:232)

10. The normal value for intravascular colloidal osmotic (oncotic) pressure is approximately:
    A. 15 mm Hg
    B. 25 mm Hg
    C. 35 mm Hg
    D. 10 mm Hg
    E. 5 mm Hg
       (1:437) (42)

11. The respiratory therapy practitioner is reviewing a patient's chart prior to therapy. The practitioner notices that the bacteriology report on a sputum sample sent 24 hours previously states that the sample contained numerous squamous epithelial cells and a wide variety of Gram-positive organisms. From this information the practitioner may safely conclude that:
    A. The patient has lung cancer.
    B. The laboratory report is in error.
    C. The sample contained excessive saliva.
    D. The patient has extrinsic asthma.
    E. The patient should be started on aminoglycoside therapy.
       (2:431)

12. In reviewing a patient's chart prior to therapy, the respiratory therapist notices that the latest chest roentgenogram revealed a diffuse bilateral alveolar filling pattern with increased vascular markings and prominent Kerley-B lines. These findings are most consistent with:
     A.   Pulmonary embolus
     B.   Bronchiectasis
     C.   Cardiogenic pulmonary edema
     D.   Bronchial asthma
     E.   Pulmonary fibrosis
          (2:284–286)

13. In reading a patient's chart prior to IPPB, the respiratory therapy practitioner notes that the patient had a permanent pacemaker implanted several months ago. Development of which of the following arrhythmias would most likely have been responsible for pacemaker placement?
     A.   Sinus tachycardia
     B.   Sinus arrhythmia
     C.   Third-degree (complete) heart block
     D.   Multifocal premature ventricular contractions
     E.   Atrial tachycardia
          (25: Chap 6, p 27)

14. A patient with chronic obstructive pulmonary disease who is on a Bennett MA-I ventilator has a pulmonary artery (Swan-Ganz) catheter in place. In reading the patient's chart, the respiratory therapy practitioner notes that the patient's mean pulmonary pressures have consistently been around 35 mm Hg. This value most likely represents:
     A.   Pulmonary hypotension
     B.   Pulmonary hypertension
     C.   Normal study
     D.   Adult respiratory distress syndrome
     E.   Right ventricular failure
          (11:182) (61)

15. A patient in the intensive care unit is noted to have a serum potassium concentration of 2.6 mEq/L. This value most likely indicates the presence of:
     A.   Metabolic alkalosis
     B.   Hypocalcemia
     C.   Hypokalemia
     D.   Normal study
     E.   Hypercalcemia
          (7:254)

16. In reading a patient's chart, the respiratory therapy practitioner notes that the patient's Ca_{O_2} is 18 vol% and the $C\bar{v}_{O_2}$ is 11 vol%. These findings most likely indicate the presence of which of the following?
     A.   Normal cardiac output
     B.   Increased cardiac output

C. Need for PEEP therapy
D. Low cardiac output
E. Hypometabolic state
   (5:232)

Answer Key

1. B	4. B	7. C	10. B	13. C
2. B	5. B	8. D	11. C	14. B
3. E	6. B	9. B	12. C	15. C
				16. D

B. Collect and Evaluate Clinical Information

Questions in this category are designed to assess the candidate's ability to obtain additional pertinent clinical information prior to performing diagnostic or therapeutic procedures. In the clinic this information can be obtained in one of four ways:

1. By performing a chest physical examination
2. By interviewing the patient
3. By performing and evaluating bedside pulmonary function tests
4. By inspecting the patient's chest roentgenogram

The candidate should note here that these methods are all assessed on the Entry Level Examination, whereas on the Advanced Practitioner Examination this category consists *entirely* of questions assessing the candidate's ability to evaluate the patient's chest roentgenogram.

Entry Level Pretest

According to the NBRC, 10.5% of the questions on the Entry Level Examination are from the collect and evaluate clinical information category. In addition, the Composite Examination Matrix (see reference 80) states that the questions in this category will assess the following competencies:

1. Perform all four phases of a chest physical assessment:
   a. Assess the patient's overall respiratory status by inspection of the patient in general and the thorax in particular
   b. Assess the patient's overall respiratory status by palpation of the thorax
   c. Assess the patient's overall respiratory status by percussion of the thorax
   d. Assess the patient's overall respiratory status by auscultation of the thorax

2. Interview the patient to determine:
    a. Level of consciousness
    b. Orientation to time and place
    c. Patient's emotional state
    d. Patient's ability to cooperate
    e. Presence of dyspnea and/or orthopnea
3. Perform and evaluate bedside pulmonary function tests to determine:
    a. Tidal volume
    b. Minute volume
    c. Forced vital capacity
    d. Timed forced expiratory volumes
    e. Negative inspiratory force
    f. Maximum expiratory force
    g. Peak flow
4. Inspect and evaluate the patient's chest roentgenogram to determine:
    a. Presence of or changes in consolidation and/or atelectasis
    b. Position of endotracheal or tracheostomy tube
    c. Presence of or changes in pneumothorax or subcutaneous emphysema

The following self-study questions were developed from the NBRC Composite Examination Matrix:

1. The presence of which of the following when noted on a chest roentgenogram is *most* suggestive of the presence of consolidated lung tissue?
    A. Blunting of the costophrenic angles
    B. Multiple reticulonodular densities that do not coalesce
    C. Areas of increased radiolucency
    D. Areas of increased opacification
    E. Increased vascular markings
    (1:105–107)

2. The presence of which of the following physical findings is *least* suggestive of the presence of consolidated lung tissue?
    A. Whispered pectoriloquy
    B. Wheezing
    C. Dull percussion note
    D. Egophony
    E. Bronchial breath sounds
    (95:83–95)

3. Which of the following statements about the technique of percussion are true?
    I.   A dull note is heard over the normal lung fields.
    II.   Emphysema is associated with a hyperresonant note.
    III. Areas of consolidation usually yield a resonant note.
    IV.   Percussion over the liver will yield a flat note.
        A. II and III
        B. I and IV

C. II and IV
D. III and IV
E. I and III
(95:87 and 92)

4. Which of the following is (are) most frequently used to describe the sputum of patients with lung abscess?
I. Mucoid
II. Bloody
III. Copious
IV. Purulent
A. II and III
B. I and IV
C. III and IV
D. I and II
E. III only
(11:114) (2:262)

5. A routine chest roentgenogram when performed in the radiology department consists of which of the following views?
A. Posteroanterior projection only
B. Anteroposterior projection only
C. Anteroposterior and lateral projections
D. Posteroanterior and lateral projections
E. Oblique and lateral projections
(2:106)

6. Which of the following disorders is most frequently associated with the term *orthopnea?*
A. Idiopathic respiratory distress syndrome
B. Congestive heart failure
C. Bronchial asthma
D. Bronchiolitis
E. Pulmonary fibrosis
(2:259)

7. The phrase "episodic shortness of breath in which sleep is interrupted" best defines:
A. Orthopnea
B. Paroxysmal nocturnal dyspnea
C. Dyspnea
D. Biot's breathing
E. Sleep apnea
(2:259)

8. Which of the following chest physical findings may be ascertained through palpation of the chest wall?
A. Rales
B. Tactile fremitus
C. Whispered pectoriloquy
D. Bronchophony
E. Egophony
(95:83)

9. The presence of which of the following chest physical findings suggests the presence of pulmonary consolidation?
     I. Vocal or tactile fremitus
    II. Vesicular breath sounds
   III. Bronchophony
    IV. Egophony
        A. I, III, and IV
        B. II, III, and IV
        C. III and IV
        D. I, II, III, and IV
        E. I and IV
     (95:83–95)

10. Patients who are deeply comatose would be *least* likely to exhibit which one of the following signs and symptoms?
    A. Absence of tracheal or carinal reflexes
    B. Soft tissue obstruction of upper airway tissues
    C. Purposeful response to pain
    D. Abnormal peripheral muscle tone
    E. Lack of corneal reflexes
       (93)

11. The phrase "a nasal bleating quality of spoken voice sounds when heard through the stethoscope" best describes:
    A. Bronchovesicular breath sounds
    B. Whispered pectoriloquy
    C. Egophony
    D. Bronchophony
    E. Tactile fremitus
       (95:95)

12. Pink-tinged pulmonary secretions have been associated with:
    A. Asthma
    B. Left ventricular failure
    C. Cor pulmonale
    D. Use of isoetharine
    E. B and D are correct.
       (17:280) (2:273)

13. The decision to intubate and initiate continuous ventilatory support in patients with acute neuromuscular disorders is most reliably made on the basis of which of the following clinical determinations?
    A. Arterial blood gas analysis
    B. History and physical examination
    C. Serial vital capacity measurements
    D. Peak expiratory flow rates
    E. Chest roentgenogram
       (2:761)

14. Which of the following physical findings are *most* likely to be seen in a patient with a large tension pneumothorax?
     I. Hyperresonant percussion note over the affected area

II. Mediastinal shift to the unaffected side
III. Increased breath sounds over the affected area
IV. Bronchophony over the affected area
    A. I, II, and IV
    B. I, III, and IV
    C. II, III, and IV
    D. I, II, III, and IV
    E. I and II
   (32:212) (2:272)

15. The hemoptysis that is sometimes noted by the respiratory therapy practitioner while performing IPPB therapy is most frequently due to:
    A. Mitral stenosis
    B. Tearing of mucosa during a coughing spell
    C. Pulmonary embolus
    D. Bronchogenic carcinoma
    E. Pulmonary infection
   (1:191)

16. Which of the following chest physical findings is most frequently associated with partial upper airway obstruction?
    A. Tracheal shift
    B. Inspiratory stridor
    C. Harsh dry cough
    D. Dullness to percussion
    E. Tactile fremitus
   (95:343)

17. Which of the following disorders is most likely to be associated with the presence of Kussmaul's type breathing?
    A. Postanoxic encephalopathy
    B. Damage to the medulla oblongata
    C. Pulmonary emphysema
    D. Diabetic acidosis
    E. Subphrenic abscess
   (17:228)

18. The phrase "periods of hyperpnea that wax and wane and are frequently separated by apneic spells" most accurately describes:
    A. Hyperventilation
    B. Biot's breathing
    C. Obstructive breathing
    D. Cheyne-Stokes respirations
    E. Kussmaul's breathing
   (95:94)

19. For which of the following disorders is the presence of very large quantities of putrid-smelling sputum a common clinical finding?
    A. Anaerobic lung abscess
    B. Extrinsic asthma
    C. Pulmonary emphysema

D.   Pulmonary interstitial fibrosis
E.   Intrinsic asthma
     (11:69–72) (2:262)

20. Which of the following auscultatory findings is *most* likely to become evident after an effective cough maneuver has been performed?
A.   Amphoric breathing sounds
B.   Rales
C.   Wheezes
D.   Bronchophony
E.   Bronchial breath sounds
     (17:250)

21. The following are the four most important aspects of a chest physical assessment:
I.   Inspection
II.   Palpation
III. Percussion
IV.   Ausultation
Under most clinical circumstances the respiratory therapy practitioner should perform them in which of the following orders?
A.   I, III, IV, and II
B.   II, IV, III, and I
C.   I, III, II, and IV
D.   I, IV, II, and III
E.   I, II, III, and IV
     (17:226–251) (2:99)

22. Patients with which of the following conditions would be most likely to exhibit cyanosis?
I.   Anemia
II.   Low cardiac output
III. Polycythemia
IV.   High cardiac output
     A.   I and IV
     B.   II only
     C.   I and II
     D.   II and III
     E.   III and IV
     (17:200–202)

23. Which of the following is the most common abnormal hematologic finding in a patient with extrinsic asthma?
A.   Decreased red blood cell count
B.   Leukocytopenia
C.   An increase in eosinophils
D.   Massive increase in neutrophils
E.   Agammaglobulinemia
     (2:797) (17:299)

24. Which of the following is *least* likely to occur following slippage of a patient's endotracheal tube into the right mainstem bronchus during continuous ventilatory support?
A. Left-sided pneumothorax
B. Increased aeration on the right side
C. Increased ventilator plateau pressure
D. Dull percussion note on the left side
E. Hyperresonant right-sided percussion note
     (32:209–210) (34:122–128)

25. The presence of which of the following is *least* likely to be associated with the term *hyperventilation?*
A. Bradypnea and hypopnea
B. Hyperpnea and tachypnea
C. Hyperpnea with a normal V_D/V_T
D. Arterial hypocapnia
E. Hyperpnea with a decreased V_D/V_T
     (2:203) (95:94)

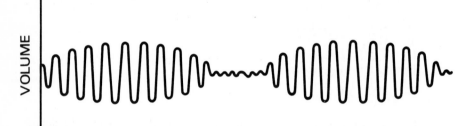

TIME
Figure IV-1.

26. The above illustration may best be described as:
A. Cheyne-Stokes respirations
B. Biot's breathing
C. Hyperventilation
D. Hyperpnea
E. Apneustic breathing
     (95:94)

Answer Key

1. D	6. B	11. C	16. B	21. E
2. B	7. B	12. E	17. D	22. D
3. C	8. B	13. C	18. D	23. C
4. C	9. A	14. E	19. A	24. A
5. D	10. C	15. B	20. B	25. A
				26. A

Advanced Practitioner Pretest

According to the NBRC, 5% of the questions on the Advanced Practitioner Examination are from the collect and evaluate clinical information content category. In addition, the Composite Examination Matrix (see reference 80) states that questions in this category assess the advanced practitioner's competency in inspecting and evaluating the patient's chest roentgenogram to determine:

1. Position of chest tubes
2. Position and presence of foreign bodies
3. Presence of or changes in consolidation and/or atelectasis
4. Position of or changes in the hemidiaphragms
5. Presence of or changes in hyperinflation
6. Presence of or changes in pleural fluid
7. Presence of or changes in pulmonary edema and/or opacification

The following self-study questions were developed from the NBRC Composite Examination Matrix:

1. In which of the following disorders is the classic radiologic appearance that of reticulogranular infiltrates distributed throughout the lung fields with a pronounced air bronchogram?
   A. Cystic fibrosis
   B. Bronchiolitis
   C. Idiopathic respiratory distress syndrome
   D. Emphysema
   E. Bronchiectasis
   (4:244)

2. Which of the following statements about the chest roentgenogram is *not* true?
   A. Adult respiratory distress syndrome is associated with increased radiopacity.
   B. The cardiac shadow is usually smaller in the portable chest film.
   C. Radiolucent structures tend to be black in appearance.
   D. An area of calcification will be white in appearance.
   E. An air bronchogram is often seen when diffuse alveolar filling processes exist.
   (1:105–108) (2:276–283)

3. The roentgenographic changes most frequently seen in patients with pulmonary emphysema include:
   I.   Increased radiolucency
   II. Widened cardiac shadow
   III. Flattened diaphragms
   IV. Decreased anteroposterior diameter
       A. I and IV
       B. I and III
       C. II and IV
       D. III only

E.   I, III, and IV
(11:97) (2:714–715)

4.   The appearance of a thick-walled round shadow containing an air-fluid level on a chest roentgenogram is most suggestive of which of the following disorders?
A.   Pulmonary infarct
B.   Pulmonary emphysema
C.   Pulmonary abscess
D.   Werdnig-Hoffmann disease
E.   Bronchiectasis
(2:294)

5.   Which of the following disorders is known to produce characteristic bronchographic evidence of a lack of the normal tapering of the medium-sized airways?
A.   Bronchiolitis
B.   Cystic fibrosis
C.   Bronchiectasis
D.   Bronchogenic carcinoma
E.   Dermatomycosis
(11:114–115)

6.   All of the following disorders are known to lead to an abnormal pulmonary perfusion scan. Which is *least* likely to be accompanied by a "matched" abnormality in the pulmonary ventilation scan?
A.   Emphysema
B.   Pulmonary embolism
C.   Cystic fibrosis
D.   Chronic bronchitis
E.   A and C are correct.
(2:284 and 740)

7.   Which of the following radiologic findings would *most* likely be seen in a patient who has cor pulmonale?
I.   Left ventricular hypertrophy
II.   Increased pulmonary vascular markings
III.   Right ventricular hypertrophy
IV.   Compensatory hyperinflation
A.   I and III
B.   III and IV
C.   I and II
D.   II and III
E.   I and IV
(11:183–184) (2:284–285)

8.   The chest roentgenogram of a patient who received a pneumonectomy several years ago is *most* likely to reveal which of the following abnormalities?
A.   Large wedge-shaped densities
B.   Diffuse bilateral reticular granular pattern
C.   Compensatory emphysema involving the remaining lung tissue

D.   Left ventricular hypertrophy
E.   Widespread miliary atelectasis
     (2:712)

9.   For which of the following disorders is the presence of an increased anteroposterior diameter on the lateral chest film a common clinical finding?
     I.   Hamman-Rich syndrome (idiopathic pulmonary fibrosis)
     II.   Emphysema
     III. Bacterial pneumonia
     IV.   Cystic fibrosis
           A.   I and IV
           B.   II and III
           C.   I and III
           D.   III only
           E.   II and IV
     (11:96–97 and 120–121) (95:93) (2:146–187 and 714)

10. Which of the following roentgenologic studies would be most beneficial in quantitating the extent of diaphragmatic involvement in a patient with a neurologic disorder affecting the phrenic nerve?
     A.   Ventilation-perfusion lung scintiscanning
     B.   Computerized axial tomography
     C.   Fluoroscopy
     D.   Posteroanterior and lateral chest films
     E.   Angiography
          (2:283)

11. The presence of which of the following, when noted on a chest roentgenogram, is *most* suggestive of a fluid within the pleural space?
     A.   Mediastinal shift to the affected side
     B.   Areas of increased radiolucency
     C.   Multiple small densities that coalesce into larger densities
     D.   Blunting of the costophrenic angles
     E.   Presence of the silhouette sign
          (2:279–280)

12. On viewing a lateral chest roentgenogram, the respiratory therapy practitioner would most frequently note the presence of pleural fluid in which one of the following locations?
     A.   Anterior costophrenic sulcus
     B.   Posterior costophrenic sulcus
     C.   Mediastinum
     D.   Thoracic duct
     E.   Right middle lobe
          (3:326–328) (2:300–304)

13. Which of the following is *least* likely to be associated with radiologic evidence of tracheal deviation?
     A.   Pleural fluid
     B.   Pneumonectomy

C. Patient rotation
D. Lobar atelectasis
E. Roentgenogram film underexposure
(3:312)

14. A poor inspiraton on a chest roentgenogram is said to exist if the diaphragm does not descend to the bottom of which ribs anteriorly and posteriorly?
A. Sixth and tenth
B. Eighth and twelfth
C. Fourth and tenth
D. Fourth and twelfth
E. Eighth and tenth
(3:328)

15. Scalloping of the right hemidiaphragm is said to be part of the normal chest film of what percentage of cases?
A. 5%
B. 25%
C. 40%
D. 60%
E. 90%
(3:314)

16. The phrase "a localized area of overaeration caused by destruction of pulmonary tissue" most correctly describes:
A. A pneumatocele
B. A pulmonary abscess
C. A solitary nodule
D. A Gohne's complex
E. A granuloma
(3:325)

17. Which of the following correctly describes the appearance of cavities as seen on chest films?
A. A fine, lacelike pattern
B. A solid, white patch
C. A round, radiopaque mass
D. A black hole on the film
E. A poorly circumscribed area of infiltration
(3:311)

18. Which of the following is *not* a density that is seen on the normal chest roentgenogram?
A. Bone
B. Hard tissue
C. Air
D. Soft tissue
E. Fat
(3:310)

19. In which of the following conditions would hemidiaphragm elevation *not* be noted while viewing the chest film?
A. Phrenic nerve paralysis
B. Pulmonary emphysema

C. Subphrenic abscess
D. Old lobectomy
E. Right middle lobe collapse
   (3:314)

20. Which of the following signs would *not* typically be noted while viewing the chest film of a patient in congestive heart failure?
A. A cardiothoracic ratio shadow greater than 50%
B. Left ventricular enlargement
C. Presence of Kerley-B lines
D. A diffuse bibasal alveolar filling process
E. Diminished pulmonary vascular markings
   (3:Chap 9) (2:304–307)

21. The chest roentgenogram of which of the following disorders does *not* typically reveal an alveolar filling pattern?
A. Cardiogenic pulmonary edema
B. Noncardiogenic pulmonary edema
C. Near drowning
D. Hamman-Rich syndrome
E. Viral pneumonia
   (3:319)

22. Which of the following is (are) true statements regarding Kerley-B lines as seen while viewing the chest?
I. They are part of the classic radiologic picture of cor pulmonale.
II. They are believed to be indicative of pulmonary underperfusion.
III. They are a type of pulmonary vascular marking.
   A. I and II
   B. III only
   C. I only
   D. II only
   E. I and III
   (3:320)

23. Which of the following radiologic signs would alert the respiratory therapy practitioner to the presence of pneumomediastinum?
A. Elevation of the left hemidiaphragm
B. Tracheal shift to the left side
C. Presence of fine linear streaks around the heart
D. Presence of cardiomegaly
E. Increased pulmonary vascular markings
   (3:324) (2:299)

24. Which of the following statements are true regarding the solitary pulmonary nodule?
I. It is often noted to be a roughly spherical radiopaque mass.
II. It may be confused with breast shadows.
III. It cannot be caused by a benign tumor.
IV. It often indicates the presence of bronchogenic carcinoma.

    A.   II and IV
    B.   III and IV
    C.   II and III
    D.   I and III
    E.   I and IV
(3:325) (2:290)

25. The radiologic picture of which of the following disorders would most likely be associated with a honeycombed interstitial pattern?
    I.   Idiopathic pulmonary fibrosis
    II.   Congestive heart failure
    III. Adult respiratory distress syndrome
    IV.   Scleroderma
        A.   II and IV
        B.   III and IV
        C.   I and IV
        D.   I and III
        E.   II only
    (3:319)

26. Which of the following statements is (are) true regarding a so-called coin lesion seen while viewing a chest roentgenogram?
    I.   It usually appears as a large cavity with an air-fluid interspace.
    II.   It may be confused with nipple shadows.
    III. It may be described as a large, solitary nodule.
    IV.   Its presence is usually suggestive of benign neoplastic disease.
        A.   II, III, and IV
        B.   III only
        C.   I and II
        D.   II and III
        E.   I and IV
    (3:325)

27. Which of the following statements regarding chest roentgeno-grams is *not* true?
    A.   Breast shadows may be confused with increased interstitial markings.
    B.   Female nipple shadows may be mistaken for solitary nodules.
    C.   The scapulae may appear to be pleural lesions.
    D.   Very large breasts may cause the costophrenic angle to exceed 90°.
    E.   The carina may usually be located at the level of the fifth to sixth intercostal space.
    (2:277–278) (3:333)

28. Indirect signs of atelectasis that may be noted on the chest roent-genogram include all of the following *except:*
    A.   Elevation of the diaphragm on the affected side
    B.   Narrowing of the intercostal spaces on the affected side

C. Flattening of the hemidiaphragms bilaterally
D. Compensatory overinflation of adjacent lung tissue
E. Shifting or displacement of the hilum
(2:291–292) (3:Chap 9)

29. Which of the following most accurately represents the typical radiologic picture of widespread pneumonias caused by viral organisms?
A. A diffuse alveolar filling process
B. Multiple nodules along with a honeycombed interstitial pattern
C. Dense consolidation involving the right middle lobe, usually accompanied by prominent Kerley-B lines
D. Blunting of the costophrenic angle with an absent silhouette sign
E. Discrete areas of calcification involving primarily the apical segments
(2:304–307)

30. When viewing a chest roentgenogram, noting the presence of Westermark's sign would be most indicative of the presence of which of the following?
A. Cor pulmonale
B. Kyphoscoliosis
C. Pulmonary embolus
D. Congestive heart failure
E. Pulmonary hypertension
(3:331)

31. Which of the following disorders is *least* likely to be associated with radiologic evidence of overaeration?
A. Emphysema
B. Cystic fibrosis
C. Acute bronchial asthma
D. Kyphoscoliosis
E. Alveolar proteinosis
(3:325)

32. Which of the following disorders is *not* associated with radiologic evidence of calcified pulmonary tissue?
A. Bronchiectasis
B. Silicosis
C. Tuberculosis
D. Coccidioidomycosis
E. Asbestosis
(3:331)

Answer Key

1. C	8. C	15. A	22. B	29. A
2. B	9. E	16. A	23. C	30. C
3. B	10. C	17. D	24. E	31. E
4. C	11. D	18. B	25. C	32. A
5. C	12. B	19. B	26. D	
6. B	13. E	20. E	27. D	
7. D	14. A	21. D	28. C	

C. Recommend and Obtain Diagnostic Procedures (Entry Level Only)

According to the NBRC, this category is *only* assessed on the Entry Level Examination. Questions in this category are designed to assess the ability of the candidate to recommend and/or obtain additional diagnostic data that may be pertinent in the management of patients requiring respiratory care. It should be pointed out that this category is used to assess the candidate's competency in performing arterial puncture techniques and in handling the sample once it is obtained. Questions on arterial blood gas analysis and arterial blood gas analyzers appear in other categories.

Entry Level Pretest

According to the NBRC, 3% of the questions on the Entry Level Examination are from the recommend and obtain diagnostic procedures category. In addition, the Composite Examination Matrix (see reference 80) states that questions in this category assess the ability of the candidate to obtain or recommend the following laboratory tests:

1. Obtain a sputum sample
2. Obtain an arterial blood sample
3. Recommend electrolytes and other blood chemistries
4. Recommend an electrocardiogram
5. Recommend a chest roentgenogram
6. Recommend spirometry and/or before and after bronchodilator studies

The following self-study questions were developed from the NBRC Composite Examination Matrix:

1. Which of the following diagnostic procedures would be most valuable in establishing the diagnosis of bronchial asthma?
   A. Simple spirometry
   B. Flow-volume loop analysis
   C. Before and after bronchodilator study

D. History and physical examination
E. Presence of neutrophils in sputum
   (2:709)

2. All of the following solutions have been recommended for aerosolization to help the respiratory therapy practitioner induce sputum specimens. Which has been shown to inhibit the growth of *Mycobacterium tuberculosis?*
   A. 10% NaCl
   B. Distilled water
   C. Propylene glycol
   D. Acetylcysteine
   E. A and D are correct.
   (3:226)

3. For which of the following reasons should arterial blood samples be placed in an ice bath immediately after being drawn?
   A. To prevent air bubbles in the sample from coalescing
   B. To decrease red blood cell metabolism *in vivo*
   C. To decrease red blood cell metabolism *in vitro*
   D. To allow for more efficient use of computer time
   E. A and B are correct.
   (5:158)

4. True statements regarding the brachial artery include:
   I. It lies in close proximity to the medial nerve.
   II. Venipuncture cannot occur at this site.
   III. It usually does not have collateral blood flow.
   IV. It is less superficial than the dorsalis pedis artery.
      A. I and III
      B. II and IV
      C. I and IV
      D. II, III, and IV
      E. I, III, and IV
   (5:146–147) (97:615)

5. When obtaining an arterial sample from a patient who is being treated with sodium warfarin (Coumadin®), the *most* important action for the respiratory therapy practitioner to take is which of the following?
   A. Perform the Allen test
   B. Inform the physician that arterial puncture is contraindicated in this patient
   C. Infiltrate the puncture site with 2% lidocaine (Xylocaine®)
   D. Analyze the sample immediately
   E. Take extra precautions to prevent postpuncture bleeding
   (2:235)

6. The use of excessive quantities of sodium heparin in preparing a syringe for sampling of arterial blood may result in which of the following blood gas data errors?
   I. Low pH
   II. High P_{CO_2}

III. High P_{O_2}
IV. Low P_{O_2}
V. Low P_{CO_2}
    A. I, II, and IV
    B. I, II, and III
    C. I, III, and V
    D. II and III
    E. I, IV, and V
(5:156–157)

7. Which of the following determinations would be most beneficial in establishing the presence of respiratory failure?
A. $C(a\text{-}\bar{v})_{O_2}$
B. $P\bar{v}_{O_2}$
C. Pa_{CO_2}, Pa_{O_2}, and pH
D. $P(A\text{-}a)_{O_2}$
E. V_D/V_T
(1:300)

8. Which of the following tests should the respiratory therapist recommend to help establish the diagnosis of cystic fibrosis?
A. Talk test
B. Methylene blue test
C. Sweat chloride test
D. Allen test
E. Tensilon test
(11:121)

9. Which of the following radiologic studies should the respiratory therapy practitioner recommend to help establish the presence of bronchiectasis?
A. Ventilation-perfusion lung scan
B. Bronchogram
C. Air bronchogram
D. Fluoroscopy
E. Tomography
(11:115)

10. Which of the following determinations is considered most useful in establishing the presence or absence of tissue hypoxia?
A. Pa_{O_2}
B. $S\bar{v}_{O_2}$
C. $C(a\text{-}\bar{v})_{O_2}$
D. PWP
E. Systemic vascular resistance
(2:240)

11. Which of the following statements regarding arterial blood sampling from the femoral artery is (are) true?
    I. Venipuncture cannot occur at this site.
    II. It is not believed to have adequate collateral blood flow.
    III. It is considered the most hazardous of sampling sites.
    IV. It is generally the least superficial sampling site.

A. II, III, and IV
B. I, III, and IV
C. I and III
D. II and IV
E. III only
(97:659) (5:146–147 and 151)

12. Failure to immediately send a sputum sample to the laboratory for examination is known to allow which of the following bacteria to overgrow and thus appear to be the dominant flora?
A. Gram-negative anaerobes
B. Gram-positive cocci
C. *Candida* species
D. Gram-negative aerobic rods
E. *Mycobacterium tuberculosis*
(2:431)

13. Which of the following tests is usually considered *most* beneficial in establishing the diagnosis of pulmonary fibrosis?
A. Arterial blood gas analysis
B. Simple spirometry
C. Full-body plethysmography
D. Lung biopsy
E. Flow-volume loop analysis
(11:124–125)

14. Which of the following should the practitioner recommend as being *most* beneficial in helping to establish the diagnosis of acute pulmonary embolus in a patient with sudden dyspnea and chest pain?
A. Serum enzyme studies
B. Coagulation studies
C. Ventilation-perfusion lung scan
D. 12 lead electrocardiogram
E. Chest roentgenogram
(11:181) (2:229)

15. Which of the following would be the most useful in distinguishing allergic from nonallergic asthma?
A. Before and after bronchodilator tests
B. History and physical examination
C. Monitoring patient eosinophil concentrations
D. Patient response to systemic corticosteroids
E. Chest roentgenogram
(11:103–105)

Answer Key

1. C	4. C	7. C	10. B	13. D
2. C	5. E	8. C	11. A	14. C
3. C	6. C	9. B	12. B	15. C

D. Perform and Evaluate Laboratory Procedures

Questions in this category are designed to assess the candidate's ability to perform and/or evaluate the tests that are performed in blood gas laboratories and/or pulmonary function laboratories.

Entry Level Pretest

According to the NBRC, 6% of the questions on the Entry Level Examination are from the perform and evaluate laboratory procedures category. In addition, the Composite Examination Matrix (see reference 80) states that questions in this category will assess the candidate's ability to perform and evaluate the following pulmonary laboratory tests on a *basic* level:

1. Spirometry and/or before and after bronchodilator studies
2. Blood gas and acid-base analysis

The following self-study questions were developed from the NBRC Composite Examination Matrix:

1. A 25-year-old patient is admitted to the emergency department in a coma. She has tachypnea and tachycardia, and her breath is noted to have an acetone odor. Arterial blood obtained at this time reveal the following data:

FI_{O_2}	0.21
Pa_{O_2}	106 mm Hg
Pa_{CO_2}	24 mm Hg
pH	7.18
Base excess	-22 mEq/L
Hb	15 g/dL

Which of the following is the correct interpretation of the above acid-base information?
    A. Partially compensated metabolic acidosis
    B. Overcompensated respiratory alkalosis
    C. Respiratory acidosis and metabolic acidosis
    D. Uncompensated metabolic acidosis
    E. Partially compensated respiratory acidosis
       (5:195–196)

2. The term *pH* may be accurately defined as:
    A. The negative log of the hydrogen ion concentration
    B. The negative log of the reciprocal of the hydrogen ion concentration
    C. The log of the reciprocal of the hydrogen ion concentration

P.69-D

D. The ratio of carbonic acid to the bicarbonate ion
E. A and C are correct.
(2:243) (25:Chap 10, p 5)

3. For each 1.0 change in pH (e.g., from 6.4 to 7.4), the hydrogen ion concentration of the body fluids will change by which of the following factors?
A. 2
B. 5
C. 10
D. 20
E. 100
(25:Chap 10, p 5)

handwritten: $PH \ 8 \ 7 = 100 \rangle \ 10 \times 10 \quad P.70-D$
$PH \ 8 \ 8 = 10$

4. Physiologic compensation for a primary metabolic alkalosis is accomplished through the development of a secondary or compensatory:
A. Respiratory acidosis
B. Metabolic alkalosis
C. Respiratory alkalosis
D. Respiratory and metabolic acidosis
E. Metabolic acidosis
(2:252–255)

5. An unconscious fireman with suspected carbon monoxide poisoning is brought to the emergency department where he is intubated and placed on a volume-cycled ventilator. Twenty minutes later, arterial blood is analyzed at an FIo_2 of 1.0. This information is presented below:

Pao_2	490 mm Hg
$Paco_2$	36 mm Hg
pH	7.36
HCO_3	18.2 mEq/L
HbCO	32%
Hb	14 g/dL

handwritten: comp. metab acid

Which of the following represents the approximate amount of oxygen dissolved in this patient's plasma?
A. 0.4 vol%
B. 0.8 vol%
C. 1.3 vol%
D. 1.5 vol%
E. 1.7 vol%
(5:84)

handwritten: $490 \times .003 = 1.47$ 5.67

6. The expiratory reserve volume normally represents what percentage of an individual's vital capacity?
A. 10%
B. 25%
C. 35%

D.   40%
E.   50%
     (16:4)

7. Which of the following represents the normal value for the residual volume to tidal volume ratio (RV/TLC) in healthy young subjects?
    A.   20-40%
    B.   25-60%
    C.   40-60%
    D.   50-60%
    E.   60-70%
         (16:13)

8. Which of the following is *not* considered an obstructive lung disorder?
    A.   Chronic bronchitis
    B.   Pickwickian syndrome
    C.   Emphysema
    D.   Bronchiectasis
    E.   Asthma
         (11:196)

9. Which of the following blood gas results would most likely be reported for a patient who has severe chronic bronchitis?

	pH	Pao_2 (mm Hg)	$Paco_2$ (mm Hg)
A.	7.32	53	76
B.	7.43	76	90
C.	7.16	43	62
D.	7.51	71	54
E.	7.36	60	45

         (2:1009)

10. Pulmonary function tests are performed on a 53-year-old woman prior to undergoing upper abdominal surgery. The results appear below:

Test	Predicted	Observed
FVC	3.4 L	2.8 L
$FEV_1\%$ FVC	80%	39%
$FEF_{200-1200}$	6.3 L/sec	1.8 L/sec
FEF_{25-75}	3.1 L/sec	0.7 L/sec

    The most likely diagnosis for this patient would be:
    A.   Histoplasmosis
    B.   Chronic bronchitis
    C.   Acute pulmonary embolus
    D.   Alveolar proteinosis
    E.   Normal study
         (2:215 and 705)

11. A young, healthy individual is generally expected to exhale approximately what percentage of his forced vital capacity in 1 second (FEV_1)?
   A. 50%
   B. 60%
   C. 75%
   D. 90%
   E. 97%
   (16:30)

12. A 45-year-old patient with a history of gastric distress is admitted to the hospital for an exploratory laparotomy. Arterial blood analyzed preoperatively reveals the following data:

FIo_2	0.21
Pao_2	121 mm Hg
$Paco_2$	22 mm Hg
pH	7.30
Base excess	−5.8 mEq/L

   (handwritten annotations: add them together; (metab) acid)

   Which of the following is the *most* likely reason for the above information?
   A. Venous sample
   B. Physiologic overcompensation
   C. Too much sodium heparin in sample
   D. Delay in running sample
   E. A normal study exists.
   (5:156) (2:1010)

   (handwritten annotations: makes it acid; $PCO_2 + PO_2$ would approach rm air values; AIR IN SAMPLE ↓PCO_2 + ↑PO_2 150 ↑pH; ↓Pa O_2; 260)

13. A 63-year-old patient with a history of bronchiectasis dating to adolescence is admitted to the emergency department with a complaint of dyspnea and excessive sputum production. Arterial blood drawn at that time yields the following data:

FIo_2	0.28
Pao_2	53 mm Hg
$Paco_2$	62 mm Hg
pH	7.68
HCO_3^-	34 mEq/L
Base excess	+10 mEq/L

   (handwritten annotations: COPD → acidosis; par compensated > 40; metab alka)

   The correct interpretation of the above acid-base data would be:
   A. Fully compensated respiratory acidosis
   B. Fully compensated metabolic alkalosis
   C. Partially compensated metabolic alkalosis
   D. Laboratory error exists
   E. Respiratory acidosis and metabolic alkalosis
   (5:Chap 12) (2:246)

The next two questions pertain to the following illustration:

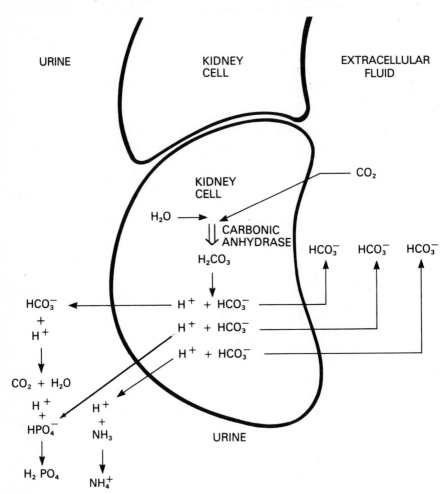

Figure IV-2.

14.   The urine buffers play an important role in the kidneys':
      A.   Ability to excrete large amounts of HCO_3^-
      B.   Ability to secrete large amounts of CO_2
      C.   Ability to secrete large amounts of H^+
      D.   Ability to excrete large amounts of H^+
      E.   Ability to secrete large amounts of NH_3^+
           (5:94)

15.   The most important urine buffer described in the above illustration is:
      A. HPO_4^-
      B. NH_3
      C. HCO_3^-

D. CO_2
E. H_2O
(5:94)

16. Pulmonary function testing performed during an acute episode of asthma would most likely reveal all of the following *except:*
   A. Increased FRC
   B. Increased VC
   C. Decreased FEV_1
   D. Decreased $\dfrac{FEV_1}{FVC}\%$
   E. Increased RV/TLC
   (2:705–712)

17. Which of the following lung volumes or capacities cannot be determined directly from analysis of spirometric (time–volume) data? $P. 119-D$
   I. Tidal volume
   II. Residual volume
   III. Inspiratory capacity
   IV. Total lung capacity
      A. II and III
      B. I and III
      C. II and IV
      D. III and IV
      E. I and IV
   (16:4–8)

18. The vital capacity when measured on both men and women may vary as much as which of the following percentages from predicted normal values?
   A. Plus or minus 5%
   B. Plus or minus 10%
   C. Plus or minus 20%
   D. Plus or minus 30%
   E. Plus or minus 40%
   (16:1)

19. A patient is noted to have a Pa_{CO_2} of 50 mm Hg. Which of the following is *least* likely to be a cause of this abnormality?
   A. Alveolar hypoventilation
   B. Decreased V_D/V_T
   C. Hypermetabolism uses O_2 .. $\uparrow P_{CO_2}$
   D. Decreased minute ventilation
   E. Decreased tidal volume
   (5:207–210)

20. For every 10 mm Hg *acute* decrease in Pa_{CO_2}, the pH of the blood will increase approximately:
   A. 0.5
   B. 0.05
   C. 0.10

D.   0.15
E.   0.20
    (5:128) (2:246)

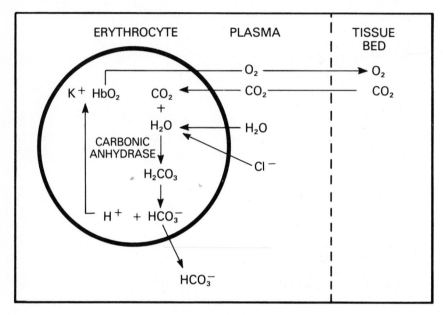

Figure IV-3.

21.   The above diagram illustrates:
      A.   Haldane effect
      B.   Carbonic anhydrase cycle
      C.   Bohr effect
      D.   Chloride shift
      E.   Bicarbonate cycle
         (5:26) (5:Chap 3) (2:Chap 12)

22.   Sampling of blood from which of the following blood vessels
      would most likely yield the highest carbon dioxide tension?
      A.   Radial artery
      B.   Pulmonary vein
      C.   Femoral artery
      D.   Pulmonary artery
      E.   Temporal artery
         (5:241–242)

23.   A 57-year-old woman is brought to the emergency department
      after suffering a cerebrovascular accident at home. Results of
      admission blood gas analysis performed while receiving 4 L oxy-
      gen via nasal cannula are revealed below: ~ 36%

                    Pa_{O_2} 182 mm Hg
                    Pa_{CO_2} 28 mm Hg ↓

$$pH \qquad 7.63$$
$$HCO_3^- \qquad 32 \text{ mEq/L}$$

Based on the above information, which of the following is the most correct interpretation of the above data?

A. Acute respiratory alkalosis
B. Partially compensated metabolic alkalosis
C. Combined respiratory and metabolic alkalosis
D. Acute metabolic alkalosis
E. Chronic respiratory alkalosis
   (2:246) (25:Chap 10, pp 2–6) (5:128–130)

24. A patient in the intensive care unit is noted to have the following arterial blood gas values:

pH	7.59
$Paco_2$	21
HCO_3^-	22 mEq/L
Base excess	+0.7 mEq/L

Which of the following is the most correct interpretation of the above data?

A. Respiratory alkalosis and metabolic acidosis
B. Uncompensated respiratory alkalosis
C. Fully compensated respiratory alkalosis
D. Partially compensated respiratory alkalosis
E. Laboratory error exists
   (5:128)

25. Which of the following acid-base abnormalities would most likely be present in a 35-year-old patient who is in a diabetic coma?

A. Partially compensated metabolic acidosis
B. Partially compensated respiratory acidosis
C. Fully compensated metabolic alkalosis
D. Partially compensated respiratory alkalosis
E. Fully compensated respiratory acidosis
   (5:195–196)

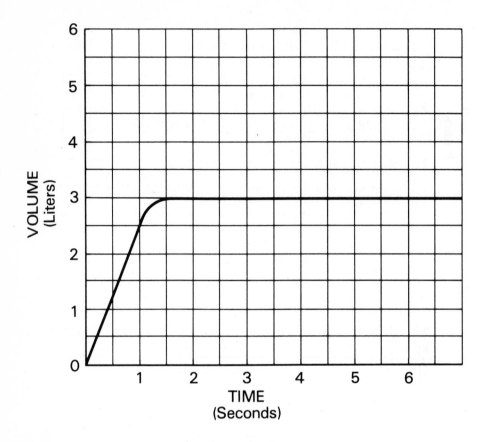

Figure IV-4.

26. The above time-volume tracing was performed on a 42-year-old former professional football player. He is 78 inches tall and weighs 235 lbs. What is the best interpretation?   6'6"
    A. Obstructive disease – flat line
    B. Restrictive disease ↓ vol
    C. Combined obstructive and restrictive disease
    D. Chronic bronchitis
    E. Bronchial asthma
    (2:221)

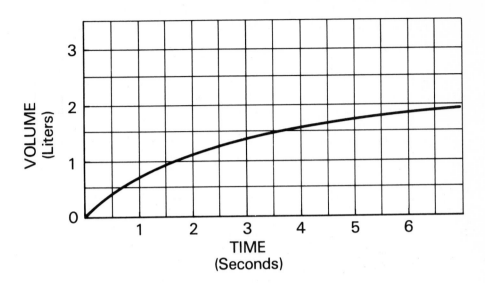

Figure IV-5.

27. The above spirometric data were most likely obtained from a 70-kg patient with which of the following disorders?
    A. Obstructive disease
    B. Restrictive disease
    C. Normal study
    D. Inconsistent patient effort
    E. Poor response to bronchodilator administration
    (70:174)

28. A before and after bronchodilator (BD) test is performed on a 23-year-old woman. The results appear below:

Test	Predicted	Pre BD Observed	Post BD Observed
FVC	3.8 L	2.6 L	3.7 L
FEV_1	3.1 L	1.1 L	3.1 L
FEF_{25-75}	3.6 L/sec	0.5 L/sec	3.2 L/sec
$FEF_{200-1200}$	5.7 L/sec	2.4 L/sec	5.4 L/sec

Based on the above information, which of the following most accurately describes this patient's response to aerosolized sympathomimetics?
    A. None noted
    B. Mild
    C. Modest
    D. Moderate
    E. Excellent
    (16:94–95) (2:705 and 996)

29. Which of the following may be used in the treatment of metabolic alkalosis?

   I.   KCl

   II. Acetazolamide (Diamox®)

   III. NH_4Cl

   IV. HCl

depends on cause

     A. I and III

     B. II, III, and IV

     C. I, II, III, and IV

     D. I, III, and IV

     E. II and III

  (5:195–196) (33:277–280)

30. A 53-year-old woman with a history of psychotic polydipsia is transferred directly to the intensive care unit from the psychiatric wing after being found in a coma. On admission the following arterial blood gas data are obtained with the patient receiving 3 L oxygen via nasal cannula:

Pa_{O_2}	127 mm Hg
Pa_{CO_2}	20 mm Hg
pH	7.47
HCO_3^-	17 mEq/L
Base excess	−6.3 mEq/L

Based on the above information, which of the following is the most correct interpretation of the above arterial blood gas information?

  A. Acute metabolic alkalosis

  B. Partially compensated metabolic acidosis

  C. Acute respiratory alkalosis with acute metabolic alkalosis

  D. Partially compensated respiratory alkalosis

  E. Fully compensated metabolic acidosis

    (5:175–176)

31. In which of the following conditions would alveolar hyperventilation *without* hypoxemia be a clinical finding?

   I.   Carbon monoxide poisoning

   II. Adult respiratory distress syndrome

   III. Cyanide poisoning

   IV. Bacterial pneumonia

     A. I and III

     B. II and III

     C. II and IV

     D. I and IV

     E. I and II

  (5:50 and 207) (2:241)

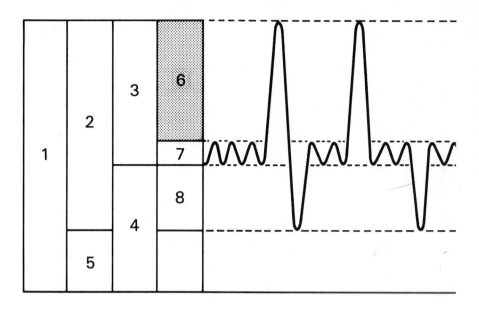

Figure IV-6.

32. The above illustration shows lung volumes and capacities. The only volume that cannot be measured with simple spirometry is:
    A. 6
    B. 7
    C. 8
    D. 5
    E. 2
       (2:206)

Answer Key

1. A	8. B	15. A	22. D	29. C
2. E	9. A	16. B	23. C	30. D
3. C	10. B	17. C	24. B	31. A
4. A	11. C	18. C	25. A	32. D
5. D	12. C	19. B	26. B	
6. B	13. D	20. C	27. A	
7. A	14. D	21. D	28. E	

$$\frac{22}{31} = 71\%$$

Advanced Practitioner Pretest

According to the NBRC, 10% of the questions on the Advanced Practitioner Examination are from the perform and evaluate laboratory procedures category. In addition, the Composite Examination Matrix (see reference 80) states that questions in this category assess the candidate's ability to perform and evaluate the following *advanced* pulmonary laboratory tests:

1. Advanced spirometry and/or before and after bronchodilator studies
2. Diffusing capacity
3. Measurement of the FRC by helium dilution method
4. Deadspace calculations (V_D/V_T)
5. Intrapulmonary shunt calculations (Q_S/Q_T)
6. Flow-volume loop studies
7. Lung thorax compliance studies
8. Electrocardiography

The following self-study questions were developed from the NBRC Composite Examination Matrix:

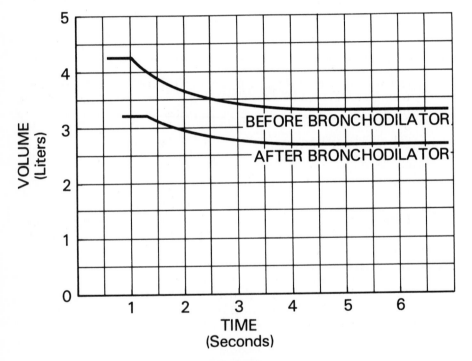

Figure IV-7.

1. The above tracing was performed on a 53-year-old man. It is most likely that this patient suffers from which of the following disorders?
    A. Pulmonary fibrosis
    B. Severe emphysema
    C. Adult respiratory distress syndrome
    D. Asthmatic bronchitis
    E. Bronchial asthma
       (2:241)

2. When performing helium dilution and/or nitrogen washout residual volume determinations, the test should begin when the patient is:
   A. At the end of a normal inspiration
   B. At the end of a normal expiration
   C. At the end of a forced expiration
   D. In the middle of a normal tidal volume
   E. During a maximal voluntary ventilation (MVV) procedure
   (16:4–8) (2:972)

3. Pulmonary function tests performed on a patient with chronic obstructive pulmonary emphysema would most likely reveal all of the following *except:*
   A. Decreased FEV_1
   B. Decreased VC
   C. Increased FEF_{50}
   D. Decreased D_LCO
   E. Decreased FEF_{25-75}
   (2:221)

4. A 24-year-old man is rescued after nearly drowning. On admission to the emergency department, the patient's rectal temperature is 92°F. Arterial blood is sampled at that time with the patient breathing room air. Uncorrected *in vitro* blood gas data appear below:

Pa_{O_2}	103 mm Hg
Pa_{CO_2}	52 mm Hg
pH	7.32
HCO_3^-	24 mEq/L

   If the above information were to be corrected back to the patient's *in vivo* temperature, which of the following would most likely be noted?
   A. The Pa_{O_2} would be below 40 mm Hg.
   B. The Pa_{O_2} would be somewhat lower.
   C. The Pa_{O_2} would be slightly higher.
   D. The pH would show severe alkalosis.
   E. The Pa_{O_2} would remain unchanged.
   (84)

The next four questions refer to the illustration shown below:

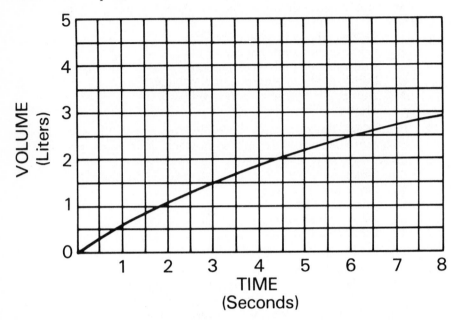

Figure IV-8.

5. The preceding time-volume tracing was obtained from an 80-kg, 32-year-old **male**. Which of the following is the most correct interpretation?
    A.   Restrictive disorder
    B.   Mild obstructive disorder
    C.   Moderate obstructive disorder
    D.   Upper airway obstruction
    E.   Severe obstructive disorder
        (16:34)

6. Which of the following most accurately represents this patient's FEV_1 at ATPS?
    A.   0.2 L
    B.   0.3 L
    C.   0.6 L
    D.   1.0 L
    E.   1.2 L
        (2:971)

7. Which of the following most accurately represents this patient's $\dfrac{FEV_1 \%?}{FVC}$
    A.   5%
    B.   12%
    C.   20%

    D. 28%
    E. 32%
      (2:271)

8. Which of the following most accurately represents this patient's FEF_{25-75} at ATPS?
    A. 0.1 L/sec
    B. 0.25 L/sec
    C. 0.4 L/sec
    D. 1.0 L/sec
    E. 1.4 L/sec
      (2:971)

9. When pulmonary disease is a result of inhalation of particulate matter during the performance of one's occupation, it is most commonly referred to as:
    A. Black lung disease
    B. Hypersensitivity pneumonitis
    C. Nosocomial disease
    D. Industrial morbidity
    E. Pneumoconiosis
      (89:642)

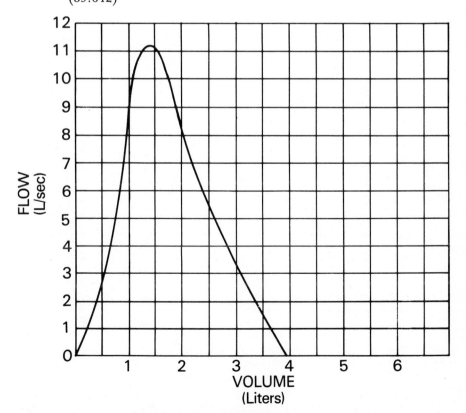

Figure IV-9.

10. The preceding flow-volume tracing was obtained from a 25-year-old pharmacist. He is 79 inches tall and weighs 250 lbs. What is the best interpretation for this flow-volume study?
   A. Obstructive pulmonary disease
   B. Restrictive pulmonary disease
   C. Severe obstructive pulmonary disease
   D. Poor patient effort
   E. Fixed large airway obstruction
   (2:221)

11. Which of the following disorders are known to frequently result in marked to severe decreases in the diffusion capacity of the lung (D_{LCO})?
   I.   Bronchial asthma
   II. Emphysema
   III. Idiopathic pulmonary fibrosis
   IV. Small airways disease
      A. I, III, and IV
      B. II, III, and IV
      C. I, II, and IV
      D. I, II, and III
      E. II and III
   (16:75) (2:217 and 705)

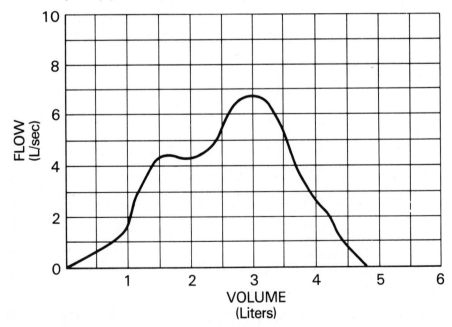

Figure IV-10.

12. The above flow-volume tracing was performed on a 27-year-old woman who works in a supermarket as a checker. She is 64 inches

tall and weighs 110 lbs. What is the best interpretation of the above study?

A. Early obstructive pulmonary disease
B. Restrictive pulmonary disease
C. Combined obstructive and restrictive pulmonary disease
D. Severe obstructive pulmonary disease
E. Variable effort by the patient
   (2:221)

13. Which of the following can be determined from a flow-volume loop study?
   I. Maximal expiratory flow rate (MEFR)
   II. Forced expiratory flow rate at 75% of the vital capacity (FEF_{75})
   III. Average flow rate of the middle 50% of the vital capacity
   IV. Maximal inspiratory flow rate (MIFR)
      A. I, II, and IV
      B. II and III
      C. I, II, and III
      D. II, III, and IV
      E. III and IV
   (16:45–48)

14. Pulmonary function tests are performed on a 48-year-old patient prior to upper abdominal surgery. These data appear below:

Test	Predicted	Observed
FVC	4.5 L	4.4 L
FEV_1	3.5 L	3.6 L
$\dfrac{FEV_1\%}{FVC}$	80%	77%
$FEF_{25\text{-}75}$	4.1 L/sec	2.5 L/sec
RV/TLC%	28%	30%

True statements regarding the above information include:
   I. The patient has a restrictive lung disorder.
   II. Surgery should be postponed.
   III. Early chronic obstructive pulmonary disease may exist.
   IV. Postoperative pulmonary complications should be minimal.
      A. III and IV
      B. II and III
      C. I and IV
      D. I and III
      E. II and IV
   (1:463–465) (2:211 and 994)

15. Which of the following pulmonary function determinations is known to yield the largest value for total lung capacity when performed on patients with emphysema?
A. Time-volume studies
B. Flow-volume loop

C.   Open analysis circuit nitrogen washout method
D.   Full body plethysmography
E.   Closed circuit helium dilution method
     (16:12–13)

The next four questions refer to the illustration shown below:

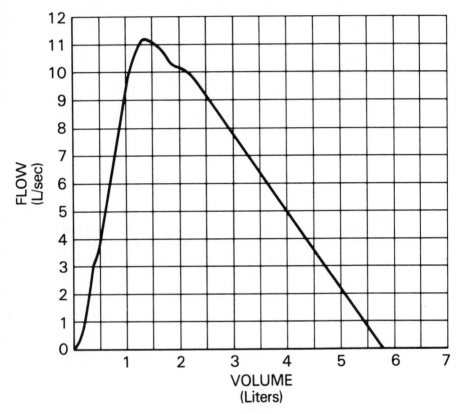

Figure IV-11.

16. The preceding flow-volume tracing was performed on a 70-kg,
     32-year-old man. Which of the following is the most correct
     interpretation?
     A.   Normal tracing
     B.   Obstructive defect
     C.   Restrictive defect
     D.   Small airways disease
     E.   Combined obstructive and restrictive defect
          (2:221)

17. From the preceding tracing calculate the forced vital capacity at
     ATPS.
     A.   6.08 L
     B.   11.39 L

C.   4.52 L
D.   5.19 L
E.   5.75 L
   (16:45–48)

18. From the preceding tracing calculate the peak expiratory flow rate at ATPS.
     A.   9 L/sec
     B.   8 L/sec
     C.   11.3 L/sec
     D.   10.6 L/sec
     E.   12 L/sec
        (16:45–48)

19. From the preceding tracing calculate the forced expiratory flow at 50% vital capacity (FEF_{50}) at ATPS.
     A.   6 L/sec
     B.   8.3 L/sec
     C.   5 L/sec
     D.   4 L/sec
     E.   9 L/sec
        (16:45–48)

20. Results of pulmonary function tests performed on a 55-year-old patient are as follows:

Test	Predicted	Observed
FVC	4.8 L	2.9 L
$\dfrac{FEV_1\%}{FVC}$	↑ 80%	88%
$FEF_{200\text{-}1200}$	6.8 L/sec	6.1 L/sec
$FEF_{25\text{-}75}$	3.3 L/sec	3.1 L/sec
D_{LCO}	25 mL/min/mm Hg	12 mL/min/mm Hg

Based on the above information, the most accurate interpretation is:
     A.   Obstructive pattern
     B.   Restrictive pattern
     C.   Mixed obstructive and restrictive pattern
     D.   Upper airway obstruction
     E.   Poor patient effort
        (2:216)

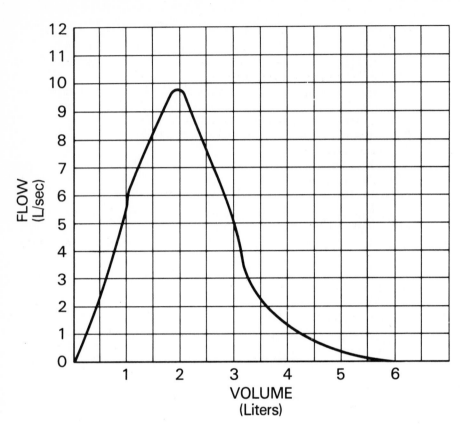

Figure IV-12.

21. The above flow-volume tracing was obtained from a 56-year-old man. He is 72 inches tall and weighs 195 lbs. He has a 20 pack-year history of cigarette smoking. The best interpretation for this loop would be:
    A. Small airways disease
    B. Early restrictive lung disease
    C. Severe combined obstructive and restrictive pulmonary disease
    D. Typical Hamman-Rich configuration
    E. Poor patient effort
    (2:221)

22. Which of the following gases is administered in calculating the residual volume using the open circuit (nonrebreathing) method?
    A. Helium
    B. Xenon
    C. Nitrogen
    D. Oxygen
    E. Carbon monoxide
    (16:5)

23.   Lung volumes and flow rates obtained while performing spirome-
      try or flow-volume studies must be corrected for the differential
      that exists between ambient and body temperatures. Which of the
      following statements regarding this is (are) true?
      I.   It is an application of Charles's law.
      II.   Volumes at BTPS must be corrected to ATPS.
      III. Volumes are larger at ATPS than at BTPS.
      IV.   It is also used to correct leaks in the circuit.
            A.   II and III
            B.   I and III
            C.   I, II, and III
            D.   I and IV
            E.   I only
      (2:1015–1016)

24.   Direct measurement of which of the following types of compliance
      requires the use of an esophageal balloon?
      A.   Static effective
      B.   Static lung (C_L)
      C.   Static lung-thorax (C_{LT})
      D.   Static thorax (C_T)
      E.   Dynamic effective
      (16:38)

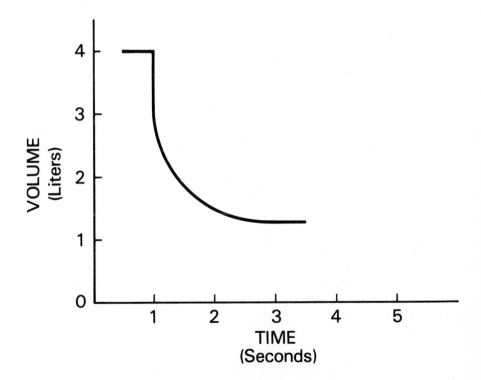

Figure IV-13.

25. The above spirometric data were obtained from a 15-year-old, 35-kg girl. Which of the following is the most correct interpretation?
    A. Obstructive disease
    B. Restrictive disease
    C. Normal study
    D. Mixed obstructive and restrictive disease
    E. Poor patient effort
       (70:174)

26. The FEF_{25-75} is known to be a measurement of which of the following?
    A. The maximum volume of gas expired within the middle 50% of a vital capacity effort
    B. The peak flow rate of the middle 50% of the vital capacity
    C. The mean maximal time segment of the middle 50% of the vital capacity
    D. The average flow rate of the middle 50% of the vital capacity
    E. The instantaneous flow rate of the middle 50% of the vital capacity
       (16:33)

Answer Key

1. B	6. C	11. B	16. A	21. A
2. B	7. C	12. E	17. E	22. D
3. C	8. C	13. A	18. C	23. E
4. B	9. E	14. A	19. B	24. B
5. E	10. E	15. D	20. B	25. C
				26. D

E. Assess Therapeutic Plan (Entry Level Only)

According to the NBRC, this content category is assessed only on the Entry Level Examination. This category is designed to assess the candidate's ability to determine the appropriateness of the prescribed respiratory care plan and to recommend modifications in this plan where indicated. For example, the respiratory therapy practitioner is asked to perform therapy on a patient with long-standing chronic obstructive lung disease whose baseline arterial carbon dioxide tension is well in excess of 60 mm Hg. In reading this patient's chart, the practitioner notes that part of the physician's care plan involves placing this patient on 6 L oxygen by simple oxygen mask. The respiratory therapy practitioner should thus be prepared to recommend modifications involving the administration of oxygen to this patient.

In addition, questions in this category deal with the ability of the respiratory therapy practitioner to identify the patient's pathophysiologic state based on available information. For example, a 22-year-old man is admitted to the emergency department in severe hemorrhagic shock following a motorcycle accident. The patient is resuscitated and successfully treated in the emergency department and subsequently transferred to the intensive care unit. Twelve hours later, the patient has tachypnea, tachycardia, and hypertension. Arterial blood gas analysis performed at that time with the patient receiving 8 L oxygen by simple mask revealed an arterial oxygen tension of 40 mm Hg. Based on the foregoing information, the respiratory therapy practitioner should be able to identify that the most likely cause of this patient's symptoms is adult respiratory distress syndrome.

Entry Level Pretest

According to the NBRC, 6% of the questions on the Entry Level Examination are from the assess therapeutic plan category. In addition, the Composite Examination Matrix (see reference 80) states that questions in this category assess the ability of the candidate to:

1. Determine the appropriateness of prescribed therapy and goals for identified pathophysiologic states
2. Analyze available data to determine the pathophysiologic state
3. Review planned therapy to establish therapeutic goals
4. Recommend changes in therapeutic plan
5. Participate in the development of respiratory care plans

The following self-study questions were developed from the NBRC Composite Examination Matrix:

1. The risk of oxygen-induced hypoventilation is apparently minimal in patients with steady-state arterial CO_2 tensions less than:
   A. 50–60
   B. 60–70
   C. 70–80
   D. 80–90
   E. A and B are correct.
   (1:483)

2. PEEP therapy is believed to be most effective in the management of which one of the following?
   A. Status asthmaticus
   B. Cardiogenic pulmonary edema
   C. Adult respiratory distress syndrome
   D. Unilateral aspiration pneumonitis
   E. Guillain-Barré syndrome
   (45)

3. Which of the following statements is (are) true regarding cyanide poisoning?
   I.   It is invariably accompanied by arterial hypoxemia.
   II. It is an example of anemic hypoxia.
   III. It is known to result in abnormally high mixed venous oxygen tensions.

IV. Its primary pathology involves leftward shifts in the oxyhe-
moglobin dissociation curve.
A. I and III
B. II and IV
C. I and IV
D. III and IV
E. III only
(2:241) (5:50)

4. The presence of which of the following is believed to be necessary
for sustained maximal inspiratory maneuvers to be effective in
preventing postoperative atelectasis?
I. Vital capacity less than 20 mL/kg
II. Patient ability to cooperate
III. Respiratory rate greater than 20/min
IV. Effective patient instruction
A. II and IV
B. I and IV
C. III only
D. II and III
E. III and IV
(1:195)

5. The administration of low concentrations of oxygen is believed to
be of greatest therapeutic benefit when administered to patients
with which of the following pulmonary disorders?
A. Guillain-Barré syndrome
B. Adult respiratory distress syndrome
C. Congestive heart failure
D. Chronic bronchitis
E. Narcotic overdose
(5:176)

6. Continuous positive airway pressure (CPAP) is believed to be of
greatest benefit when employed in the treatment of which of the
following disorders?
A. Refractory hypoxemia with hypercarbia
B. Advanced chronic obstructive pulmonary disease with right
ventricular failure
C. Diffuse microatelectasis with upper airway obstruction
D. Refractory hypoxemia with hypocarbia
E. Acute ventilatory failure superimposed on chronic hypoxemia
(1:325–384)

7. Depression of the peripheral respiratory drive is a known compli-
cation when excessive concentrations of oxygen are administered
to patients with which of the following pulmonary disorders?
I. Cystic fibrosis
II. Pickwickian syndrome
III. Asphyxia neonatorum
IV. Infant respiratory distress syndrome

A. I and II
B. I and IV
C. III and IV
D. II and III
E. II and IV
(11:119–122 and 196–199)

8. A tall, thin 20-year-old man presents to the emergency department with a complaint of sharp chest pain and difficulty in breathing. The patient states these symptoms began half an hour previously during a game of racquetball. Chest physical examination reveals a hyperresonant percussion note over the left lung fields and a tracheal shift toward the right thorax. Based on the above information, the most likely cause of this patient's distress is:
A. Myocardial infarct
B. Pulmonary embolus
C. Spontaneous tension pneumothorax
D. Congenital lobar emphysema
E. Traumatic pneumothorax
(11:170–193)

9. A 40-year-old man with a history of alcoholism is admitted to the emergency department. He has tachypnea and tachycardia and is febrile. Cough efforts are productive of copious amounts of putrid-smelling sputum. Physical examination also reveals extremely poor dental hygiene. Based on the above information, the most likely cause of this patient's distress is:
A. Cystic fibrosis
B. Pulmonary tuberculosis
C. Anaerobic lung abscess
D. Chronic bronchitis
E. Bronchiectasis
(11:69–72)

10. Seventy-two hours after being subjected to an exploratory laparotomy, a 30-year-old man is noted to have both tachypnea and tachycardia. His temperature at this time is 37.5°C. Breath sounds are diminished bibasally, and coughing yields small amounts of mucopurulent sputum. The white blood cell count is noted to be 7000/μL. Based on the above information, the most likely cause of this patient's distress is:
A. Gram-negative nosocomial pulmonary infection
B. Pulmonary embolus
C. Aspiration pneumonia
D. Postoperative atelectasis
E. Pulmonary edema
(1:160, 263, and 463–464)

11. Five days following hip surgery, a 74-year-old woman develops acute dyspnea accompanied by sharp chest pain. Later that afternoon the patient has an episode of hemoptysis. Arterial blood gas analysis at this time reveals arterial hypoxemia with hypocarbia.

Which of the following disorders is most likely to be responsible for this patient's distress?
A. Spontaneous pneumothorax
B. Pleural effusion
C. Pulmonary embolus
D. Massive pulmonary atelectasis
E. Myasthenia gravis
   (2:312) (11:179–181)

12. A 60-year-old woman is admitted to the hospital after falling at home and fracturing her tibia and femur. Twelve hours later she has tachycardia and tachypnea and is dusky in appearance. Arterial blood is analyzed with the patient receiving 8 L oxygen via simple oxygen mask:

$$Pa_{O_2} \qquad 42 \text{ mm Hg}$$
$$Pa_{CO_2} \qquad 32 \text{ mm Hg}$$
$$pH \qquad 7.40$$
$$HCO_3^- \qquad 20 \text{ mEq/L}$$

Based on the above information, the most likely cause of this patient's distress is:
A. Fat embolus with adult respiratory distress syndrome
B. Viral pneumonia
C. Cervical spine transection
D. Tension pneumothorax
E. Cardiogenic pulmonary edema
   (2:890) (11:181–182)

13. Which of the following statements regarding carbon monoxide poisoning is *not* true?
A. It is considered an indication for the administration of 100% oxygen.
B. It is associated with smoke inhalation.
C. It frequently results in a decreased P_{50}.
D. The rate of carbon monoxide excretion is highest on 21% oxygen.
E. It may be an indication for hyperbaric oxygen administration.
   (1:497–498)

Answer Key

1. A	4. A	7. A	10. D	13. D
2. C	5. D	8. C	11. C	
3. E	6. D	9. C	12. A	

Part II
Equipment

According to the NBRC, 25% of the Entry Level and 10% of the Advanced Practitioner Examinations are devoted to assessing the candidate's knowledge of respiratory care equipment. Questions in this area are broken down into four subcategories on the examinations:

1. *Select equipment.* These questions assess the candidate's knowledge of the classification, principles of operation, and clinically significant design characteristics of all equipment used in respiratory care.
2. *Assemble, note operation, and correct equipment malfunctions.* Questions in this category assess the candidate's ability to ensure the proper operation of all equipment in the performance of respiratory diagnostic and therapeutic procedures.
3. *Ensure the cleanliness of all equipment.* Here, the candidate's knowledge of sterilization and disinfection techniques is assessed.
4. *Perform calibration and quality control procedures.* Knowledge of the procedures as applied to blood gas analyzers, pulmonary function equipment, and gas metering devices is assessed in this category.

As stated previously, the major purpose of the NBRC Examination is to determine whether the candidate is competent to perform as a respiratory therapy practitioner. To ensure its validity in this regard, the examination is constructed around the 1981 Respiratory Therapy Task Analysis Survey (see reference 45). Statistical analysis has established a positive correlation between performance on these examinations and job performance.

This book is an educational tool. Its goals and mine are twofold. First, I wish to make the candidate familiar with the structure of the examinations; second, I want to help him or her review the fundamental and essential aspects of respiratory therapy that are assessed on these examinations. I believe then that classification of respiratory therapy equipment according to *task* (i.e., select, assemble, note operation, correct malfunction) has its greatest validity as a testing tool. A *generic* (i.e., according to name, as in oxygen administration devices) classification system on the other hand excels for an instructional guide like this if for no other reason than its almost universal employment in respiratory therapy textbooks.

201

In summary, I am going to *drop* the following two task-oriented categories:

1. Select equipment
2. Assemble, note operation, and correct equipment malfunctions

I will *replace* them with the following seven generic categories:

1. Medical gas therapy devices
2. Oxygen administration devices
3. Humidity and aerosol therapy devices
4. Airway care and resuscitation devices
5. Hyperinflation therapy devices
6. Continuous mechanical ventilator devices
7. Cardiopulmonary function monitoring devices

I will, because of their specific nature, retain the following two categories as they are reflected in the NBRC Composite Examination Matrix:

8. Ensure the cleanliness of all equipment
9. Perform calibration and quality control procedures

These nine categories are further described in the self-study sections that follow.

A. Medical Gas Therapy Devices (Entry Level Only)

Questions in this category assess the candidate's ability to select and assemble all medical gas therapy equipment prior to performing respiratory care procedures. These questions also test the candidate's understanding of the principles of proper operation and his or her ability to correct all malfunctions of selected equipment.

Entry Level Pretest

According to the NBRC Composite Examination Matrix (see reference 80), questions in this category assess the candidate's understanding of the following types of respiratory care equipment:

1. Oxygen analyzers
2. Regulators, reducing valves, and all miscellaneous connectors and adaptors
3. Flowmeters
4. Air/oxygen proportioners (blenders)
5. Oxygen concentrating devices
6. Gas cylinders, bulk systems, and manifolds
7. Air compressors

The following are self-study questions developed from the NBRC Composite Examination Matrix:

1. A device that registers flow rate as a result of backpressure created by a fixed orifice is:
   A. A Thorpe tube
   B. A kinetic flowmeter
   C. A rotameter
   D. A thermistor
   E. A Bourdon gauge
   (4:70 and 71)

2. Which of the following statements is (are) true regarding the non-backpressure-compensated Thorpe tube type flowmeter?
   I. The needle valve is downstream from the Thorpe tube.
   II. The needle valve is upstream from the Thorpe tube.   P. 199-D
   III. In response to backpressure, indicated flow may be lower than actual flow.
   IV. In response to backpressure, indicated flow may be higher than actual flow.
   A. II and III
   B. II and IV
   C. I, III, and IV
   D. IV only
   E. I and III
   (4:75–77)

3. When full, cylinders of gaseous oxygen usually contain a pressure of:
   A. 1100 psig
   B. 1000 psig
   C. 2500 psig
   D. 1500 psig
   E. 2200 psig
   (3:253)

4. The respiratory therapy practitioner can most readily identify the number of stages a given reducing valve has by:
   A. Looking at the pressure gauge
   B. Counting the number of frangible disks
   C. Counting the number of pressure gauges
   D. Counting the number of pop-off valves
   E. Reading the information on the back of the device
   (4:72)

5. Which of the following safety systems was designed for use with the connecting valves of large medical gas cylinders (F–H)?
   A. Pin Index Safety System (PISS)
   B. Diameter Index Safety System (DISS)
   C. Color Code Safety System
   D. American Standard Safety System (ASSS)
   E. Frangible Disk/Fusible Metal Safety System
   (4:37)

The next two questions refer to the following illustration:

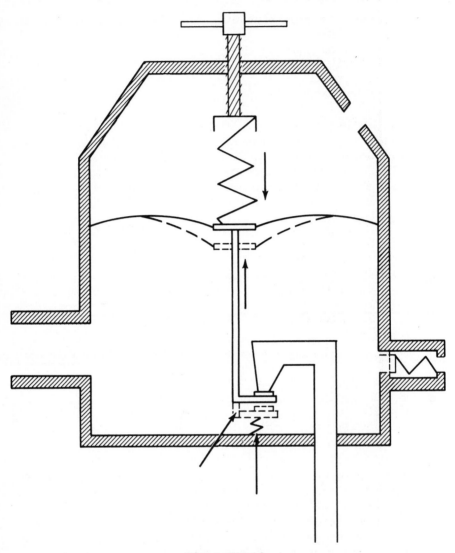

Figure IV-14.

6. The above diagram illustrates:
   - I.   A single-stage reducing valve
   - II. The inner mechanism of the Bourdon gauge
   - III. A simple example of an oxygen blender
   - IV. An adjustable pressure regulator
   - V.   A DISS wall outlet
       - A. I, II, and III
       - B. II, III, and IV

       C.   I, III, and IV
       D.   I and IV
       E.   II, IV, and V
   (4:71)

7. The diaphragm in the above illustration:
    I.   Separates the high pressure from the low pressure side of the regulator
    II.   Opens the poppet valve when the low pressure side loses pressure
    III.   Closes the poppet valve when the low pressure side gains pressure
    IV.   Allows for the pressure needed to move it to be varied by the user
       A.   I, II, and III
       B.   III and IV
       C.   I, II, III, and IV
       D.   I and III
       E.   II only
   (4:71)

8. Which of the following safety systems was designed for use on small medical gas cylinders (A–E) with post-type valves:
       A.   Pin Index Safety System (PISS)
       B.   Diameter Index Safety System (DISS)
       C.   American Standard Safety System (ASSS)
       D.   Color Code Safety System
       E.   Frangible Disk/Fusible Metal Safety System
   (4:36)

9. The Pin Index code that has been designated for use on oxygen cylinders is:
       A.   2–6
       B.   2–4
       C.   3–5
       D.   2–5
       E.   4–6
   (4:38)

10. Which of the following organizations is responsible for regulating the purity of compressed medical gases?
       A.   Compressed Gas Association
       B.   National Formulary
       C.   United States Pharmacopeia
       D.   Food and Drug Administration
       E.   Department of Transportation
   (4:38)

11. When a medical gas cylinder has been designated and stamped with the symbol 3AA, which of the following is true?
       A.   It is capable of containing medical quality gases.
       B.   It can withstand pressures up to 5000 psig.
       C.   It has been produced from high carbon steel.

D.   It has undergone hydrostatic testing.

E.   It has been manufactured from cast iron.
     (4:33)

12.   Federal regulations regarding the construction of cylinders used in transport of medical gases are under the jurisdiction of the:
      A.   Department of Transportation
      B.   Interstate Commerce Commission
      C.   Food and Drug Administration
      D.   Department of Commerce
      E.   Office of the Surgeon General
      (4:34)

13.   Which of the following statements regarding the design and construction of medical gas cylinders is *not* true?
      A.   Most cylinders must currently undergo hydrostatic testing every 5 years.
      B.   Cylinders must contain a pressure release mechanism to prevent explosion.
      C.   The cylinders marked maximum filling pressure may be exceeded by 50% if needed.
      D.   Hydrostatic retesting is performed at ⅗ of the cylinder service pressure.
      E.   A "+" following the hydrostatic testing date indicates that the cylinder has passed periodic cylinder retesting procedures.
      (4:35–37)

14.   The International Color Code for oxygen is:
      A.   White
      B.   Green   u.s.
      C.   Brown
      D.   Orange
      E.   Black
      (4:39)

15.   A high temperature safety release valve using "Woods" metal can be found:
      A.   On large cylinder valves
      B.   On double-stage reducing valves
      C.   On single-stage reducing valves
      D.   On small cylinder valves
      E.   On liquid bulk oxygen systems
      (3:250–251)

16.   Which of the following *most* correctly defines the minimal standard for a bulk oxygen system?
      A.   More than 50,000 cubic feet of gaseous oxygen connected and ready for use
      B.   More than 480 cylinders of oxygen connected and ready for use
      C.   More than 13,000 cubic feet of gaseous oxygen connected and ready for use

D.   More than 4000 cubic feet of liquid oxygen connected and
ready for use

E.   B and D are correct.
(4:50)

17.   The Food and Drug Administration requires that medical oxygen
be at least _____ in purity.

A.   90%

B.   99%

C.   98%

D.   99.9%

E.   99.5%
(4:44)

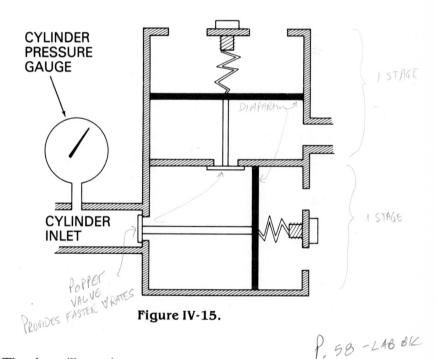

CYLINDER
PRESSURE
GAUGE

CYLINDER
INLET

Figure IV-15.

18.   The above illustration:

I.   Shows a triple-stage pressure regulator

II.   Shows two poppet valves

III.   Shows a double-stage pressure regulator

IV.   Shows two diaphragms

V.   Shows five pop-off valves

A.   I, II, and IV

B.   II, III, and IV

C.   I, II, IV, and V

D.   I, III, IV, and V

E.   I, II, III, and IV
(4:72)

19. Which of the following devices/systems does *not* use a compressor as part of its principle of operation?
    A. Piped vacuum systems
    B. Bennett MA-I ventilator
    C. Molecular sieve type oxygen concentrators
    D. Piped 100% oxygen
    E. Piped room air
       (4:65–67)

20. The compressor on the Bennett MA-I ventilator may be described as being which of the following types?
    A. A diaphragm compressor
    B. A rotary compressor
    C. A vacuum compressor
    D. A piston compressor
    E. None of the above
       (4:66)

The next two questions refer to the following illustration:

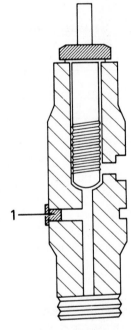

Figure IV-16.

21. The above diagram illustrates:
    A. A cylinder valve for sizes A–E cylinders
    B. A single-stage reducing valve
    C. A cylinder valve of cylinder sizes larger then E cylinders
    D. A 50 psi wall outlet
    E. The ceramic switch for a Bird® Mark 7
       (3:427)

22. The number "1" in the above illustration refers to:
    A. The example of color coding
    B. The outlet of the yoke
    C. The Woods metal relief valve
    D. Female adaptor for PISS system
    E. A Venturi valve
    (3:427)

23. Which of the following statements regarding backpressure-compensated Thorpe tube type flowmeters is *not* true?
    A. They are calibrated at 50 psig and 70°F.
    B. Their accuracy is not significantly affected by changes in backpressure.
    C. Their accuracy may be affected by changes in gas density.
    D. Their accuracy is not affected by changes in wall pressure.
    E. Their accuracy is affected by changes in position.
    (4:74–78)

24. Which of the following may be considered an example of an electrochemical type oxygen analyzer?
    A. Paramagnetic type analyzer
    B. Thermal conductivity type analyzer
    C. Polarographic devices
    D. Scholander device
    E. A and B are correct.
    (4:153–157)

P. 18 notes

P. 415-K

25. Which of the following types of oxygen analyzers cannot be used in the presence of flammable gases owing to their use of heated wires?
    A. Paramagnetic types
    B. Galvanic cell types
    C. Scholander types
    D. Polarographic types
    E. Wheatstone bridge types (thermal conductivity)
    (4:156)

26. Which of the following types of oxygen analyzers are believed to be accurate in the presence of other than oxygen/nitrogen atmospheres?
    I. Paramagnetic devices
    II. Wheatstone bridge devices
    III. Galvanic cell devices
    IV. Polarographic devices
        A. II, III, and IV
        B. I and II
        C. I, II, and IV
        D. II and IV
        E. I, III, and IV
    (51)

27. The respiratory therapy practitioner is asked to assist in the transport of a critically ill patient from one hospital to another. Which

of the following flowmeter type devices should the practitioner
select to best assist in the administration of oxygen to this patient
via nasal cannula?
A.   A kinetic flowmeter
B.   A nonbackpressure-compensated flowmeter
C.   A backpressure-compensated flowmeter
D.   A Bourdon gauge
E.   A Bird Mark 7
   (4:69-71)

28. Which of the following is (are) true statements regarding kinetic
     type flowmeters?
     I.   Their accuracy is not affected by changes in position.
     II.   They cannot be backpressure compensated.
     III. They use a plunger type device to indicate flow.
        A.   I and II
        B.   II only
        C.   I, II, and III
        D.   II and III
        E.   III only
     (4:76-78)

29. After attaching a regulator to a medical gas cylinder, the respira-
     tory therapy practitioner must open the cylinder valve slowly.
     Which of the following best explains the rationale for this
     procedure?
     A.   The cylinder will explode.
     B.   The flow rate will be inaccurate.
     C.   The cylinder valve handle may not be calibrated properly.
     D.   Heat from the recompression of gases in the regulator should
          be allowed to dissipate.
     E.   The cylinder valve is prevented from being stuck in the open
          position.
     (4:46)

30. Which of the following types of oxygen analyzers does (do) not
     have to be recalibrated for use at high altitudes?
     I.   Paramagnetic devices
     II.   Thermal conductivity devices
     III. Galvanic cell devices
     IV.   Polarographic devices
        A.   I and III
        B.   II and IV
        C.   II only
        D.   I and II
        E.   I and IV
     (51)

31. A so-called universal adaptor has which of the following inside
     and outside diameters?
     A.   51 mm I.D./33 mm O.D.
     B.   12 mm I.D./22 mm O.D.

C. 15 mm I.D./22 mm O.D.
D. 15 mm I.D./24 mm O.D.
E. 22 mm I.D./33 mm O.D.
    (2:Chap 21)

32. The Diameter Index Safety System would be used on which of the following gas systems?
    A. Those with pressures greater than 2200 psig
    B. Those with pressures greater than 500 psig
    C. Those with pressures less than 500 psig
   —D. Those with pressures less than 200 psig
    E. Those with pressures greater than 200 psig
    (4:41)

33. Which of the following types of oxygen analyzers consume oxygen as part of their functioning process?
    I.   Paramagnetic type devices
    II.   Thermal conductivity type devices
   —III. Galvanic cell type devices
   —IV.   Polarographic type devices
        A. I and II
        B. II and III
        C. II and IV
       —D. III and IV
        E. I and IV
    (51) (4:153–158)

34. Which of the following types of oxygen analyzers generate an electrical current as part of their functioning process?
    A. Paramagnetic type devices
    B. Thermal conductivity type devices
   —C. Polarographic type devices
   —D. Galvanic cell type devices
   →E. C and D are correct.
    (51)

35. A regulator that has been designed to attach to a 95% oxygen and 5% carbon dioxide medical gas cylinder cannot be attached to a cylinder that contains 90% oxygen and 10% carbon dioxide. This safety provision is enforced by which of the following regulating agencies?
    A. Department of Transportation
    B. United States Pharmacopeia
    C. Food and Drug Administration
   — D. Compressed Gas Association
    E. National Fire Protection Association
    (4:41)

36. The respiratory therapy practitioner notices the numbers DOT-3AA-2015 on the shoulder of an H cylinder of oxygen. These last four numbers indicate:
    A. The Department of Transportation code number
    B. The FDC purity control number

C.   That the cylinder is over 15 years old
—D.   The standard filling pressure of this cylinder
E.   The serial number of the manufacturing company
     (4:35)

INDICATOR

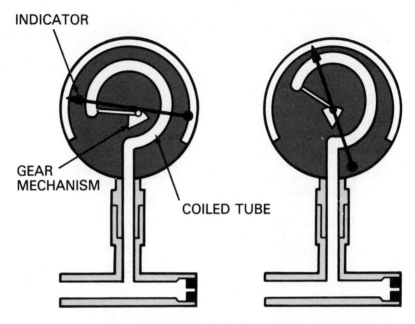

GEAR
MECHANISM

COILED TUBE

Figure IV-17.

37. True statements regarding the above illustration include:
    I.   A Thorpe tube is illustrated.
   —II.   A Bourdon gauge is illustrated.
   III.   A single-stage regulator is shown.
  —IV.   The coiled tube will straighten with increasing pressure.
   V.   The coiled tube will curl with increasing pressure.
     A.   I, II, and IV
     B.   I, II, and III
   — C.   II and IV
     D.   III, IV, and V
     E.   II, III, and IV
  (4:9)

38. Which of the following statements regarding the color coding of
     medical gases are correct?
    I.   The code for a cylinder containing helium and oxygen is
          grey and green.
    II.   The color code for a cylinder containing oxygen and carbon
          dioxide is brown and green.
  —III.   The color code for a cylinder of compressed air is yellow.
  —IV.   The color code for a cylinder of nitrous oxide is blue.

A. I and III
B. II and III
C. I and IV
D. I, III, and IV
—E. III and IV
(4:39)

39. True statements regarding the Bird oxygen blender include which of the following?
   I. An air entrainment device is used to equalize the pressures of the gases being blended.
— II. The gases being blended must have similar inlet pressures.
— III. The device proportions the gases through a valve designed so that as one side opens the other closes.
   IV. If the inlet pressure on one side drops slightly, the delivered FIo_2 will change substantially.
— V. The device's alarm is pneumatically powered.
      A. I, II, and III
      B. III, IV, and V
      ✗ C. I, IV, and V
   —→D. II, III, and V
      E. II, III, and IV
      (4:142–152)

40. A threaded male outlet on a backpressure-compensated compressed air flowmeter is an example of which of the following safety systems?
   A. American Standard
— B. Diameter Index
   C. Pin Index
   D. Fire Protection
   E. Threaded Outlet
   (4:41)

41. The first stage of a multiple-stage pressure regulator will generally lower cylinder pressure to around _____ psig.
   A. 200–1500
   B. 1200–1500
   C. 700–1200
   D. 300–1800
—E. 200–700
   (3:444)

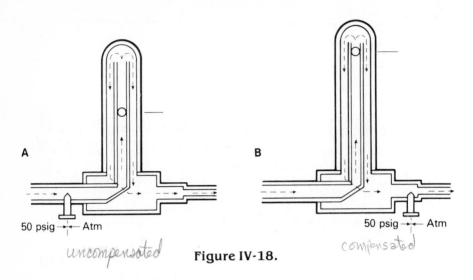

A

B

50 psig →▪◂— Atm   50 psig →▪◂— Atm

uncompensated   **Figure IV-18.**   *compensated*

42. The following statements about the flowmeters illustrated above
    are all true *except:*
    A. If the outlets of *A* and *B* are occluded, flowmeter *A* will read
       incorrectly.
    B. These are Thorpe tube flowmeters.
    C. Proper or true flow rate will be shown for only one medical
       gas.
    D. Flowmeter *A* is not backpressure compensated.
    E. In response to backpressure, flowmeter *A* will record a
       higher than actual flow.
       (3:446) *lower flow*

Answer Key

1. E	10. D	19. D	28. E	37. C
2. A	11. C	20. B	29. D	38. E
3. E	12. A	21. A	30. C	39. D
4. D	13. C	22. C	31. C	40. B
5. D	14. A	23. D	32. D	41. E
6. D	15. D	24. C	33. D	42. E
7. C	16. C	25. E	34. E	
8. A	17. B	26. E	35. D	
9. D	18. B	27. D	36. D	

B. Oxygen Administration Devices (Entry Level Only)

Questions in this category assess the candidate's ability to select and
assemble all oxygen administration devices and equipment prior to per-

forming respiratory care procedures. These questions will also test the candidate's understanding of the principles of proper operation and his or her ability to correct all malfunctions of any selected equipment.

Entry Level Pretest

According to the NBRC, the oxygen administration devices content category is assessed only on the Entry Level Examination. According to the Composite Examination Matrix (see reference 80), questions in this category assess the candidate's understanding of the following types of respiratory therapy equipment:

1. Oxygen cannulas and catheters
2. Oxygen masks
    a. Simple oxygen masks
    b. Reservoir type oxygen masks (partial rebreathing and non-rebreathing types)
    c. Face tents
3. Air entrainment devices (e.g., masks)
4. Environmental oxygen systems (oxygen hoods and tents)
5. Tracheostomy collars and T-adaptors (Briggs)

The following are self-study questions from this category:

1. Which of the following most correctly defines a high flow oxygen delivery system?
    A. One that has a flow rate greater than 30 L/min
    B. One that requires more than one flowmeter to drive the system properly
    C. One whose flow rate is sufficient to meet all patient inspiratory demands
    D. A system that is present only on ventilators that are true constant-flow generators
    E. A system that contains a partial rebreathing valve and a reservoir bag
    (1:136–138)

2. For which of the following reasons should toys with metal gears be kept out of oxygen tents?
    A. The high oxygen contents will make the toys rust.
    B. They are considered a fire hazard.
    C. Children should be resting in the tent, not playing with toys.
    D. The toys can tear the tent canopy, compromising the oxygen-enriched atmosphere.
    E. C and D are correct.
    (4:92)

3. Which of the following statements regarding the nonrebreathing type oxygen mask is (are) true?
    I. It incorporates its own flow-regulating device.

II.   It is believed to be capable of delivering concentrations of oxygen that approach 100%.
III. It uses a one-way valve between the reservoir bag and the mask.
IV.   It should not be operated with flow rates greater than 8 L/min.
   A.   I and III .
   B.   II and III
   C.   III and IV
   D.   I and IV
   E.   II only
   (4:85–86) (1:Chap 7)

4. The respiratory therapy practitioner is administering 5 L oxygen via a nasal cannula to a 70-kg patient with a normal ventilatory pattern. Which of the following most closely approximates this patient's FI_{O_2}?
   A.   30%
   B.   35%
   C.   40%
   D.   45%
   E.   50%
   (1:134)

5. The most common method of administering oxygen to a newborn is via which of the following?
   A.   Nasal cannula
   B.   Nasal CPAP prongs
   C.   Face tent
   D.   Oxygen hood
   E.   Nasal catheter
   (2:Chap 27)

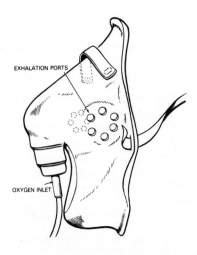

EXHALATION PORTS

OXYGEN INLET

Figure IV-19.

6. The above illustration shows a:
   A. Simple aerosol mask
   B. Oxygen-powered breathing device
   C. Anesthesia mask
   D. Nonrebreathing oxygen mask
   E. Simple oxygen mask
   (4:84)

7. An air entrainment type mask would most likely be used on a patient suffering from which of the following disorders?
   A. Advanced stage emphysema
   B. Bronchial asthma
   C. Carbon monoxide poisoning
   D. Adult respiratory distress syndrome
   E. Idiopathic pulmonary fibrosis
   (4:Chap 3)

8. Which of the following is (are) true about the Air Shields Croupette® tent?
   I.   It employs refrigeration coils.
   II. It should be able to provide a high humidity environment.
   III. It should be able to provide a cool environment.
   IV. It should be employable on both adult and pediatric populations.
       A. I, II, and IV
       B. I and IV
       C. III and IV
       D. II and III
       E. II only
   (4:Chap 3)

9. If the air entrainment port of an air entrainment type oxygen mask were to become occluded, which of the following would apply?
   I.   The FIo_2 would decrease.
   II. Gas flow to the patient would cease completely.
   III. The FIo_2 would increase.
   IV. Gas flow to the patient would decrease.
       A. I and II
       B. II and III
       C. III and IV
       D. I and IV
       E. I only
   (4:76–78)

10. Which of the following statements is (are) true regarding partial rebreathing masks?
   I.   There is an air entrainment mechanism built into the reservoir system.
   II. There is a one-way valve between the reservoir system and the mask.
   III. FIo_2s between 60% and 80% are believed to be obtainable.

A. I only
B. II only
C. III only
D. I and III
E. I, II, and III
(4:Chap 3)

11. Disposable oxygen administration devices are most frequently composed of:
A. Polycarbonate plastic
B. Polyvinyl chloride
C. Polypropylene
D. Polyester
E. Polyurethane
(4:Chap 3)

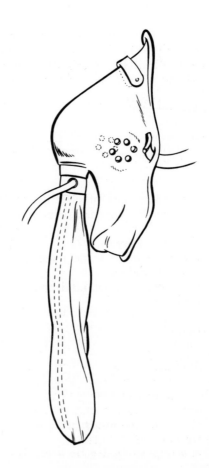

Figure IV-20.

12. The above diagram shows which of the following?
    A. Simple mask
    B. Face tent
    C. Partial rebreathing mask
    D. Aerosol mask
    E. Air entrainment mask
       (4:85)

13. Which of the following best describes the range of oxygen concentration available with a standard croup type tent?
    A. Less than 50%
    B. Less than 30%
    C. 21-35%
    D. 21-60%
    E. 21-70%
       (4:Chap 3)

14. The major disadvantage associated with the use of oxygen hoods is:
    A. The oxygen concentration cannot be controlled.
    B. The temperature inside the hood cannot be controlled.
    C. The absolute humidity within the hood cannot be controlled.
    D. The hood must be removed for feeding.
    E. B and C are correct.
       (4:Chap 3)

15. Which of the following actions should the respiratory therapy practitioner take to help maintain a constant FI_{O_2} within an oxygen tent?
    I.   Use a canopy that can ensure an enclosed environment.
    II.   Avoid opening the canopy unnecessarily.
    III. Use the smallest canopy that is practical.
    IV.   Periodically analyze the tent gas at the patient's proximal airway.
       A. I, III, and IV
       B. II, III, and IV
       C. I, II, and IV
       D. I, II, and III
       E. I, II, III, and IV
    (4:Chap 3)

16. During oxygen rounds, the respiratory therapy practitioner discovers a humidifier that is producing a high-pitched whistle. What is the most likely cause of this?
    A. The humidifier is empty.
    B. The cannula is disconnected from the humidifier.
    C. The delivery tubing is crimped.
    D. The cannula is off the patient.
    E. The heater on the humidifier is malfunctioning.
       (4:Chap 4)

17. All of the following concerning disposable simple oxygen masks are true *except:*
    A. They are made of polyvinyl chloride.
    B. They are as effective as nondisposable masks if used properly.
    C. They can be autoclaved.
    D. They may reduce nosocomial infections.
    E. They may be relied on to deliver oxygen concentrations from 40% to 60%.
    (1:Chap 7)

18. Which of the following represents the average volume of an adult patient's anatomic reservoir that must be taken into account when considering low-flow oxygen systems?
    A. 25 cc
    B. 50 cc
    C. 75 cc
    D. 100 cc
    E. 150 cc
    (1:139) 183-S

19. The partial rebreathing mask is designed to:
    I. Collect the first two thirds of the exhaled gas in the reservoir bag
    II. Allow the patient to draw room air in through the exhalation ports on the side of the mask
    III. *Not* deliver FIo_2s in excess of 0.5
        A. I and II
        B. II only
        C. III only
        D. I and III
        E. I, II, and III
    (4:73)

20. Isolettes® (incubators) are designed to allow the operator to provide all of the following except:
    A. Control of environmental humidity
    B. Control of environmental temperature
    C. Control of inspired oxygen concentration
    D. Control of alveolar ventilation
    E. Control of an isolated or filtered-gas environment
    (4:97)

21. When administering oxygen to newborns via hood devices, important considerations include which of the following?
    I. Providing sufficient gas flow to prevent carbon dioxide buildup
    II. Adequately heating and humidifying therapeutic gases
    III. Keeping the FIo_2 below 0.4
    IV. Periodically monitoring the FIo_2 with an oxygen analyzer
        A. I, III, and IV
        B. I, II, and IV

   C. I and IV
   D. II, III, and IV
   E. I, II, III, and IV
  (4:97)

22. Which of the following is (are) believed to be an advantage of the nasal cannula as compared with air entrainment mask devices?
  I. The cannula does not have to be removed when the patient is eating.
  II. It may be safely used on patients with irregular ventilatory patterns.
  III. It is generally more comfortable for the patient.
  IV. It eliminates fluctuations in inspired oxygen concentration.
   A. I and III
   B. II and III
   C. II and IV
   D. I, III, and IV
   E. III only
  (1:132–134)

23. Which of the following is the best method for controlling the inspired oxygen concentration in Isolette (incubator) devices?
  A. Keeping the red flag down
  B. Using precise liter flows
  C. Monitoring arterial oxygen tension
  D. Adequately monitoring the oxygen concentration at the patient's proximal airway
  E. Bagging the newborn whenever diapers have to be changed
  (13:294–295)

24. Which of the following oxygen liter flow rates is recommended when the respiratory therapy practitioner is employing a partial or nonrebreathing type oxygen mask?
  A. 6–8 L/min
  B. 6–12 L/min
  C. 8–15 L/min
  D. Adjusted so the bag does not collapse during expiration
  E. Adjusted so the bag does not collapse during inspiration
  (4:83–88)

25. Which of the following will result in reduction of the amount of ambient gas entrained by an air entrainment type mask device? *venti mask*
  I. A reduction in valve orifice size
  II. A decrease in the FIo_2 of the source gas
  III. An increase in valve orifice size
  IV. An increase in entrainment port size
   A. I and III
   B. II and III
   C. I and IV
   D. III and IV
   E. III only
  (4:83–86)

Answer Key

1. C	6. E	11. B	16. C	21. B
2. B	7. A	12. C	17. C	22. A
3. B	8. D	13. A	18. B	23. D
4. C	9. C	14. D	19. B	24. E
5. D	10. C	15. E	20. D	25. E

C. Humidity and Aerosol Therapy Devices (Entry Level Only)

According to the NBRC, questions in this category are designed to assess the candidate's ability to select and assemble all humidity and aerosol therapy devices prior to performing respiratory care procedures. These questions will also test the candidate's understanding of the principles of proper operation and his or her ability to correct all malfunctions of any selected equipment.

Entry Level Pretest

According to the NBRC Composite Examination Matrix (see reference 80), questions in this category assess the candidate's understanding of the following types of respiratory therapy equipment:

1. Humidifiers (e.g., bubble, passover, Cascade® type)
2. Aerosol generators
   a. Pneumatic nebulizers (including Babington type)
   b. Ultrasonic nebulizers

The first two questions refer to the following illustration:

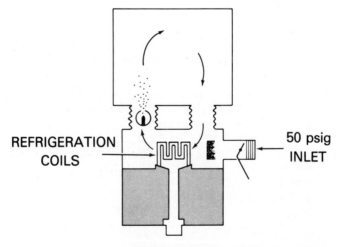

Figure IV-21.

1.   The above illustration shows:
     A.   A molecular sieve oxygen concentrator
     B.   The oxygen accumulator of the Bennett MA-I ventilator
     C.   The Babington nebulizer
     D.   An oxygen tent
     E.   An oxygen blender
        (4:83)

2.   The item referred to in the above question:
     I.   Is used to deliver 100% body humidity at BTPS
     II.   Can deliver particulate water to the patient
     III. Cannot be used to administer FIo_2s greater than 21%
     IV.   May be considered a high-flow system
        A.   I and III
        B.   I, III, and IV
        C.   II only
        D.   I and IV
        E.   II and IV
        (4:94–95)

3.   Which of the following factors will influence the absolute humidity
     of therapeutic gases that are delivered by a bubble type humid-
     ifier?
     I.   The size of the liquid/gas interface
     II.   Gas exposure time (unit liter flow)
     III. Type of medical gas administered
     IV.   Temperature within the humidifier device
        A.   I, II, and IV
        B.   III and IV
        C.   I, II, and III
        D.   II and IV
        E.   III only
        (4:105)

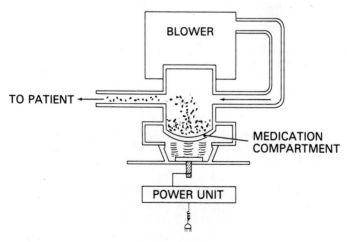

Figure IV-22.

4. The above illustration shows a(n):
   A. All-purpose jet nebulizer
   B. Hydronamic nebulizer
   C. Croup tent
   D. Ohio® Delux nebulizer
   E. Ultrasonic nebulizer
      (1:179)

5. The device on an ultrasonic nebulizer that converts electrical energy to mechanical/vibrational energy is called a(n) _____ .
   A. Electric transducer
   B. Condenser module
   C. Piezoelectric transducer
   D. Aerosol generator
   E. Mechanical transducer
      (4:134–135)

6. Which of the following are true statements regarding the Cascade type humidifier?
   I. It is used to deliver gases at APTD.
   II. It is a type of jet humidifier.
   III. It is not capable of delivering particulate water.
   IV. It has been implicated in the transmission of nosocomial infection.
      A. I and II
      B. III and IV
      C. I, III, and IV
      D. II, III, and IV
      E. I and IV
   (4:109–111)

7. The size of the aerosolized particles that are generated by an ultrasonic nebulizer is believed to be determined by which of the following factors?
   A. Unit ultrasonic frequency
   B. Unit amplitude
   C. Type of solution nebulized
   D. Shape of the ceramic disk
   E. Level of water within the nebulizer chamber
      (4:136)

8. The quantity of aerosol produced by an ultrasonic nebulizer is most directly related to:
   A. The type of solution in the nebulizer cup
   B. The shape of the ceramic disk
   C. The setting on unit amplitude control
   D. The device's ultrasonic frequency
   E. The amount of current flowing from the electrical outlet to the nebulizer
      (4:136–137)

The next two questions refer to the following illustration:

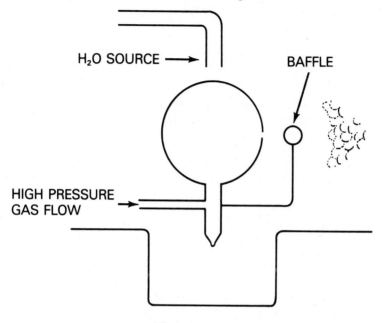

Figure IV-23.

9. The above illustration shows a(n):
    A. Ultrasonic nebulizer
    B. Intermittent sidestream jet nebulizer
    C. Jet nebulizer
    D. Hydronamic or Babington nebulizer
    E. Spinning disc nebulizer
        (1:178)

10. The majority of particles aerosolized by this device is believed to be in the range of:
    A. Less than 10μ
    B. 10–20μ
    C. 20–30μ
    D. 30–40μ
    E. 40–50μ
        (1:177–180)

11. The respiratory therapy practitioner would be most concerned about the transmission of nosocomial infection when using which of the following aerosol and/or humidity therapy devices?
    A. A jet nebulizer
    B. An ultrasonic nebulizer
    C. A Cascade humidifier
    D. A hydronamic nebulizer
    E. A jet humidifier
        (1:180)

12. The baffle in a nebulizer serves which of the following purposes?
    A. It increases the aerosol output.
    B. It decreases the aerosol output.
    C. It increases gas density.
    D. It breaks up the larger particles into smaller particles.
    E. It increases aerosol density.
    (4:122–123)

13. Which of the following is (are) known to occur when water inside a pneumatic nebulizer is heated through the use of an immersion heater?
    I. An increase in aerosol density
    II. An increase in nebulizer flow rate
    III. An increase in absolute humidity
    IV. An increase in delivered oxygen concentration
       A. II and IV
       B. III and IV
       C. I and III
       D. I, II, and III
       E. III only
    (4:109 and 131)

14. The respiratory therapy practitioner is operating an all-purpose type nebulizer on the 100% oxygen setting using a flow rate of 10 L/min to drive the jet. If he or she were to place this nebulizer on the 40% setting, which of the following would occur?
    I. The aerosol density (mg/L) would increase.
    II. The aerosol output (mL/min) would increase.
    III. The total flow rate delivered by the apparatus would double.
    IV. The total flow rate delivered by the apparatus would quadruple.
       A. I and III
       B. II and III
       C. I and IV
       D. II and IV
       E. II only
    (4:131)

15. Which of the following aerosol therapy devices is reportedly capable of aerosolizing up to 6 cc of liquid per minute?
    A. Hydronamic (Babington) nebulizer
    B. Pneumatic all-purpose nebulizer
    C. Ultrasonic nebulizer
    D. Bird micronebulizer
    E. Bennett twin jet nebulizer
    (4:136)

16. Which of the following aerosol therapy devices are reportedly able to deliver aerosols the majority of whose particles are less than 10μ in diameter?
    I. Pneumatic jet nebulizers

II.   Atomizers
III. Ultrasonic nebulizers
IV.   Hydronamic (Babington) nebulizers
   A.   I and II
   B.   I and III
   C.   III and IV
   D.   I, II, and IV
   E.   III only
(4:122–137)

17. In any given nebulizing device, which of the following may act to baffle the aerosolized particles?
I.   The surface of the water
II.   The sides of the container
III. A sphere placed in the path of the aerosol's flow
IV.   A bend in the aerosol tubing
   A.   I and III
   B.   II and III
   C.   I, II, and III
   D.   I, III, and IV
   E.   I, II, III, and IV
(4:122)

18. Assuming an optimal ventilatory pattern, what is the fate of most aerosolized particles smaller than 10μ in diameter?
   A.   They will be deposited in the upper airways.
   B.   They will not be deposited; they will be exhaled.
   C.   They will be deposited in the mainstem bronchi.
   D.   They will be deposited in the smaller airways.
   E.   They will be deposited in the trachea.
(4:122)

19. The functioning of which of the following types of aerosol generators is dependent on the effects of the lateral negative pressure and surface tension to pull fluid over a sphere so it may be exposed to a high-velocity jet?
   A.   Pneumatic jet
   B.   Spinning disk
   C.   Hydronamic (Babington)
   D.   Ultrasonic
   E.   An atomizer
(4:133)

20. The air entrainment port on a pneumatic jet nebulizer serves which of the following purposes?
I.   Increases aerosol density
II.   Increases total system flow
III. Decreases the delivered FIo_2
IV.   Provides a larger particle size
   A.   I and III
   B.   III and IV
   C.   I and II

    D. I and IV
    E. II and III
  (4:129–131)

21. Which of the following respiratory therapy devices is known to use a heated passover humidifier?
    A. Bennett MA-I ventilator
    B. Baby Bird® ventilator
    C. Emerson postoperative ventilator
    D. Bennett PR-II ventilator
    E. Bourns BP-200 ventilator
  (4:105–106)

Answer Key

1. D	5. C	9. D	13. C	17. E
2. E	6. B	10. A	14. D	18. D
3. A	7. A	11. B	15. C	19. C
4. E	8. C	12. D	16. C	20. E
				21. C

D. Airway Care and Resuscitation Devices

Questions in this category assess the candidate's ability to select all airway care devices and equipment prior to performing related respiratory care procedures. These questions also test the candidate's understanding of the principles of operation and his or her ability to correct all malfunctions of any selected equipment.

Entry Level Pretest

According to the NBRC Composite Examination Matrix (see reference 80), questions in this category assess the candidate's understanding of the following types of respiratory care equipment:

1. Artificial airways
    a. Oropharyngeal and nasopharyngeal airways
    b. Endotracheal tubes (oral and nasal)
    c. Tracheostomy tubes and buttons
    d. Mechanical percussors and vibrator devices
2. Resuscitation devices
    a. Manual resuscitators (bag-valve units)
    b. Pneumatic resuscitators (demand-valve devices)

The following self-study questions were developed from the NBRC Composite Examination Matrix:

1. A double-lumen endotracheal tube with two cuffs attached that, when inflated, may allow for differential lung ventilation most correctly describes which of the following types of endotracheal tubes?
   A. Jackson®
   B. Fome-Cuff®
   C. Cole®
   D. Carlens®
   E. National Catheter®
   (4:174)

2. Which of the following statements is (are) true regarding the oro-pharyngeal airway?
   I.   It is well tolerated by all patients.
   II.   It is designed to prevent soft tissue upper airway obstruction.
   III. It may be used on semiconscious patients.
   IV.   It may induce vomiting.
      A. III and IV
      B. I, II, and III
      C. II, III, and IV
      D. II and IV
      E. IV only
   (1:237)

3. Which of the following is the most common material used in the manufacture of endotracheal and tracheostomy tubes?
   A. Natural rubber
   B. Teflon™
   C. Polyvinyl chloride
   D. Polyurethane
   E. Silicone rubber
   (4:167)

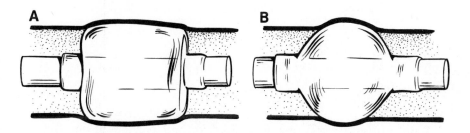

A   **B**

Figure IV-24.

4. The above illustration shows:
   I.   A high volume, low pressure cuff and a low volume, high pressure cuff
   II.   A low volume, high pressure cuff and a high volume, high pressure cuff

See p. 501.E

III. A high volume, high pressure cuff and a low volume, low pressure cuff

IV. A nasotracheal tube and an anesthesia tube
  A. III and IV
  B. III only
  C. II and IV
  D. I and IV
  E. I only
(4:170)

5. Which of the following is *not* a disadvantage of a Cole type pediatric endotracheal tube?
  A. Has high resistance to gas flow
  B. Is easily obstructed by secretions
  C. May not be able to provide deep tracheal suction
  D. Presents potential for damage to tracheal tissue
  E. May kink at the tube shoulder
(25:Chap 16, p 4)

6. Which of the following statements regarding esophageal obturator airways is *not* true?
  A. Their removal is frequently followed by vomiting.
  B. They should not be removed before endotracheal intubation is performed.
  C. They require visualization of the larynx for insertion.
  D. Tracheal intubation is a recognized hazard.
  E. Esophageal damage is a recognized hazard.
(25:Chap 4, pp 2–3)

7. Which of the following are true statements regarding the nasopharyngeal airway?
  I.   It is indicated to relieve soft tissue obstructions.
  II. It should be used only in comatose patients.
  III. It may be used to facilitate nasotracheal suctioning.
  IV. Epitaxis is a known hazard.
  A. I and III
  B. II and III
  C. II, III, and IV
  D. I, III, and IV
  E. III and IV
(25:Chap 4, p 2) (1:237–238)

8. Which of the following types of endotracheal tubes uses an external pressure regulating valve and control balloon device that if properly used prevent intercuff pressures from exceeding 20 mm Hg to 25 mm Hg?
  A. Hollinger®
  B. Fome-Cuff
  C. Lanz®
  D. Shiley®
  E. Foregger®
(4:171)

The next two questions refer to the following illustration:

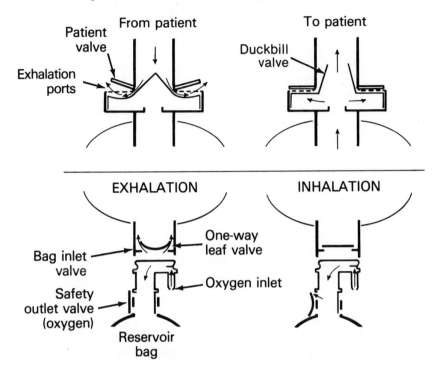

Figure IV-25.

9. The above illustration is a schematic representation of:
   A. Puritan® PMR-II bag-valve unit
   B. Ambu® bag-valve unit
   C. Laerdal® bag-valve unit
   D. Ohio® Hope II bag-valve unit
   E. Air Bird® bag-valve unit
   (4:183)

10. True statements regarding the illustrated device include:
   I. It can deliver up to 100% O_2 at the proper flow rate and with the proper reservoir bag.
   II. The valve reportedly will not clog easily.
   III. The valve will *not* allow for spontaneous ventilation.
   IV. It has a stroke volume of approximately 1 L.
       A. I, II, and IV
       B. II, III, and IV
       C. III and IV
       D. I, III, and IV
       E. I, II, III, and IV
   (4:183)

11. The respiratory therapy practitioner is asked to select an airway care device for a patient with a permanent tracheostomy who is to

be discharged. The physician's orders stipulate that the patient's device have the following characteristics: (1) allow the patient to communicate; (2) provide for administration of IPPB therapy; and (3) provide a patent suction port. Which of the following devices should the practitioner select?

   I.   Olympic® tracheostomy button
   II.   Olympic Trach-Talk
   III.   Kistner® valve
   IV.   Shiley tracheostomy tube with a fenestrated outer cannula

     A.   I and III
     B.   II and IV
     C.   IV only
     D.   I, II, and III
     E.   I, II, III, and IV

   (2:506 and 670)

12. Which of the following is *not* thought be be a hazard associated with the use of the esophageal obturator airway?

     A.   Tracheal intubation
     B.   Regurgitation following removal
     C.   Esophageal rupture
     D.   Alveolar hyperventilation
     E.   B and C are correct.

   (1:249–250) (25:Chap 4, pp 2–4)

13. Which of the following features distinguishes the esophageal gastric airway from the esophageal obturator airway?

     A.   Direct laryngoscopy is not necessary.
     B.   Alveolar ventilation is usually improved.
     C.   A gastric tube may be passed following proper insertion.
     D.   The technique for placement is simpler.
     E.   The device does not have an inflatable cuff.

   (25:Chap 4, pp 3–4)

14. Which of the following methods does the American National Standards Institute's Z-79 Committee use to ensure that intratracheal tubes are not composed of toxic material?

   I.   Implementation of tube materials into animal tissue
   II.   Mass spectrometry
   III.   Placing actual tube materials in a live-cell culture

     A.   I and III
     B.   I, II, and III
     C.   II and III
     D.   III only
     E.   I only

   (2:517–518)

15. True statements regarding low pressure type tracheal tube cuffs include:

   I.   They are necessary to provide a seal during positive pressure ventilation.
   II.   They generally use a large residual volume.

    III.   They frequently decrease the extent of tracheal necrosis.
    IV.   They are associated with cuff herniation over the end of the
         tube.
       A.   I, II, and III
       B.   II, III, and IV
       C.   I, III, and IV
       D.   III and IV
       E.   I, II, and IV
    (4:169–172) (32:211)

16. Which of the following statements is (are) true regarding Kamen-
    Wilkenson (Fome-Cuff) type endotracheal tubes?
    I.   They are a type of low pressure cuff.
    II.   They need to be inflated with 5 cc of air to function
         properly.
    III. Placement of too small a tube may result in excessive cuff-
         to-wall pressure.
    IV.   They are not considered suitable for use during prolonged
         mechanical ventilation therapy.
       A.   I and III
       B.   I, II, III, and IV
       C.   I only
       D.   I and II
       E.   II, III, and IV
    (1:293–294) (4:171–172)

17. When the respiratory therapy practitioner is referring to the vari-
    ous portions of an endotracheal tube, use of the term *inflating tube*
    would most likely be associated with which of the following
    statements?
    A.   A small balloon that indicates the inflation of the tube cuff
    B.   The endotracheal tube itself
    C.   The inflatable sleeve that is used to provide an effective,
         leak-resistant fit between the tube and the trachea
    D.   The tube provided for inflating the tracheal tube cuff
    E.   The transparent reservoir that houses the pilot balloon and
         the pressure regulating valve
    (2:515)

18. On endotracheal tubes the markings that indicate the tube length
    from the bevel tip are in which of the following units?
    A.   Millimeters
    B.   Centimeters
    C.   Inches
    D.   Angstroms
    E.   None of the above
    (4:168)

19. Which of the following markings is *least* likely to be found on a
    standard endotracheal tube?
    A.   I.D. size
    B.   Z-79

C. I.T.
D. R.T.
E. French size
(4:168)

20. Which of the following statements regarding pneumatically pow-
ered demand valve type resuscitation devices is (are) true?
I.   They are not capable of delivering high concentrations of
O_2 to the patient.
II. They usually have a 100 cm H_2O pressure pop-off.
III. They are designed to provide inspiratory flow rates of
approximately 100 L/min.
IV. They are satisfactory only if manual triggering is available.
A. I and IV
B. II and III
C. III and IV
D. I, II, and III
E. III only
(25:Chap 4, p 7)

21. The respiratory therapy practitioner is asked to select an adult
manual resuscitator device for use on his hospital's emergency
crash carts. Which of the following features would be *least* advisable for this unit?
A. A self-expanding bag
B. A pop-off valve
C. The ability to deliver FIo_2s greater than 80% with appropriate reservoir system
D. Use of standard 15 mm to 22 mm universal type adaptor
system
E. A patient ventilating valve that is unaffected by high flow
rates
(25:Chap 4, p 7)

22. Most adult manual resuscitator units have a total volume of which
of the following ranges?
A. 0–500 cc
B. 500–1000 cc
C. 1000–1500 cc
D. 1500–2000 cc
E. Greater than 2000 cc
(4:194–196) (8:189–190)

23. Which of the following types of manual resuscitators employs a
diaphragm and duckbill type patient valve?
A. Ambu E-2
B. Puritan PMR
C. Laerdal infant unit
D. Ohio Hope II
E. Air Bird
(4:194)

24. Which of the following manual resuscitators is notable because of the fact that oxygen flows greater than 10–15 L/min can force the patient valve to "jam" in the open position leading to excessive pressures within the patient's airway?
    A. Ohio Hope II
    B. "Early" Ambu model
    C. Laerdal RFB-II
    D. Puritan PMR
    E. Ambu E-2
       (4:176)

25. Which of the following pediatric manual resuscitators has the smallest total volume?
    A. Ohio Hope II pediatric model
    B. Ambu E-2 infant model
    C. Penlon infant model
    D. Laerdal infant model
    E. Air Bird pediatric model
       (4:194)

Answer Key

1. D	6. C	11. C	16. C	21. B
2. D	7. D	12. D	17. D	22. D
3. C	8. C	13. C	18. B	23. C
4. E	9. C	14. A	19. D	24. B
5. D	10. A	15. B	20. C	25. D

Advanced Practitioner Pretest

According to the NBRC Composite Examination Matrix (see reference 80), questions in this category assess the candidate's understanding of the following types of respiratory care equipment:

1. Artificial airways (all intubation equipment [laryngoscope blades, laryngoscope handles, and stylets])
2. Suctioning devices
   a. Suction catheters
   b. Specimen collectors
   c. Oropharyngeal suctioning devices

The following self-study questions were developed from the NBRC Composite Examination Matrix:

1. Which of the following laryngoscope blades is (are) generally preferred when performing neonatal endotracheal intubation?
   I.   A No. 2 or No. 3 curved laryngoscope blade
   II. A No. 0 straight laryngoscope blade
   III. A No. 1 straight laryngoscope blade
   IV. A No. 0 or No. 1 curved laryngoscope blade

A. II and III
B. I and IV
C. I and III
D. IV only
E. I, II, III, and IV
(25:Chap 16, p 4) (36:53) (29:32–33)

2. A grasping instrument with a right-angle bend incorporated into its design that is particularly useful in guiding the tracheal tube tip into the larynx during nasal intubation best describes which of the following pieces of equipment?
A. The curved laryngoscope blade
B. A malleable metal stylet
C. A Magill forcep
D. A Kelly forcep
E. An obturator device
(36:34)

3. Which of the following statements is true regarding placement of the curved laryngoscope blade during endotracheal intubation of the adult?
A. It is placed under the epiglottis so that it may be lifted.
B. It is placed above the epiglottis in the vallecula.
C. It is placed between the adenoidal tissues.
D. It is placed between the base of the tongue and the epiglottis.
E. B and D are correct.
(25:Chap 4, p 5) (36:33–34) (1:242–244)

4. A laryngoscope that is used for the technique of endotracheal intubation consists of which of the following parts?
I. A blade
II. A handle
III. A light source
IV. A malleable stylet
A. I and III
B. II and III
C. II, III, and IV
D. I, II, III, and IV
E. I, II, and III
(25:Chaps 4 and 5)

5. Which of the following statements is (are) true regarding the use of a malleable stylet during endotracheal intubation?
I. It is used to help the tube conform to a desired configuration.
II. It should be attached to a fiberoptic light source for direct laryngoscopy.
III. For optimal performance, the end of the stylet should be advanced approximately one-half inch beyond the opening of the endotracheal tube.
A. I and III
B. II and III

C. I and II
D. I only
E. I, II, and III
    (25:Chap 4, p 4)

6. Which of the following types of airway suctioning devices should
    the respiratory therapy practitioner select to aid in the removal of
    very thick oropharyngeal secretions during attempts at intuba-
    tion?
    A. Coudé type
    B. Ring tip type (Argyle Aeroflow)
    C. Metal or plastic (Yankaur type)
    D. Whistle tip type
    E. Rusch red rubber type
        (25:Chap 4, p 8) (36:32 and 37)

7. The respiratory therapy practitioner is asked to select an endotra-
    cheal suction catheter to prevent airway occlusion during endotra-
    cheal suctioning attempts. The *maximum* allowable outer diameter
    of the suction catheter selected should be:
    A. No more than 50% of the inner diameter of the tube being
        suctioned
    B. No more than 50% of the outer diameter of the tube being
        suctioned
    C. No more than two thirds of the inner diameter of the tube
        being suctioned
    D. No more than two thirds of the outer diameter of the tube
        being suctioned
    E. No more than 50% of the outer diameter French size
        (2:527)

8. Which of the following is the major purpose of the multiple side
    holes near the tip of some suction catheters?
    A. They allow greater volumes of secretions to be aspirated.
    B. They are less expensive to manufacture.
    C. Their presence ensures that the catheter is made of toxic
        materials.
    D. They reportedly help reduce mucosal trauma.
    E. They facilitate the instillation of irrigating solutions.
        (1:268)

9. The respiratory therapy practitioner would theoretically be able to
    aspirate tracheobronchial secretions most rapidly with which one
    of the following hypothetical suction catheter devices?
    A. 14 French O.D. 60 cm length
    B. 14 French O.D. 40 cm length
    C. 12 French O.D. 40 cm length
    D. 12 French O.D. 60 cm length
    E. 14 French O.D. 50 cm length
        (2:523–524)

10. When a straight laryngoscope blade is being used to intubate the trachea of an adult patient, which of the following should *not* be done?
    A. The patient's head and neck should be hyperextended.
    B. The tip of the blade should be placed under the epiglottis.
    C. The patient's teeth should not be used as a fulcrum.
    D. The blade should be inserted into the left side of the patient's mouth.
    E. The patient should be hyperoxygenated prior to performing the procedure.
       (25:Chap 4, pp 4–5) (1:244–246)

11. Which of the following laryngoscope blades would most likely be selected for intubating the trachea of an 1100-g newborn?
    A. A No. 0 (7 cm) straight Miller blade
    B. A No. 1 (10 cm) straight Miller blade
    C. A No. 2 straight Miller or curved MacIntosh
    D. A No. 2 curved MacIntosh
    E. A No. 1 curved Miller blade
       (25:Chap 15, p 5)

Answer Key

1. A	3. E	5. D	7. C	9. B
2. C	4. E	6. C	8. D	10. D
				11. A

E. Hyperinflation Therapy Devices (Entry Level Only)

Questions in this category assess the candidate's ability to select and assemble all hyperinflation therapy devices and equipment prior to performing respiratory care procedures. These questions also test the candidate's understanding of the principles of operation and his or her ability to correct all malfunctions of any selected equipment.

Entry Level Pretest

According to the NBRC, questions in this category are assessed only on the Entry Level Examination. Also, according to the Composite Examination Matrix (see reference 80), questions in this category assess the candidate's understanding of the following types of respiratory care equipment:

1. Pneumatic pressure-cycled ventilators (Bird and Bennett type)
2. Sustained maximal inspiratory therapy devices (incentive spirometers)

3. Patient breathing circuits
    a. Intermittent positive pressure breathing type
    b. Sustained maximal inspiratory type (incentive spirometry)

The following are self-study questions from this category:

1. The respiratory therapy practitioner, by performing which of the following actions, would be most successful in making the Bird Mark 7 ventilator more responsive to patient inspiratory efforts?
    A. Turning the dial marked "expiratory time for apnea"
    B. Moving the sensitivity magnet closer to the soft metal plate
    C. Moving the sensitivity magnet away from the soft metal plate
    D. Increasing the cycling pressure
    E. Moving the pressure magnet closer to the soft metal plate
    (4:249-252)

2. Which of the following controls on the Bennett PR-II ventilator functions to add flow to the backside of a vane on the Bennett valve and thus causes the ventilator to initiate inspiration at preset intervals?
    A. Pressure control
    B. Terminal flow control
    C. Rate control
    D. Peak flow control
    E. Sensitivity control
    (4:309-313)

3. During the administration of IPPB with a Bird Mark 8 ventilator, the respiratory therapy practitioner notices that the ventilator repeatedly cycles ON shortly after the patient has begun his expiratory phase. In order to correct this malfunction the practitioner should check which of the following controls?
    I.   The flow rate control
    II.   The expiratory time for apnea control
    III. The sensitivity control
    IV.   The peak flow control

        A. I and III
        B. II, III, and IV
        C. I, II, and IV
        D. I, II, and III
        E. II and III
    (4:249-259)

4. Which of the following ventilators is (are) known to be capable of administering a constant inspiratory flow pattern despite changes in patient lung characteristics?
    I.   Bird Mark 7
    II.   Bennett PR-II
    III. Bennett AP-5
    IV.   Bird Mark 8

        A. I, III, and IV
        B. II, III, and IV

C.   I and IV
D.   IV only
E.   I only
(4:223)

5.   Which of the following is *not* present on the Bird Mark 7 ventilator?
A.   Ceramic switch assembly
B.   Spring-loaded gate
C.   Inspiratory nebulizer line
D.   Expiratory nebulizer control
E.   Expiratory time for apnea control
(4:249–260)

6.   All of the following are commonly referred to as pressure-cycled ventilators. Which of these may be time cycled into expiration?
I.   Bennett PR-II
II.   Bird Mark 7
III. Bennett PR-I
IV.   Bird Mark 7A
A.   I only
B.   I and III
C.   II and III
D.   II, III, and IV
E.   I and IV
(4:249–260) (4:314–319)

7.   Which of the following ventilators is (are) sometimes referred to as being pressure/flow cycled?
I.   Bennett PR-II
II.   Bird Mark 7
III. Bennett PR-I
A.   I and II
B.   II only
C.   II and III
D.   I and III
E.   I only
(4:249–260 and 314–329)

8.   In the face of high resistance and/or low compliance, the inspiratory flow pattern generated by the Bennett PR-I ventilator will _____ from beginning to end of inspiration.
A.   Accelerate slightly
B.   Decrease severely
C.   Decrease slightly
D.   Accelerate rapidly
E.   Remain constant and unchanged
(4:309–321)

9.   Which of the following terms most correctly describes the Bennett valve?
A.   Flow adjustable
B.   Flow restrictive

C. Flow sensitive
D. Pneumatically sensitive
E. Flow injectable
    (4:301–305)

10. The respiratory therapy practitioner is *not* capable of adjusting the peak inspiratory flow rate on which of the following ventilators?
    A. Bird Mark 7
    B. Bennett PR-II
    C. Bird Mark 8
    D. Bennett PR-I
    E. Bird Mark 7A
    (4:323–324)

11. Which of the following ventilators incorporates a mechanism designed to compensate for leaks in the patient's circuit?
    A. Bennett PR-I
    B. Bennett AP-5
    C. Bird Mark 7
    D. Bird Mark 8
    E. Bird Mark 14
    (4:266–268)

12. Which of the following features characterizes the Bird Mark 7 ventilator?
    I.   Pressure cycled
    II.   Flow adjustable
    III. Single circuit
    IV.   Time cycled into exhalation
        A. I and III
        B. II, III, and IV
        C. II and IV
        D. I, II, and III
        E. I, III, and IV
    (4:249–260)

13. Which of the following ventilators has separate controls that allow the respiratory therapy practitioner to vary the amount of aerosolization during both the inspiratory and expiratory phases?
    A. Bennett AP-5
    B. Bird Mark 7
    C. Bird Mark 8
    D. Bennett PR-I
    E. Bennett PR-II
    (4:309)

14. Which of the following controls are present on the Bennett PR-II ventilators but *not* the Bennett PR-I?
    I.   Flow control
    II.   Air dilution control
    III. Rate control
    IV.   Terminal flow control
    V.   Sensitivity control

A. I, III, and IV
B. II, III, and IV
C. I and IV
D. III, IV, and V
E. I, II, and V
   (4:309, 323, and 328)

15. Which of the following ventilators is *not* capable of administering positive pressure greater than 30 cm H_2O pressure?
    A. Bennett PR-II
    B. Bennett PR-I
    C. Bennett AP-5
    D. Bird Mark 7
    E. Bird Mark 8
       (4:328)

16. Which of the following best describes the function of the terminal flow control on the Bennett PR-II ventilator?
    A. Allows the ventilator to function as a constant flow generator
    B. Allows the ventilator to deliver an inspiratory positive pressure plateau
    C. Allows the ventilator to cycle off in the presence of leaks in the patient circuit
    D. Allows the operator to retard and prolong the expiratory phase
    E. Allows the operator to administer NEEP
       (4:312)

17. While using a Bird Mark 7 ventilator, should the respiratory therapy practitioner wish to increase the inspiratory time during the administration of intermittent positive pressure breathing but *not* increase the delivered tidal volume appreciably, he should adjust which of the following controls?
    A. Expiratory time for apnea
    B. Ventilator sensitivity
    C. Pressure control
    D. Flow rate control
    E. Air mix control
       (4:229)

18. On the Bennett PR-II ventilator, activation of which of the following controls will tend to decrease the FI_{O_2} when the ventilator is on the 100% source gas setting?
    A. Inspiratory nebulizer control
    B. Expiratory nebulizer control
    C. Flow control
    D. Terminal flow control
    E. Sensitivity control
       (4:312)

19. During the inspiratory phase of positive pressure ventilation, which of the following ventilators when operated in the air mix

Venturi mode will deliver oxygen concentrations that may range from 40% to 100%?
I.   Bennett PR-I
II. Bird Mark 8
III. Bird Mark 7
IV. Bennett PR-II
   A.   I, III, and IV
   B.   II, III, and IV
   C.   I, II, and III
   D.   I and III
   E.   I, II, III, and IV
  (4:258)

20. Which of the following is a design characteristic that is shared by all currently employed incentive breathing devices?
   A.   The use of a bellows type volume metering device
   B.   The use of a piston type volume metering device
   C.   The use of an electronic volume metering device
   D.   The use of a weighted sphere metering device
   E.   None of the above
  (4:Chap 7)

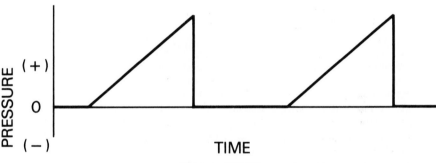

Figure IV-26.

21. The above pressure waveform would most likely be generated by which of the following ventilators?
   A.   Bennett PR-II
   B.   Bird Mark 7
   C.   Bennett AP-5
   D.   Bird Mark 7A
   E.   Bennett PR-I
  (4:257)

Answer Key

1. C	5. D	9. C	13. E	17. D
2. C	6. B	10. D	14. C	18. D
3. E	7. D	11. E	15. C	19. E
4. C	8. B	12. D	16. C	20. E
				21. B

F. Continuous Mechanical Ventilator Devices

Questions in this category assess the candidate's ability to select and assemble all continuous mechanical ventilatory equipment prior to performing respiratory care procedures. These questions also test the candidate's understanding of the principles of operation and his or her ability to correct all malfunctions of any selected equipment.

Entry Level Pretest

According the the NBRC Composite Examination Matrix (see reference 80), questions in this category assess the candidate's understanding of the following types of volume-, pressure-, or time-cycled continuous mechanical ventilatory equipment on a basic level:

1. Electronically powered ventilators
2. Pneumatically powered, electronically controlled ventilators
3. Fluidic ventilators
4. Ventilator circuits

The following are self-study questions from this category:

1. Which of the following most correctly describes the principle of operation of the rate control mechanism employed by the Bennett MA-I ventilator?
   A. A vortex-shedding device
   B. A reference potentiometer
   C. An electronic timer
   D. A pneumatic timer
   E. A 64K microprocessor
   (4:401)

2. Pneumatically powered, pneumatically controlled, time-cycled controller best describes which of the following ventilators?
   A. Sechrist infant ventilator
   B. Engström ventilator
   C. Bourns BP-200 infant ventilator
   D. Baby Bird ventilator
   E. Bennett MA-II ventilator
   (4:280–285)

3. The respiratory therapy practitioner is monitoring a patient in the intensive care unit who is on a Bennett MA-I ventilator in the assist/control mode. The physician asks that the patient be placed on 10 cm PEEP. At the same time the respiratory therapy practitioner should:
   A. Ask the physician to paralyze the patient pharmacologically
   B. Increase the ventilator sensitivity

    C.   Adjust the low exhaled tidal volume alarm

    D.   Recommend fluid administration to prevent arterial hypertension

    E.   Increase the tidal volume 200 cc to compensate for volume lost in the tubing circuit

    (4:402)

4.   If a volume-cycled ventilator has its inspiratory time and inspiratory flow rate held constant, then the respiratory rate becomes a function of which of the following controls?

    A.   Tidal volume

    B.   Expiratory timer

    C.   Pressure limit

    D.   I:E ratio

    E.   B and D are correct.

    (4:228–230)

5.   If a ventilator is *only* capable of initiating the inspiratory phase as a result of the action of an electronic or pneumatic timing device, then this ventilator must be classified as a (an):

    A.   Assister

    B.   Assist/controller

    C.   Controller

    D.   Time-cycled assister

    E.   Volume-cycled, pressure-limited assister

    (4:218)

6.   The pressure manometer on the control panel of which of the following ventilators is factory designed to be referenced to the proximal airway?

    I.   Bennett MA-I

    II.   Bourns Bear I

    III.   Bennett MA-II

    IV.   Siemens Servo 900 C

        A.   I, III, and IV

        B.   II, III, and IV

        C.   I, II, and IV

        D.   I, II, III, and IV

        E.   I, II, and III

    (4:280, 404, and 474)

7.   Electrically powered, single circuit, and rotary piston driven best describes which of the following ventilators?

    A.   Engström

    B.   Bourns LS-104 infant

    C.   Emerson 3P-V postoperative

    D.   Bennett MA-I

    E.   Ohio CCV

    (4:336–337)

8.   The physician wants to provide continuous ventilatory support for a very small child who weighs approximately 25 lbs. It would be

least advisable for the respiratory therapy practitioner to select
which one of the following ventilators?
A. Bennett MA-I
B. Baby Bird
C. Bourns BP-200
D. Bourns Bear I
E. Sechrist
   (4:479)

9. Which of the following best describes the Bennett MA-I's exhaled
    tidal volume monitor?
    A. A vortex-shedding device
    B. A wedge spirometer
    C. A bellows spirometer
    D. A pressure drop pneumotachometer
    E. A thermistor bead device
       (4:409)

10. Which of the following alarms is *not* available on the Bourns Bear
     I ventilator as it comes from the factory?
     A. Low inspiratory pressure
     B. Low source gas pressure
     C. Ventilator inoperative
     D. Low delivered FI_{O_2}
     E. Low PEEP and CPAP
        (4:477–479)

11. Which of the following is the principle of operation of the PEEP
     control employed by the Bennett MA-I?
     A. Adjustable reducing valve
     B. Venturi system
     C. Fluidic valve
     D. Needle valve
     E. Demand valve
        (4:405–407)

12. Which of the following ventilators are capable of delivering an
     accelerating flow pattern?
     I.   Emerson 3P-V
     II.   Bennett MA-I
     III. Siemens Servo 900 C
     IV.   Bourns Bear I
          A. I and III
          B. II and III
          C. III and IV
          D. I and IV
          E. III only
        (4:337)

13. With which of the following ventilators is the respiratory therapy
     practitioner capable of administering SIMV?
     I.   Bourns Bear I
     II. Siemens Servo 900 C

III.   Bennett MA-II
IV.   Bennett 7200
    A.   I, II, and III
    B.   II and IV
    C.   I, III, and IV
    D.   I and III
    E.   I, II, III, and IV
  (4:416–417)

14. When used as an assister, the Bennett 7200 ventilator will initiate the inspiratory phase:
A.   Automatically as a result of a timer
B.   In response to the patient's inspiratory efforts
C.   When there is a change in the patient's mean airway pressure
D.   If the expiratory phase becomes prolonged
E.   If the ventilator does not sense the termination of expiration
  (4:395)

15. The Baby Bird ventilator, when used to mechanically ventilate newborns, is usually set to operate as a (an):
A.   Time-cycled, pressure-limited assister
B.   Pressure-cycled, time-limited controller
C.   Assist/controller
D.   Time-cycled, pressure-limited controller
E.   Time-cycled assister with a variable inspiratory apneustic plateau
  (4:280)

16. Which of the following is (are) known to occur when the set pressure limit on a Bourns Bear I ventilator and a Bennett MA-I ventilator is reached?
  I.   An audible alarm will sound.
  II.   The inspiratory phase will be terminated.
  III. The pressure will be held at the airway until the set volume is delivered.
  IV.   Time cycling will occur.
    A.   II only
    B.   II and IV
    C.   I, II, and IV
    D.   I and II
    E.   I and III
  (4:404 and 474)

17. Subsequent to placing a 58-year-old patient with chronic obstructive pulmonary disease pneumonia on a Bennett MA-I ventilator, the respiratory therapy practitioner notes that the monitoring bellows spirometer fills only during the inspiratory phase. Which of the following is most likely to be responsible for this?
A.   There is a leak in the ventilator circuit.
B.   The spirometer line is disconnected.
C.   The exhalation line is disconnected.

D.   The exhalation valve is not seating properly
E.   C and D are correct.
     (4:329–332)

18. Which of the following mechanical ventilators is capable of developing an inspiratory flow pattern that most closely resembles a sine wave?
     A.   Bennett MA-I
     B.   Bourns BP-200
     C.   Bourns Bear II
     D.   Bennett 7200
     E.   Bourns LS-104 infant
          (4:336–338)

19. Which of the following *best* describes the inspiratory flow pattern of the Bennett MA-I ventilator when used to ventilate patients with very noncompliant lungs?
     A.   A sine wave flow pattern
     B.   A constant flow pattern
     C.   A downward, tapered (decelerating) flow pattern
     D.   A modified sine wave flow pattern
     E.   An accelerating flow pattern
          (4:395–400)

20. Which of the following ventilators should the respiratory therapy practitioner select to provide continuous mechanical ventilation for a 66-year-old obese postoperative patient?
     A.   A pressure-cycled ventilator
     B.   A negative-pressure ventilator
     C.   A volume-cycled ventilator
     D.   A time-cycled ventilator
     E.   A pressure flow-cycled ventilator
          (4:216–248)

21. During controlled mechanical ventilation, the inspiratory phase may be initiated by:
     I.   An inspiratory timer
     II.   An expiratory timer
     III. A pneumatic timer
     IV.   An electronic timer
           A.   I, III, and IV
           B.   I, II, III, and IV
           C.   II, III, and IV
           D.   I and IV
           E.   IV only
     (4:216–248)

22. On a volume-cycled ventilator the development of an episode of bronchospasm will most likely result in which of the following occurrences?
     A.   A decrease in the delivered tidal volume
     B.   An increase in respiratory rate
     C.   An increase in the ventilator peak pressure

D.   Altered ventilator sensitivity
E.   Activation of the ventilator's low pressure alarm
(4:216–248)

23.   Under which of the following conditions will the low FI_{O_2} alarm be activated on the Bennett MA-I ventilator?
A.   If O_2 inlet pressure falls below 30 psig
B.   When the oxygen accumulator is empty and the oxygen control percentage is set at 21%
C.   If the oxygen accumulator empties with the oxygen percentage control set at greater than 21%
D.   If the ventilator is connected to a gas source other than oxygen
E.   If concentrations of oxygen greater than 80% are being used
(4:403–404)

24.   Which of the following is the most fundamental consideration in determining how a mechanical ventilator is *cycled?*
A.   That which initiates inspiration
B.   That which terminates expiration
C.   That which terminates inspiration
D.   That which initiates apneusis
E.   C and D are correct.
(4:218–220)

25.   Which of the following are true statements regarding activation of the ratio alarm on the Bennett MA-I ventilator?
I.   The inspiratory phase has exceeded 50% of the cycle time.
II.   Correction may be achieved by increasing the respiratory frequency.
III. It can only occur during the assist/control mode.
IV.   Correction may be achieved by increasing the inspiratory flow rate.
A.   II and IV
B.   III and IV
C.   I and IV
D.   I, III, and IV
E.   I, II, and IV
(4:401–402)

26.   The respiratory therapy practitioner is operating a Bennett MA-I ventilator in the control mode with a respiratory rate of 18, a tidal volume of 700 cc, and a peak flow rate of 40 L/min. Which of the following would be *least* likely to occur if the inspiratory flow rate were increased to 60 L/min?
A.   The peak inspiratory pressure would increase.
B.   The exhalation time would increase.
C.   The I:E ratio would change.
D.   The inspiratory time would decrease.
E.   The minute ventilation would increase.
(4:401)

27. Which of the following ventilators is (are) double circuit?
     I.   Bennett 7200
     II. Bennett MA-II
     III. Bourns Bear I
          A. II and III
          B. I and III
          C. II only
          D. I, II, and III
          E. III only
     (4:395)

28. On the Baby Bird ventilator, the inspiratory phase is initiated by which of the following mechanisms?
     A. The patient creating a subatmospheric airway pressure
     B. Delivering a burst of gas to the assist-sensitivity mechanism
     C. Interrupting gas flow through the patient's circuit
     D. The result of an electronic timer
     E. C and D are correct.
     (4:280–285)

29. With which of the following types of ventilators will the delivered tidal volume be directly proportional to the patient's lung-thorax compliance?
     A. Pressure cycled
     B. Volume cycled
     C. Time cycled
     D. Flow cycled
     E. B and C are correct.
     (4:226–230)

30. A ventilator that is classified as a constant-flow generator will most likely produce:
     A. A saw-toothed shaped pressure waveform
     B. A sharply decelerating pressure waveform
     C. An upward tapering and rounded pressure waveform
     D. An inspiratory positive pressure plateau type waveform
     E. A parabolic pressure waveform
     (4:222–230)

31. Which of the following correctly describes the Bennett MA-I ventilator?
     I.   Single circuit
     II. Volume cycled
     III. Flow adjustable
     IV. Turbine bellows driven
     V.   Pneumatically powered
          A. I, III, and V
          B. II, III, IV, and V
          C. II and III
          D. I, II, III, IV, and V
          E. I and V
     (4:395)

32.   The flow control on the Bennett MA-I ventilator consists of:
    A.   A scissors valve
    B.   An adjustable needle valve
    C.   A butterfly valve
    D.   A zone valve
    E.   A gate valve
        (4:395–400)

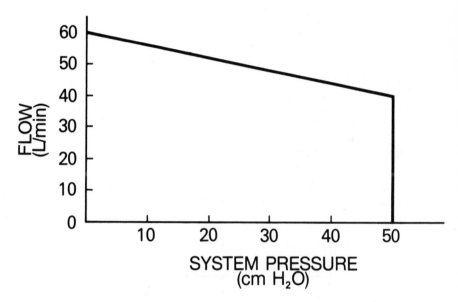

Figure IV-27.

33.   The above pressure waveform would most likely be generated by which of the following ventilators during actual patient care conditions?
    A.   Baby Bird
    B.   Bennett PR-II
    C.   Emerson 3P-V
    D.   Bourns BP-200
    E.   Bennett MA-I
        (4:226 and 400)

Answer Key

1. C	8. D	15. D	22. C	29. A
2. D	9. C	16. D	23. C	30. A
3. B	10. D	17. E	24. C	31. C
4. E	11. A	18. D	25. C	32. B
5. C	12. A	19. C	26. E	33. E
6. B	13. E	20. C	27. C	
7. C	14. B	21. C	28. C	

Advanced Practitioner Pretest

According to the NBRC Composite Examination Matrix (see reference 80), questions in this category assess the candidate's understanding of the following types of respiratory care equipment:

1. Fluidic ventilators
2. External negative pressure, rocking bed, and other miscellaneous types of ventilators
3. All volume- and time-cycled ventilators on an *advanced* level

The following are self-study questions from this category:

1. The phenomenon whereby an airstream passing by a wall will tend to adhere to that wall refers to the:
   A. Schmitt effect
   B. Coanda effect
   C. Flip-flop phenomenon
   D. AND/NAND effect
   E. OR/NOR effect
   (4:235)

The next two questions refer to the following illustration:

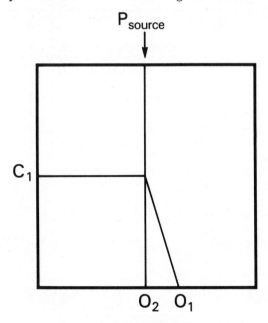

P_{source}

C_1

O_2 O_1

Figure IV-28.

2. Which of the following correctly describes the fluidic element pictured in the previous diagram?
   A. OR/NOR gate
   B. AND/NAND gate

C. Flip-flop component
D. Schmitt trigger
E. Backpressure switch
    (4:235–237)

3. In the fluidic element pictured previously, if gas is supplied at point Ps (Psource) only, the port of exit will be:
    A. O_1 and C_1
    B. O_2 only
    C. O_2 and C_1
    D. O_1 only
    E. C_1 only
        (4:235–237)

The next three questions refer to the following illustration:

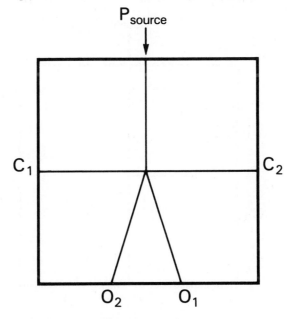

Figure IV-29.

4. If gas is supplied under pressure at Ps and C_1, gas will exit at which of the following points?
    A. O_2 and O_1
    B. O_1 only
    C. O_2 only
    D. Ps
    E. C_2 and O_1
        (4:235–237)

5. In the fluidic element pictured above, if gas flow were to be supplied to Ps and C_2, the port of exit would be at point(s):
    A. C_1 and O_2
    B. O_1 only

    C. C_2 and O_1
    D. O_2 only
    E. O_1 and O_2
    (4:235–237)

6. Which of the following terms best describes the previous fluidic element?
    A.   OR/NOR gate
    B.   Backpressure switch
    C.   Coanda gate
    D.   AND/NAND gate
    E.   Flip-flop element
    (4:235–237)

The next two questions refer to the following illustration:

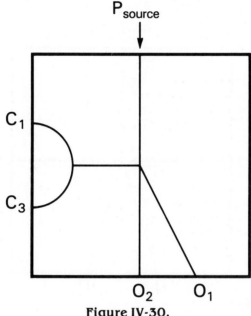

Figure IV-30.

7. Which of the following best describes the fluidic element pictured above?
    A.   OR/NOR gate
    B.   Schmitt trigger
    C.   AND/NAND gate
    D.   Bistable flip-flop element
    E.   Bistable NOR gate
    (4:235–237)

8. If the previous fluidic element were to have gas under pressure supplied to points Ps, C_1 and C_3, gas will exit from tract:
    A. O_2
    B. O_1 and O_2

C. O_1, O_2, and C_3
D. O_1, O_2, and C_1
E. O_1
     (4:235–237)

9. Which of the following correctly describe the Siemens Servo 900 B
    and 900 C ventilators?
    I.   Pneumatically powered, pneumatically controlled
    II.   Single circuit
    III. Minute volume preset
    IV.   Time-cycled controller
          A.   I and IV
          B.   II and IV
          C.   I, II, and III
          D.   II and III
          E.   III and IV
     (4:457–459)

10. The drive mechanism of the Siemens Servo 900 B and 900 C con-
    sists of:
    A.   A weighted bellows
    B.   A double-circuit bellows
    C.   A spring-driven bellows
    D.   A compressor-driven bellows
    E.   A turbine-driven bellows
     (4:459)

11. Which of the following inspiratory waveforms may be adminis-
    tered with the Siemens Servo 900 B and 900 C ventilators?
    I.   Constant flow pattern
    II.   Sine wave type pattern
    III. Decelerating flow pattern
          A.   I and III
          B.   II and III
          C.   I and II
          D.   I only
          E.   I, II, and III
     (4:459–460)

12. The assist and sensitivity mechanism of the Bourns Bear I and
    Bear II ventilators incorporates which of the following mecha-
    nisms?
    A.   A spring-loaded diaphragm
    B.   A Venturi device
    C.   A heat transfer transducer
    D.   A pressure drop transducer
    E.   An ultrasonic transducer
     (4:472–473)

13. The tidal volume control on the Bourns Bear I and Bear II venti-
    lators is referenced to:
    A.   A vortex-shedding device
    B.   A strain gauge

C.   A pressure drop pneumotachometer
D.   An ultrasonic transducer
E.   A and D are correct.
   (4:471)

14. The respiratory therapy practitioner is operating a Siemens Servo
     900 C in the control mode with the following settings:

Minute volume	12 L
Control rate	12
Inspiratory time percentage	33%

Based on this information, which of the following most accurately
represents the average inspiratory flow rate?
A.   24 L/min
B.   36 L/min
C.   60 L/min
D.   80 L/min
E.   90 L/min
   (4:461)

15. The respiratory therapy practitioner is operating a Siemens Servo
     900 C ventilator in the control mode with the following settings:

Minute ventilation	12 L
Set rate	12
Inspiratory time percentage	50%

Based on this information, what is the I:E ratio?
A.   1:1
B.   1:2
C.   1:2.5
D.   1:3
E.   2:1
   (4:461)

16. The respiratory therapy practitioner is operating a Siemens Servo
     900 C ventilator in the control mode with the following settings:

Minute ventilation	10 L
Set rate	10
Inspiratory time percentage	20%
Pause time percentage	5%

Based on the above information, what is the I:E ratio?
A.   1:1
B.   1:2
C.   1:3
D.   1:4
E.   1:5
   (4:463)

17. The Siemens Servo 900 B and 900 C are:
     A. Pneumatically powered, pneumatically controlled
     B. Pneumatically powered, electrically controlled
     C. Electrically powered, pneumatically controlled
     D. Electrically powered, fluidically controlled
     E. Fluidically powered, electrically controlled
     (4:457)

18. A respiratory therapy practitioner is operating a Siemens Servo
     900 C in the control mode with the following settings:

Set rate	12
Minute volume	9 L

     Shortly after switching to the assist/control mode, the practitioner
     notes a mechanical respiratory rate of 22 breaths per minute.
     Based on the above information, which of the following most
     accurately represents this patient's expired minute volume?
     A. 10 L
     B. 16 L
     C. 9 L
     D. 18 L
     E. 11.5 L
     (4:457–468)

19. The respiratory therapy practitioner is operating a Siemens Servo
     900 C ventilator in the control mode with the following settings:

Minute volume	10 L
Set rate	15
Inspiratory time percentage	33%

     Based on the above information, which of the following most
     accurately represents this patient's inspiratory time?
     A. 0.8 second
     B. 1.0 second
     C. 1.3 seconds
     D. 1.65 seconds
     E. 2.0 seconds
     (4:457–468)

20. The respiratory therapy practitioner is operating a Siemens Servo
     900 C ventilator with the following settings:

Minute volume	10 L
Set rate	12
Inspiratory time percentage	25%

     If the practitioner were to increase the minute volume to 14 L/
     min, which of the following would occur?
     I.   The I:E ratio would not change.
     II. The expiratory time would decrease.

III.   The tidal volume would increase.
IV.   The inspiratory flow rate would remain unchanged.
    A.   I and IV
    B.   III and IV
    C.   I and II
    D.   II and IV
    E.   I and III
(4:457–468)

21.   The respiratory therapy practitioner is operating a Siemens Servo ventilator with the following settings:

Minute volume	10 L
Set rate	10
Inspiratory time percentage	33%

If the practitioner were to decrease the inspiratory time percentage to 25%, which of the following would occur?
  I.   The inspiratory flow rate would increase.
  II.   The I:E ratio would change to 1:4.
III.   The inspiratory time would decrease.
IV.   The tidal volume would decrease.
    A.   I and IV
    B.   I and III
    C.   II only
    D.   III only
    E.   II and IV
(4:457–468)

Answer Key

1. B	5. D	9. D	13. E	17. B
2. A	6. E	10. C	14. B	18. B
3. B	7. C	11. E	15. A	19. C
4. B	8. E	12. C	16. C	20. E
				21. B

G. Cardiopulmonary Function Monitoring Devices

Questions in this category assess the candidate's ability to select and assemble all cardiopulmonary function monitoring devices and equipment prior to performing respiratory care procedures. These questions also test the candidate's understanding of the principles of operation and his or her ability to correct all malfunctions of any selected equipment.

Entry Level and Advanced Practitioner Pretest

According to the NBRC Composite Examination Matrix (see reference 80), this content category is assessed on both the Entry Level and Advanced Practitioner Examinations. Unlike the vast majority of the other content categories, some of the specific types of equipment (as will be noted below) are assessed on both the Entry Level Examination and the Advanced Practitioner Examination. Therefore, in the interest of simplicity, I list the equipment below as well as the specific examination(s) that they appear on; the candidate can then select appropriate questions for the examination to be taken from the single list of questions that follows.

According to the NBRC Composite Examination Matrix (see reference 80), questions in this category assess the candidate's understanding of the following respiratory care equipment:

1. Blood gas analyzers
2. Manometers and gauges
   a. Water, mercury, and sphygmomanometers (Entry Level only)
   b. Inspiratory/expiratory metering devices (Entry Level only)
   c. Transducers and strain gauges (Advanced Practitioner only)
3. Pulmonary function testing devices (respirometers)
   a. Pneumotachometers (Entry Level and Advanced Practitioner)
   b. Vane type respirometers (Entry Level and Advanced Practitioner)
   c. Positive displacement spirometers (Entry Level only)
   d. Other electronic devices (Entry Level and Advanced Practitioner)
4. Electrocardiography devices (Advanced Practitioner only)
5. Hemodynamic monitoring devices (Advanced Practitioner only)

The following are self-study questions from this category:

1. When using a Wright respirometer, the respiratory therapy practitioner should be aware of the fact that damage to the unit can occur when flow rates in excess of which of the following are measured?
   A. 100 L/min
   B. 300 L/min
   C. 400 L/min
   D. 50 L/min
   E. 600 L/min
   (4:206)

2. Devices that measure flow and/or volume by means of rotating cogs or vanes include:
   I. Wright respirometer
   II. Dräger volumeter

    III. Wright peak flowmeter
    IV. Bourns LS-75 respirometer
    V. Fleisch® pneumotachometer
       A. I, II, and III
       B. II and III
       C. IV and V
       D. I and II
       E. II and V
    (4:206–207)

3. Flow-sensing devices that employ a heat transfer (thermistor bead) transducer use which of the following principles?
    A. Spectrophotometry
    B. Pressure drop across a fixed orifice
    C. Vortex-shedding and counting mechanism
    D. Temperature drop across a variable orifice
    E. Change in current caused by a change in temperature
    (4:209)

POLYPROPYLENE
MEMBRANE

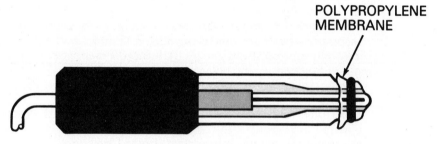

Figure IV-31.

4. The above diagram illustrates a:
    A. pH electrode
    B. Severinghaus electrode
    C. Clark electrode
    D. Spectrophotometer
    E. Scholander electrode
    (5:36)

5. The Clark type P_{O_2} electrode uses which of the following principles?
    A. Astrup
    B. Paramagnetic
    C. Polarographic
    D. Galvanic
    E. Henry
    (5:34)

6. Which of the following types of electrodes measure(s) pH?
    I. Clark type
    II. Severinghaus type

III. Galvanic type
IV. Sanz type
    A. I and IV
    B. II and III
    C. III and IV
    D. II and IV
    E. IV only
  (5:29–33)

7. The Fleisch pneumotachograph uses which of the following principles of operation to sense flow?
    A. Measures a change in electric current created by a change in temperature
    B. Measures a drop in pressure across a fixed flow-resistant element
    C. Measures a change in pressure across a variable orifice
    D. Measures a change in gas flow turbulence
    E. Uses a rotating cog assembly
  (4:210–211)

8. The Bourns LS-75 ventilation monitor uses which of the following principles of operation to measure flow?
    A. Measures a change in electrode current created by a change in temperature
    B. Measures the drop in pressure across a fixed flow-resistant element
    C. Measures a change in pressure across a variable orifice mechanism
    D. Measures a change in an ultrasonic signal
    E. Uses a rotating cog assembly
  (4:212)

9. A calomel electrode is used to create a reference current in which of the following types of electrode?
    A. Severinghaus
    B. Clark
    C. Sanz (pH)
    D. Galvanic
    E. A and C are correct.
  (5:29–35)

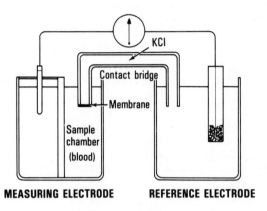

MEASURING ELECTRODE   REFERENCE ELECTRODE

Figure IV-32.

10. The above illustration:
    I.   Illustrates a pH electrode
    II.   Is the basis for the Clark electrode
    III. Measures hydrogen ion concentration
    IV.   Indirectly measures carbon dioxide tension
    V.   Is an example of an amperometric electrode
          A. I, III, and IV
          B. I, II, and III
          C. III, IV, and V
          D. I, II, and V
          E. I and III
    (5:31–32)

11. A highly specialized type of glass is used in the pH electrode to separate the known reference buffer from the sample being measured. Which of the following statements about this "pH sensitive glass" is (are) true?
    I.   It is permeable to hydrogen ions.
    ‑II.   It is permeable to electrons.
    III. It is permeable to protons.
    ‑ IV. It is responsible for the potential difference created between the two solutions.
          A. I and III
          B. I, III, and IV
          C. IV only
          D. I and IV
          ‑E. II and IV
    (4:29–31) (2:985–987 and 998–999)

12. The respiratory therapy practitioner notes that the "bell factor" for a Collins® water seal type spirometer is 41.37. This implies that:
    A. The bell will be full after approximately 41 breaths.
    B. The bell will move 1 mm for every 41.37 cc of vertical displacement.

C. The bell will move 41.37 mm for every 1000 cc of vertical displacement.
D. The bell will move 1 cm for every 41.37 cc of horizontal displacement.
E. The kymograph will make one full revolution every 41.37 seconds.
    (4:202)

13. Which of the following is an example of a bellows type spirometer?
    A. Collins underwater seal spirometer
    B. Bennett monitoring spirometer
    C. Wright respirometer
    D. Collins dry rolling seal spirometer
    E. Scott-McKesson vitalator
        (4:204–205)

14. A Tissot spirometer serves which of the following purposes?
    A. Acts as a reservoir for inspired gases
    B. Collects expired gases
    C. Measures the volume of the expired gases
    D. B and C are correct.
    E. A, B, and C are correct.
        (16:4 and 5)

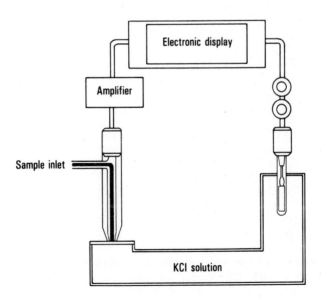

Figure IV-33.

15. The above diagram:
    I.   Illustrates a pH electrode
    II.   Illustrates a P_{CO_2} electrode
    III. Illustrates a gas chromatograph

IV.   Can measure base excess
V.   Was originally developed by Scholander
   A.   I, IV, and V
   B.   II and V
   C.   III, IV, and V
   D.   I only
   E.   IV only
(5:32)

16.   Which of the following kymograph speeds are available with the Collins underwater seal spirometer?
   I.   20 mm/min
   II.   32 mm/min
   III.   64 mm/min
   IV.   160 mm/min
   V.   1920 mm/min

   A.   I, III, and IV
   B.   II, IV, and V
   C.   I, III, and V
   D.   II and IV
   E.   IV and V
(16:107)

17.   Which of the following types of respirometers uses a lightweight plastic bell that is not counterweighted or supported by pulleys?
   A.   Collins 9-liter spirometer
   B.   Stead-Wells® spirometer
   C.   Bennett monitoring spirometer
   D.   Collins dry rolling seal spirometer
   E.   Wedge type spirometer
(16:107–108)

18.   The Severinghaus P_{CO_2} electrode most frequently uses which of the following type of membrane material?
   A.   Mylar
   B.   Polyethylene
   C.   Polyurethane
   D.   Polypropylene
   E.   Silicone
(5:33)

19.   Which of the following devices uses both a strain gauge and a heat transfer type transducer as part of its normal function and operation?
   A.   Fleisch pneumotachometer
   B.   Four-channel Swan-Ganz catheter
   C.   Variable orifice type pneumotachometer
   D.   Bourns LS-75 respirometer
   E.   Typical peripheral arterial line
(5:201–204) (2:954–955)

20. Use of a properly functioning three-channel Swan-Ganz pulmonary artery catheter gives the respiratory therapy practitioner the ability to monitor all of the following *except:*
   A. Pulmonary artery systolic pressure
   B. Central venous pressure
   C. Cardiac output
   D. Mixed venous oxygen tension
   E. Pulmonary wedge pressure
   (5:230)

21. A properly functioning indwelling *peripheral* arterial catheter gives the respiratory therapy practitioner the ability to monitor which of the following parameters?
   I. Mean arterial pressure
   II. Systolic arterial pressure
   III. Central venous pressure
   IV. Diastolic arterial pressure
      A. I, II, and IV
      B. I, II, III, and IV
      C. II, III, and IV
      D. I, II, and III
      E. I and II
   (2:952–953) (5:51–53)

22. Indwelling peripheral arterial catheters are known to use which of the following devices to measure pressure?
   A. Water column manometers
   B. Pressure drop transducers
   C. Heat transfer transducers
   D. Strain gauges
   E. Ultrasonic transducers
   (2:952–953) (33:189–190)

23. Which of the following may be used to define or describe the term *transducer?*
   A. A device used to convert one form of energy into another form
   B. A device used to convert electrical energy into mechanical energy
   C. A device used to convert pressure or temperature measurements into electrical energy
   D. A device used to convert electrical energy into ultrasonic energy
   E. All of the above
   (33:189–190) (16:114–115) (4:134–135 and 208–211)

24. A typical setup for monitoring central venous pressure involves the use of which one of the following pressure measuring devices?
   A. Thermistor bead transducer
   B. Water column manometer
   C. Mercury column manometer

D.   Sphygmomanometer
E.   Heat transfer transducer
     (33:186–187)

25.   The term *strain gauge* is most synonymous with:
      A.   A pressure transducer
      B.   A pressure drop transducer
      C.   A thermistor bead transducer
      D.   A mercury manometer
      E.   An anaroid manometer
         (69)

26.   When monitoring a patient's electrocardiogram, the respiratory
      therapist should use an electrocardiographic device that incorpo-
      rates a strip recorder to ensure that the paper travels at which of
      the following rates?
      A.   10 mm/sec
      B.   15 mm/sec
      C.   25 cm/sec
      D.   25 mm/sec
      E.   None of the above
         (1:35)

27.   A negative electrode placed in the right supermammary area and
      a positive electrode placed on the left anterior chest wall below the
      mammary area most correctly describes which of the following
      standard, electrocardiographic leads?
      A.   Lead I
      B.   Lead II
      C.   Lead III
      D.   Lead MCL-I
      E.   None of the above
         (1:37)

28.   Infrared absorption spectrometers are used frequently to measure:
      A.   pH
      B.   Nitrogen
      C.   Oxygen
      D.   Helium
      E.   Carbon monoxide
         (16:121)

29.   Giesler® tube ionizers (emission spectrometers) are most fre-
      quently used to measure which of the following?
      A.   Helium
      B.   Oxygen
      C.   Nitrogen
      D.   Carbon dioxide
      E.   Xenon
         (16:117)

30. Which of the following oxygen analyzing devices uses the principle of spectrophotometry?
   A. Galvanic cell devices
   B. Scholander devices
   C. Ear oximeters
   D. Transcutaneous oxygen monitors
   E. Van Slyke devices
   (5:38)

31. Which of the following oxygen monitoring devices incorporates modifications of the Clark electrode?
   I. Polarographic analyzers
   II. Galvanic cell analyzers
   III. Transcutaneous devices
   IV. Oximeter devices
      A. I and III
      B. II, III, and IV
      C. I and IV
      D. I and II
      E. I, II, and III
   (5:Chap 4)

32. Which of the following is actually measured by ear oximeter devices?
   A. The partial pressure of oxygen dissolved in plasma
   B. The carboxyhemoglobin concentration in blood
   C. The oxyhemoglobin concentration in blood
   D. The total hemoglobin concentration in blood
   E. The reduced hemoglobin concentration in blood
   (5:38)

33. Which of the following has (have) been shown to affect the reliability of transcutaneous oxygen measurements?
   I. Shunting of blood through the ductus arteriosus
   II. Prolonged crying
   III. Increased cutaneous blood flow
      A. I and II
      B. II and III
      C. II only
      D. III only
      E. I and III
   (5:39–40) (15:216–217)

34. Kathermometers designed to measure thermal conductivity are frequently used in pulmonary function laboratories to measure which of the following gases?
   A. Helium
   B. Nitrogen
   C. Carbon dioxide
   D. Xenon
   E. A and C are correct.
   (16:118–120)

35. The statement "The test gas sample, after being ionized, is exposed to a magnetic field that causes each gas to deflect according to its molecular mass" describes the principle of operation of a:
    A. Gas chromatograph
    B. Spectrophotometer
    C. Strain gauge
    D. Infrared analyzer
    E. Mass spectrometer
       (16:120–121) (4:153)

36. The statement "an instrument that measures the absorption or transmission of a light source with a selected wavelength" most accurately describes a:
    A. Spectrophotometer
    B. Gas chromatograph
    C. Chemical analyzer
    D. Mass spectrometer
    E. Electron accelerator
       (5:38)

37. The respiratory therapy practitioner is monitoring the transcutaneous oxygen tension of a patient in the intensive care unit. The 70-kg patient's cardiac index is 1.2 L/min/m^2 body surface area. Based on this information, the practitioner would expect which of the following degrees of correlation between $Ptco_2$ and Pao_2?
    A. Poor
    B. Good
    C. Linear
    D. Excellent
    E. Sigmoidal
       (102:176–182)

38. The respiratory therapy practitioner is monitoring the transcutaneous oxygen tension of a 70-kg patient who has a cardiac index of 3.8 L/min/m^2 body surface area. Based on this information, the practitioner would expect which of the following degrees of correlation between $Ptco_2$ and Pao_2?
    A. Poor
    B. Nonlinear
    C. Marginal
    D. Very good
    E. Inverse
       (102:176–182)

39. The statement "a wire of known electrical resistance wound back and forth across a diaphragm which when stretched produces an electrical signal that can be used for physiologic monitoring" most accurately describes:
    A. A katathermometer
    B. A thermistor bead
    C. A pressure transducer

   D.   A strain gauge
   E.   C and D are correct.
      (69)

40. Which of the following is *not* measured or reported by the Instru-
    mentation Laboratories® CO–Oximeter?
    A.   Total hemoglobin
    B.   Carbaminohemoglobin
    C.   Oxyhemoglobin
    D.   Carboxyhemoglobin
    E.   Methemoglobin
       (5:38)

41. Which of the following is actually measured by indwelling pulmo-
    nary artery oximeters?
    A.   The tension of oxygen dissolved in arterial blood
    B.   The oxyhemoglobin concentration of mixed venous blood
    C.   The tension of oxygen dissolved in mixed venous blood
    D.   The oxyhemoglobin saturation of arterial blood
    E.   B and D are correct.
       (5:38) (69)

42. Strain gauges are often used to measure:
     I.   Intravascular pressures
    II.   Helium concentrations
   III.   Intrapulmonary pressures
    IV.   Mixed expiratory carbon dioxide concentration
          A.   I and III
          B.   II and IV
          C.   III and IV
          D.   II and III
          E.   I and IV
       (69)

43. Which of the following types of oxygen analyzers operates by sep-
    arating gases according to their ionic mass?
    A.   Paramagnetic
    B.   Thermal conductivity
    C.   Modified Clark cell type
    D.   Chemical absorption type
  → E.   Mass spectrometer
       (4:153) (16:120)

Answer Key

1. B	10. E	19. B	28. E	37. A
2. A	11. E	20. C	29. C	38. D
3. E	12. B	21. A	30. C	39. E
4. C	13. B	22. D	31. E	40. B
5. C	14. D	23. E	32. C	41. B
6. D	15. D	24. B	33. A	42. A
7. B	16. B	25. A	34. A	43. E
8. D	17. B	26. D	35. E	
9. C	18. E	27. B	36. A	

H. Ensure the Cleanliness of All Equipment

According to the NBRC, questions in this category assess the candidate's ability to ensure that all respiratory care equipment has been properly decontaminated, disinfected, and/or sterilized prior to being used in patient care procedures.

Entry Level Pretest

According to the NBRC's Composite Examination Matrix (see reference 80), questions in this category assess the candidate's understanding of the following related procedures:

1. Selection or determination of the appropriate agent/agents and techniques for disinfection and sterilization
2. Performance of procedures to achieve disinfection and sterilization

The following self-study questions were developed from the NBRC Composite Examination Matrix:

1. Which of the following methods can be used to sterilize the widest variety of respiratory therapy equipment?
    A. Acid glutaraldehyde
    B. Steam autoclaving
    C. Gas sterilization
    D. Alkaline glutaraldehyde
    E. Pasteurization
       (13:290)

2. Which of the following agents or methods of disinfection/sterilization is *not* considered tuberculocidal?
    A. Ethylene oxide
    B. Pasteurization
    C. 90% isopropyl alcohol
    D. Acid glutaraldehyde
    E. None of the above
       (2:418–422)

3. Which of the following is true regarding the toxic chemical ethylene glycol?
    A. Will raise the freezing point of H_2O when added to it
    B. May be formed when ethylene oxide comes in contact with water
    C. May be formed when previously gamma-irradiated items are gas sterilized
    D. Is an isomer of ethylene chlorohydrin
    E. Is used clinically to prevent hyperthermia
       (24:338)

CIDEX

4. How long must a piece of equipment be soaked in alkaline glutar-
   aldehyde for complete sterilization to occur?
   A.   1 to 2 hours
   B.   6 to 8 hours
   C.   10 to 24 hours
   D.   48 to 72 hours
   E.   Sterilization cannot be achieved with this agent.
        (2:419)

5. Which of the following agents or methods are considered sporicid-
   al when used properly?
   I.   Alkaline glutaraldehyde CIDEX
   II.   Gamma radiation
   III. Pasteurization
   IV.   Acid glutaraldehyde — SONACIDE
   V.   90% isopropyl alcohol
         A.   I, III, and IV
         B.   II, IV, and V
         C.   II and V
         D.   I and II
         E.   I, II, and IV
   (2:418–422)

6. True statements about ethylene oxide include:
   I.   It is considered tuberculocidal.
   II.   It must be used in conjunction with heat and humidity.
   III. It is considered a means of sterilization.
   IV.   It can be employed on most types of equipment.
         A.   II, III, and IV
         B.   I, II, III, and IV
         C.   II and IV
         D.   I, III, and IV
         E.   I, II, and IV
   (13:290–291)

7. As compared with alkaline glutaraldehyde, acid glutaraldehyde is
   known to:
   I.   Have a longer shelf life
   II.   Achieve sterilization less rapidly
   III. Not be corrosive to respiratory therapy equipment
         A.   I only
         B.   II only
         C.   I and III
         D.   II and III
         E.   III only
   (24:340)

8. Which of the following statements regarding the disadvantages or
   hazards of the ethylene oxide sterilization process is (are) true?
   I.   It is expensive.
   II.   Ethylene oxide is flammable.

   III.   It cannot be used to sterilize electrical equipment.
   IV.   It is toxic to human tissues.
        A.   I and II
        B.   II and IV
        C.   I, II, and IV
        D.   I and IV
        E.   III only
    (2:419) (24:335–336) (13:290–291)

Answer Key

1. C	3. B	5. E	7. A
2. E	4. C	6. B	8. C

Advanced Practitioner Pretest

According to the NBRC Composite Examination Matrix (see reference 80), questions in this category assess the candidate's ability to monitor the effectiveness of sterilization procedures.

The following self-study questions were developed from the NBRC Composite Examination Matrix:

1. The use of spore-containing culture strips has been recommended to monitor the effectiveness of which of the following means of sterilization?
    I.   Ethylene oxide
   II.   Acid glutaraldehyde
  III.   Autoclaving
  IV.   Alkaline glutaraldehyde
        A.   I and III
        B.   II and IV
        C.   III and IV
        D.   II only
        E.   I only
    (13:289–291)

2. Which of the following statements regarding ethylene oxide indicator tape is (are) true?
    I.   A change in color indicates exposure to 50% relative humidity at a temperature of 30°C or greater.
   II.   A change in color indicates exposure to ethylene oxide gas only.
  III.   A change in color indicates that complete sterilization has been achieved.
        A.   I only
        B.   II only
        C.   III only
        D.   I and II
        E.   I and III
    (13:291)

3. Which of the following statements about the care of home respiratory therapy equipment is (are) true?
   I. Equipment should not be allowed to air dry.
   II. All equipment should be sterilized every 24 hours.
   III. All water must be drained from tubing.
   IV. Thorough cleaning and disinfection is a reasonable goal.
      A. I, II, and III
      B. I and III
      C. III and IV
      D. II and IV
      E. IV only
   (2:451–453)

4. Which of the following methods has *not* been recommended to monitor the effectiveness of a respiratory therapy department's sterilization/disinfection processes?
   A. Random culturing of equipment during its shelf life
   B. Random culturing of equipment after physical washing
   C. Random culturing of equipment while in patient use
   D. Random culturing of equipment after undergoing a sterilization process
   E. Use of spore strips when indicated
   (2:450–451)

5. Which of the following agents should the respiratory therapy practitioner recommend for sterilizing equipment used by a patient who is being treated for a pulmonary infection caused by the microorganism *Aspergillus fumigatus?*
   I. Glutaraldehyde
   II. Alcohols
   III. Ethylene oxide
   IV. Autoclaving
      A. I and III
      B. I, II, III, and IV
      C. I, II, and IV
      D. I, II, and III
      E. I, III, and IV
   (2:418–422)

Answer Key

1. A   2. B   3. C   4. B   5. B

I. Perform Calibration and Quality Control Procedures (Advanced Level Only)

This content category is assessed only on the Advanced Practitioner Examination.

Advanced Practitioner Pretest

According to the Composite Examination Matrix (see reference 80), questions in this category assess the candidate's ability to perform quality control and calibration procedures on the following types of respiratory care equipment:

1. Blood gas analyzers
2. Pulmonary function equipment
3. Gas metering devices

The following are self-study questions from this category:

1. The respiratory therapy practitioner is asked to calibrate a given spirometer to ensure that volume measurements are accurate. In order to do so the practitioner should select:
   A. A rotameter device
   B. A Bourns LS-75 spirometer
   C. A calibrated "super" syringe
   D. A biologic control subject
   E. None of the above
   (2:Chap 6)

2. The technique of tonometry may be used to establish quality control for which of the following devices?
   I. pH electrodes
   II. Clark electrodes
   III. Severinghaus electrodes
   IV. Helium meters
      A. I and III
      B. II and III
      C. I, III, and IV
      D. I, II, and III
      E. IV only
   (5:159)

3. Which of the following methods of calibration should be performed most frequently on blood gas analyzers?
   A. 1 point
   B. 2 point
   C. 3 point
   D. 3 point double blind
   E. Tonometry
   (5:160)

4. Which of the following most correctly describes the Astrup method of blood gas analysis?
   A. A method of determining P_{CO_2} using only a pH electrode
   B. A method of determining P_{O_2} using only a pH electrode
   C. A method of determining the bicarbonate level using only a pH electrode

D.   Another way of determining the base excess using only a pH electrode

E.   A method of determining the pH using a P_{CO_2} electrode
(2:998)

5.   Highly accurate samples of known calibrated gases are used to ensure the accuracy of which of the following devices?
  I.   Clark electrode
  II.   Galvanic cell devices
  III.   Sanz electrode
  IV.   Severinghaus electrode
  A.   I and IV
  B.   II and IV
  C.   I and III
  D.   III and IV
  E.   I only
(2:Appendix A)

6.   The periodic analysis of solutions or gases whose predetermined P_{O_2}, P_{CO_2}, and pH are not known to the respiratory therapy practitioner best describes:
  A.   1-point calibration
  B.   2-point calibration
  C.   Tonometry
  D.   External quality assurance
  E.   Astrup method
(5:159)

7.   The respiratory therapy practitioner is performing 1-point calibration on a Severinghaus blood gas electrode using calibration gases that contain a 4.62% CO_2. If the electrode were properly calibrated, the analyzer's carbon dioxide meter would read which of the following (assume a P_B of 760 mm Hg)?
  A.   28 mm Hg
  B.   33 mm Hg
  C.   35 mm Hg
  D.   37 mm Hg
  E.   45 mm Hg
(5:Chap 15)

8.   A 2-point calibration of the Clark blood gas electrode is most frequently performed with which of the following analyzed gas mixtures?
  A.   10% oxygen and 20% oxygen
  B.   0% oxygen and 12% oxygen
  C.   20% oxygen and 80% oxygen
  D.   78% nitrogen, 10% carbon dioxide, and 12% helium
  E.   0% oxygen and 40% oxygen
(5:35)

9.   While performing quality control procedures, the respiratory therapy practitioner correctly performs a 3-point calibration for his blood gas analyzer's polarographic electrode. He then graphs

the actual versus the measured Po_2 for all three of these points. The graphic demonstration is linear with a slope of $45°$. Which of the following is the true statement regarding this blood gas electrode?

A. Slope drift exists.
B. Balance drift exists.
C. Proper calibration exists.
D. There is a leak in the electrode membrane.
E. Electrode interference exists.
    (2:Appendix A)

10. In performing a 2-point calibration of a pH electrode, the respiratory therapy practitioner first analyzes the standard low pH buffer solution to establish a balance point. If properly calibrated, the analyzer will indicate a pH of:

A. 6.48
B. 7.384
C. 6.84
D. 6.96
E. 7.00
    (5:31)

Answer Key

| 1. C | 3. A | 5. A | 7. B | 9. C |
| 2. B | 4. A | 6. D | 8. B | 10. C |

Part III
Therapeutic
Procedures

From the standpoint of number of questions, the therapeutic procedures content category is the most important of the three major examination sections. Forty-five percent of the questions on the Entry Level Examination are drawn from this area. On the Advanced Practitioner Examination this category comprises almost two thirds of the total questions.

A convincing case can also be built that, on the whole, these questions are the most difficult on the examination. As was pointed out in the beginning of this book, NBRC examination questions as well as the ones in this book are designed to assess three levels of complexity: recall, application, and analysis. These three levels represent the hierarchy of cognitive or intellectual skills. Questions that assess analytical skills are the most difficult because they frequently require the candidate to use both abstract thinking and good judgment in their solution. From the table that follows it can be seen that the therapeutic procedures category, especially on the Advanced Practitioner Examination, contains an exceptional number of analysis type questions.

Percentage Analysis Level Questions

Examination	Clinical Data Category	Equipment Category	Therapeutic Procedures Category
Entry Level	13	6	18
Advanced Practitioner	20	10	42

In general, questions in the therapeutic procedures content category assess the candidate's ability to perform those tasks that the 1981 Job Survey identified as being essential to the practice of respiratory therapy procedures. This survey identified 12 major competencies in this area:

1. Educate patients (entry level only)
2. Control infection (entry level only)
3. Maintain airway

4. Mobilize and remove secretions (entry level only)
5. Ensure ventilation
6. Ensure oxygenation
7. Assess patient response to therapy
8. Modify therapy
9. Recommend modifications in therapy
10. Initiate cardiopulmonary resuscitation (entry level only)
11. Maintain records and communication (entry level only)
12. Assist physician with special procedures (advanced level only)

A. Educate Patients (Entry Level Only)

According to the NBRC (see reference 80), the content category educate patients is assessed only on the Entry Level Examination. Questions in this category are designed to assess the candidate's ability to explain to the patient the proper procedure for performing therapy that the physician has ordered and the specific therapeutic goals involved. These should be presented to the patient in the simplest and most easily understandable terms possible to achieve an optimal therapeutic outcome.

Entry Level Pretest

According to the NBRC, 2% of the questions on the Entry Level Examination are from the educate patients content category. The following self-study questions were developed from the NBRC Composite Examination Matrix:

1. The respiratory therapy practitioner is administering IPPB to a postoperative patient. About 3 minutes into the treatment, the patient complains of lightheadedness and tingling of the extremities. Just prior to this, the patient's cycling rate was 15/min. Which of the following actions would be most appropriate for the practitioner to take at this time?
    A. Instruct the patient to pause between each breath
    B. Employ an expiratory retard cap
    C. Instruct the patient to contract his abdominal muscles during exhalation
    D. Discontinue therapy for several hours
    E. Instruct the patient to exhale through pursed lips
        (2:578)

2. The physician asks the respiratory therapy practitioner to give preoperative instructions to a patient who is scheduled for a right pneumonectomy. In which of the following techniques would the practitioner *not* instruct this patient?
    A. Splinting of the incision while coughing
    B. IPPB

    C.   Tracheobronchial suctioning
    D.   Incentive spirometry
    E.   Diaphragmatic breathing
    (88)

3. The respiratory therapy practitioner is asked to instruct a 61-year-old patient with advanced pulmonary emphysema in breathing retraining exercises. In interviewing the patient the chief complaint was of his inability to exhale completely. In which of the following exercises should the therapist instruct this patient?
    A.   Segmental breathing exercises
    B.   Diaphragmatic breathing
    C.   Pursed lip breathing
    D.   Cough instruction
    E.   Apneustic breathing
    (1:207)

4. The respiratory therapy practitioner is asked to instruct a patient who has chronic obstructive pulmonary emphysema in breathing retraining exercises. In so doing the patient should be taught to breathe:
    I.   Using pursed lip techniques
    II.   Slowly and deeply
    III.   With abdominal muscles contracted during inspiration
    IV.   With use of the diaphragm
        A.   I, II, and IV
        B.   II, III, and IV
        C.   I, III, and IV
        D.   I, II, III, and IV
        E.   II and IV
    (85) (88)

5. Which of the following factors can act to improve the effectiveness of a patient's cough?
    I.   Placing the patient in a high Fowler's position
    II.   Supporting the patient's incision during efforts
    III.   Having the therapist demonstrate effective techniques
    IV.   Extending the trunk slightly backward while patient is coughing
        A.   II, III, and IV
        B.   I, II, and III
        C.   I and III
        D.   I, II, III, and IV
        E.   I and IV
    (85)

6. The respiratory therapy practitioner is asked to write an instructional pamphlet to be distributed to outpatients enrolled in a large pulmonary rehabilitation program. Which of the following would be the *least* appropriate topic for this paper?
    A.   Diet and fluid intake
    B.   Reconditioning exercises

C. Acid-base and electrolyte disturbances
D. Proper use and hazards of prescribed drugs
E. Postural drainage techniques
   (88)

7. The respiratory therapy practitioner is asked to teach a patient methods of caring for his home respiratory therapy equipment. Recommended instructions would include:
   I.   Culturing techniques
   II.   Proper assembly of all equipment
   III. Proper use of aldehyde sterilization agents
   IV.   Thorough washing, rinsing, and drying techniques
      A. I and IV
      B. I, II, and III
      C. II, III, and IV
      D. II and IV
      E. I, II, III, and IV
   (2:451–452)

Answer Key

1. A   3. C   5. B   7. D
2. C   4. A   6. C

B. Control Infection (Entry Level Only)

According to the NBRC, the control infection content category is assessed only on the Entry Level Examination. The questions in this category are designed to assess the candidate's ability to protect the patient from nosocomial infection through adherence to generally accepted infection control policies and procedures. For instance, if the respiratory therapist notes that a patient on whom he or she is going to perform respiratory care procedures is in strict isolation, the practitioner should be aware that before entering the patient's room, he or she must wash his or her hands and then wear an appropriate gown, gloves, and surgical mask type device.

Entry Level Pretest

According to the NBRC, 2% of the questions on the Entry Level Examination are from the control infection content category. The following self-study questions were developed from the NBRC Composite Examination Matrix (see reference 80):

1. Which of the following most correctly describes the term *nosocomial infection?*

A.   A non-hospital-acquired Gram-negative infection
B.   One that results from treatment by medical or surgical personnel
C.   One that occurs while the patient is in the hospital
D.   A Gram-negative infection that results from cross-contamination
E.   An infection that occurs through the use of respiratory therapy equipment
    (89:958)

2.   Which of the following microorganisms is most likely to contaminate the water reservoirs of respiratory therapy equipment?
A.   *Escherichia coli*
B.   *Proteus* species
C.   Beta-hemolytic *Streptococcus*   P. 290 - DESHPANDE
D.   *Candida* species
E.   *Pseudomonas aeruginosa*
    (2:406 and 420)

3.   All of the following types of respiratory therapy equipment have been associated with nosocomial pulmonary infections. Which of the following has been implicated as having the potential to cause the greatest damage?
A.   Ultrasonic nebulizers   P.243 -E.
B.   Heated pneumatic jet type nebulizers
C.   Hydronamic type nebulizers
D.   Cold bubble humidifiers
E.   Heated bubble humidifiers
    (2:441) (91)

4.   Which of the following types of respiratory therapy equipment are known to *not* transmit microorganisms to their users?
A.   Endotracheal tubes
B.   Spinning disk type nebulizers   P. 243 Eubanks
C.   Bubble type humidifiers
D.   Cascade type humidifiers
E.   None of the above
    (2:441)

5.   All of the following methods of transmitting disease have been associated with the development of nosocomial infections. Which is believed to be the single major cause?
A.   Droplet contamination by coughing and sneezing
B.   Use of respiratory therapy devices
C.   Increased resistance and virulence of hospital flora
D.   Large reservoir of defense-compromised hosts
E.   Poor handwashing technique
    (2:453)

6.   Following placement of an endotracheal or tracheostomy tube, contamination of the tracheobronchial tree can be prevented by which of the following techniques?
A.   Proper handwashing technique

B.   Sterile suctioning technique
C.   Changing all related respiratory therapy equipment at least every 8 hours
D.   All of the above
— E.   None of the above
     (1:264)

7.   Nosocomial infections occur in 5% to 15% of all hospitalized patients. Which of the following types is *most* frequently seen?
   A.   Respiratory tract
 — B.   Urinary tract
   C.   Surgical wound
   D.   Dermal
   E.   Gastrointestinal
     (2:440) (31:38)

8.   All of the following organisms are frequently implicated in the development of nosocomial respiratory tract infection. The presence of which one of the following is *most* suggestive of contamination by aerosol therapy equipment?
 — A.   *Staphylococcus aureus*
   B.   *Hemophilus influenzae*
 →C.   *Serratia* species
   D.   Pneumococcus
   E.   *Streptococcus*
     (13:286–287) (2:446–479)

9.   Which of the following is the most common fungal agent causing nosocomial pulmonary infections?
 — A.   *Candida* species
   B.   *Histoplasma capsulatum*
   C.   *Aspergillus fumigatus*
   D.   *Coccidioides immitis*
   E.   All of the above
     (2:440)

10.   Which of the following is *not* part of the normal or resident flora of the upper respiratory tract?
   A.   *Candida albicans*
   B.   *Hemophilus* species
   C.   *Staphylococcus* species
 — D.   *Klebsiella* species
   E.   Pneumococci
     (11:67) (24:332)

11.   Which of the following are most frequently implicated in the development of nosocomial pulmonary infections?
   A.   Viruses
   B.   Gram-positive bacteria
   C.   Fungi
 — D.   Gram-negative bacteria
   E.   Spores
     (11:67) (31:37–42) (8:408)

12. All of the following organisms have been held responsible for hospital-acquired pulmonary infections. Which is associated with the highest mortality rate?
    - A. *Pseudomonas aeruginosa*
    - B. *Serratia* species
    - C. *Proteus* species
    - D. *Klebsiella pneumoniae*
    - E. *Staphylococcus aureus*
      (31:37–42)

13. Patients with which of the following disorders/conditions should be placed in reverse (protective) isolation?
    - A. Small for gestational age newborns
    - B. *Pseudomonas* pulmonary infections
    - C. Extensive burns
    - D. Tuberculosis
    - E. Meningococcal meningitis
      (2:45)

14. The respiratory therapy practitioner *must* wear which of the following articles when entering the room of a patient who is in respiratory isolation?
    - I. Gown
    - II. Mask
    - III. Gloves
        - A. I and III
        - B. II and III
        - C. I, II, and III
        - D. III only
        - E. II only
          (92:39)

15. The respiratory therapy practitioner should wash his or her hands on entering and leaving the rooms of patients who are in which of the following types of isolation?
    - I. Respiratory
    - II. Enteric
    - III. Wound and skin
    - IV. Strict
        - A. I, II, and III
        - B. I, II, III, and IV
        - C. I, III, and IV
        - D. II, III, and IV
        - E. II and IV
          (92:29, 39, 51, and 61)

16. The respiratory therapy practitioner should be aware that *Mycobacterium tuberculosis* is transmitted to the host primarily by:
    - A. Fomite contamination
    - B. Direct skin-to-skin contact
    - C. Inhalation of contaminated droplets

D.   Handling of infected sputum
E.   Handling of contaminated respiratory therapy equipment
     (2:438)

Answer Key

1. C	4. E	7. B	10. D	13. C
2. E	5. E	8. C	11. D	14. E
3. A	6. E	9. A	12. A	15. B
				16. C

C. Maintain Airway

According to the NBRC, questions in this category are designed to assess the candidate's ability to conduct therapeutic procedures to achieve maintenance of a patent airway. Also assessed is the candidate's knowledge of the care and placement of the various types of artificial airways. *It should be pointed out at this time that humidity therapy is assessed only on the Entry Level Examination and that the technique of endotracheal intubation is assessed only on the Advanced Practitioner Examination.*

Entry Level Pretest

According to the NBRC, 4% of the questions on the Entry Level Examination are from the maintain airway content category. In addition, the Composite Examination Matrix (see reference 80) states that questions in this category assess the candidate's ability to perform the following related tasks:

1.   Maintain adequate humidification (humidity therapy)
2.   Position patient properly to maintain airway patency
3.   Use appropriate oropharyngeal and nasopharyngeal airways
4.   Maintain proper cuff inflation and proper position of endotracheal and tracheostomy tubes within the patient's airway

The following self-study questions were developed from the NBRC Composite Examination Matrix:

1.   Which of the following statements regarding the reported advantages of nasal over orotracheal tubes is (are) true?
     I.   Less skill is required in placement.
     II.   They are preferred whenever long-term intubation is anticipated.
     III. A larger caliber tube may be used.
     IV.   They are generally tolerated better by the patient.
          A.   I, III, and IV
          B.   I, II, and IV
          C.   II only

D.   I, II, and III
E.   II and IV
(1:251–254) (8:93–99)

2. Which of the following is the correct progression of the anatomic structures of the upper airway?
   I.   Vocal cords
   II. Arytenoid cartilage
   III. Oropharynx
   IV. Epiglottis
   V.   Uvula
      A.   III, I, IV, II, and V
      B.   IV, III, II, V, and I
      C.   IV, III, II, I, and V
      D.   III, V, IV, II, and I
      E.   III, IV, II, I, and V
   (1) (25) (7)

3. Which of the following would be the preferred method of maintaining airway patency in an unconscious patient who is not in respiratory distress?
   A.   Nasopharyngeal airway
   B.   Oropharyngeal airway
   C.   Orotracheal intubation
   D.   Nasotracheal intubation
   E.   Transtracheal catheter
   (1:237–238) (25:Chap 4, p 2)

4. Postextubation complications of tracheal intubation include(s):
   I.   Tracheomalacia
   II. Tracheoesophageal fistula
   III. Glottic and subglottic edema
   IV. Mucosal ischemia
   V.   Tracheal stenosis
      A.   I, III, and V
      B.   II, III, and V
      C.   I, IV, and V
      D.   V only
      E.   I and V
   (1:Chap 17)

5. All of the following are pathophysiologic sequelae of the use of high pressure tracheal tube cuffs. Place them in their proper order.
   I.   Mucosal edema
   II. Sloughing of mucosa
   III. Necrosis of cartilaginous tissue
   IV. Ischemia to mucosal tissue
      A.   I, IV, III, and II
      B.   IV, II, I, and III
      C.   I, IV, II, and III

D.   IV, I, III, and II
E.   IV, I, II, and III
(1:289–290)

6. Which of the following complications is *not* believed to be related to the use of high pressure cuffs?
A.   Tracheal dilatation
B.   Tracheal stenosis
C.   Brachiocephalic (innominate) artery erosion
D.   Tracheoesophageal fistula
E.   Cuff herniation
(1:287–293) (32:191–193 and 211)

7. Methods of reducing the incidence of tracheal tube cuff-related side effects include:
I.   Use of pressure-limited cuffs
II.   Use of high residual volume type cuffs
III. Use of Fome type cuffs
IV.   Monitoring of intracuff pressures
A.   I, II, III, and IV
B.   I and III
C.   II, III, and IV
D.   II and IV
E.   I, II, and IV
(1:252–254) (2:521)

8. Which of the following statements regarding tracheal dilatation is (are) true?
I.   It will not occur if low intracuff pressures are used.
II.   It is not associated with positive pressure ventilation.
III. It may result in leakage of tidal gases.
IV.   It may lead to esophageal compression.
A.   I and III
B.   III only
C.   III and IV
D.   II and IV
E.   II and III
(1:292–293)

9. The respiratory therapy practitioner is called to the recovery room. The patient in question is in a deep coma and, according to the anesthesiologist, has no upper airway reflexes. As this patient regains consciousness, which of the following reflexes will return first?
A.   Gag
B.   Tracheal
C.   Carinal
D.   Swallowing
E.   Laryngeal
(1:240)

10. The trachea of the average adult is approximately _____ cm in length.
    A. 7–9 cm
    B. 8–10 cm
    C. 12–14 cm
    D. 14–16 cm
    E. 16–18 cm
    (2)

11. Which of the following is generally considered the route of *first* choice in establishing the emergency airway?
    A. Orotracheal intubation
    B. Nasotracheal intubation
    C. Tracheotomy
    D. Cricothyroidotomy
    E. Transtracheal catheter ventilation
    (1:242–251)

12. All of the following measures tend to minimize the complications associated with the use of endotracheal tubes *except:*
    A. Intubation by experienced personnel only
    B. Selection of correct tube size
    C. Deflation of cuff for 5 minutes every hour
    D. Suctioning both above and below the cuff
    E. Limiting intracuff pressures to 20 cm to 25 cm H_2O
    (31:7–11)

13. The most serious complication resulting from *anterior* tracheal wall necrosis is:
    A. Tracheoesophageal erosion
    B. Esophageal compression
    C. Innominate artery erosion
    D. Tracheoesophageal fistula
    E. C and D are correct.
    (1:256) (2:508) (31:7–11)

14. When using a nasopharyngeal airway, the distal end should:
    A. Be level with the uvula
    B. Be level with the tip of the tongue
    C. Displace the tongue forward, preventing obstruction
    D. Partially open the epiglottis
    E. Become obstructed by the soft palate only during inspiration
    (25:Chap 4, p 3)

15. In general, use of high pressure tracheal tube cuffs is *least* likely to result in which one of the following?
    A. Tracheal ischemia
    B. Tracheal necrosis
    C. Tracheal malacia
    D. Tracheal stenosis
    E. Tracheal aspiration
    (4:Chap 6)

16. Which of the following actions would *not* be performed as part of the procedure of tracheal tube cuff care?
  A. Suctioning below the cuff
  B. Suctioning above the cuff
  C. Deflating the cuff prior to suctioning the upper airways
  D. Deflating the cuff only under pressure so as to direct pooled secretions into the oropharynx
  E. Administering oxygen before and after the procedure
  (103:200–202)

Answer Key

1. E	4. A	7. A	10. C	13. C
2. D	5. C	8. C	11. A	14. C
3. B	6. E	9. C	12. C	15. E
				16. C

Advanced Practitioner Pretest

According to the NBRC, 3% of the questions on the Advanced Practitioner Examination are from the maintain airway content category. In addition, the Composite Examination Matrix (see reference 80) states questions in this category assess the candidate's ability to perform the following related tasks:

1. Select appropriate size endotracheal tubes
2. Perform endotracheal intubation and extubation
3. Change tracheostomy tubes
4. Remove an esophageal obturator airway

The following self-study questions were developed from the NBRC Composite Examination Matrix:

1. Immediate complications of endotracheal intubation may include:
      I. Laryngeal trauma
     II. Iatrogenic hypoxia
    III. Tracheal stenosis
     IV. Endobronchial intubation
      V. Subcutaneous emphysema
        A. I, II, IV, and V
        B. I, II, III, and IV
        C. I, II, III, IV, and V
        D. I, III, and V
        E. I, II, and V
    (25:Chaps 4 through 6) (1:281–286) (36:Chap 8)

2. Endotracheal intubation may facilitate the administration of emergency life support in which of the following ways?
      I. Metabolic acidosis can be successfully treated.
     II. Aspiration pneumonitis may be prevented.

  III. A possible route for sodium bicarbonate administration is assured.

  IV. Ventilation with 100% oxygen may be assured.

   A. I and III

   B. II, III, and IV

   C. II and III

   D. II and IV

   E. I, II, III, and IV

  (25:Chap 4, pp 4–6)

3. In patients with cervical spine trauma, visualization of the larynx during nasotracheal intubation may be aided by:

  I. Flexion of the head and neck

  II. Modified jaw thrust maneuvers

  III. Use of the fiberoptic laryngoscope

  IV. Hyperextension of the head and neck

   A. III only

   B. II only

   C. I and II

   D. I and III

   E. II and III

  (2:760)

4. Which of the following statements about neonatal intubation is (are) true?

  I. It should not be used when CPAP therapy is ordered.

  II. The expiratory grunt mechanism may be abolished.

  III. Cuffed tubes are not employed.

  IV. The tip of the tube should be placed approximately 2 cm from the carina.

   A. I and IV

   B. II only

   C. II and III

   D. II, III, and IV

   E. I, II, and IV

  (1:213–214) (13:153)

5. Which of the following formulas can be used to help the respiratory therapy practitioner select the proper size (internal diameter) endotracheal tube for infants and children (newborn through 16 years of age)?

A. $\dfrac{\text{Age} + \text{Body Weight (kg)}}{\text{Age}} = \text{mm I.D.}$

B. $\dfrac{\text{Vital Capacity} - \text{FRC}}{\text{FRC}} = \text{mm I.D.}$

C. $\dfrac{\text{Age} + \text{Head Circumference}}{\text{Age}} = \text{mm I.D.}$

D. $\dfrac{\text{Age} + 16}{4} = \text{mm I.D.}$

E. $\dfrac{(V_D/V_T) \times (VC)}{Age} = \text{mm I.D.}$

(10:90)

6. Which of the following hazards is not believed to be associated with the use of the esophageal obturator airway?
    A. Low delivered tidal volumes
    B. Esophageal rupture
    C. Aspiration of gastric juice
    D. Tracheal compression
    E. Hyperventilation
    (1:248–250) (25:Chap 4, pp 2–3)

7. Successful orotracheal intubation in the average adult patient is indicated by which of the following?
    I.   Bilateral chest wall movement during inspiration
    II.   The endotracheal tube's 13-cm mark at the patient's gum line
    III. Equal and bilateral breath sounds
        A. I and III
        B. II and III
        C. III only
        D. II only
        E. I, II, and III
    (7:96)

8. Which of the following statements is (are) true regarding endotracheal intubation as a means of establishing the airway during cardiopulmonary resuscitation?
    I.   It should not be attempted by untrained personnel.
    II.   Preoxygenation is not essential if personnel and equipment are immediately available.
    III. It should be performed prior to removal of an esophageal obturator airway.
        A. I only
        B. I and III
        C. II and III
        D. I, II, and III
        E. I and II
    (25:Chap 4, pp 3–4)

9. True statements regarding tracheal intubation using the straight laryngoscope blade include:
    I.   With adults, it is used to lift the epiglottis.
    II.   With newborns, placement in the vallecula is frequently recommended.
    III. Its use is contraindicated in the emergency setting.
    IV.   It is preferred for use on stout, short-necked patients.
        A. I and III
        B. II and III
        C. I, II, and IV

D.   I and II
E.   II, III, and IV
(1:242–247) (25:Chap 4, pp 4–5; Chap 16, pp 4–6)

10. Prompt neonatal intubation and supportive ventilation is indicated by which of the following?
   I.   Presence of unilateral choanal atresia
   II. Apgar score of 0–3
   III. Prolonged periods of apnea
      A.   II only
      B.   III only
      C.   I and II
      D.   II and III
      E.   I, II, and III
   (13:53–55) (29:24–25 and 29–35) (19:88)

11. Which of the following size (I.D.) endotracheal tubes should the respiratory therapy practitioner select for an average-size, 7-year-old child?
   A.   3.5–4.0 mm
   B.   4.5–5.0 mm
   C.   5.5–6.0 mm
   D.   6.5–7.0 mm
   E.   6.0–8.0 mm
   (25)

12. Which of the following statements regarding the anatomy and physiology of the neonatal upper airway as compared with that of the adult is (are) true?
   I.   The tongue is proportionately larger.
   II. The newborn is a nose breather.
   III. The cricoid is the most narrow portion.
      A.   II only
      B.   I, II, and III
      C.   I and II
      D.   II and III
      E.   I and III
   (10:84–85)

13. The respiratory therapy practitioner is monitoring the status of a 9-year-old patient who has just returned from surgery for removal of a large tumor from the left middle lobe. Suddenly, the patient becomes dyspneic. The surgeon is paged and determines that the patient is bleeding profusely into the left lung. He then asks if there is an endotracheal tube that will seal off the left mainstem bronchus and yet allow ventilation of the unaffected lung. The practitioner should supply him with a:
   A.   Reush Trachoflex tube
   B.   Lanz tube
   C.   Hollinger tube
   D.   Carlens tube
   E.   Jackson tube
   (52)

Answer Key

1. A	4. D	7. A	10. D	13. D
2. D	5. D	8. B	11. C	
3. E	6. E	9. D	12. B	

D. Mobilize and Remove Secretions (Entry Level Only)

According to the NBRC, the mobilize and remove secretions category is assessed only on the Entry Level Examination. Questions in this category are designed to assess the candidate's ability to conduct therapeutic procedures to achieve removal of bronchopulmonary secretions. *It must be pointed out at this time that this content category is meant to include not only the more traditional aspects of bronchial hygiene therapy, such as suctioning, aerosol therapy, postural drainage, and percussion, but is also meant to include the administration of pharmacologic agents via the aerosol route.*

Entry Level Pretest

According to the NBRC, 5% of the questions on the Entry Level Examination are from the mobilize and remove secretions content category. In addition, the Composite Examination Matrix (see reference 80) states that questions in this category assess the candidate's ability to perform the following related tasks:

1. Administer prescribed pharmacologic agents (bronchodilators, mucolytics, and anti-inflammatory agents)
2. Perform postural drainage
3. Perform percussion and vibration
4. Suction endotracheal and tracheostomy tubes
5. Perform nasotracheal and orotracheal suctioning
6. Encourage proper coughing techniques

The following self-study questions were developed from the NBRC Composite Examination Matrix:

1. Improving tracheobronchial hygiene is an established clinical goal of which of the following respiratory care modalities?
     I.   Aerosol therapy
     II. IPPB therapy
     III. Sustained maximal inflation therapy (incentive spirometry)
        A. I and III
        B. II and III
        C. I only
        D. I and II
        E. I, II, and III
     (1:226)

2. The strong β_2 activity of isoproterenol has been shown to directly result in which of the following unwanted actions?
    I.   Increased airway smooth muscle tone
    II. Dilatation of the pulmonary vasculature
    III. Systemic arterial hypertension
    IV. Bradyarrhythmias
        A. I and III
        B. II only
        C. II and III
        D. III and IV
        E. I and II
    (2:473)

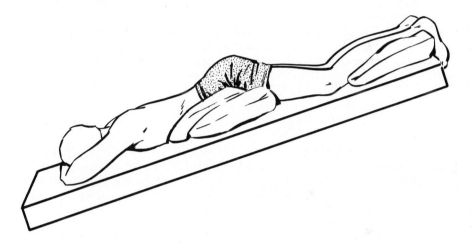

Figure IV-34.

3. The above illustration shows the patient in the prone Trendelenburg's position. In this position, which segment will drain?
    A. Lower lobe, apical basal segment, bilaterally
    B. Lower lobe, medial basal segment, bilaterally
    C. Lower lobe, posterior basal segment, bilaterally
    D. Lower lobe, anterior basal segment, bilaterally
    E. Lower lobe, lateral basal segment, bilaterally
    (7:214)

4. In general, the minimum vital capacity necessary to provide an effective cough is believed to be:
    A. 15 mL/kg
    B. 25 mL/kg
    C. 40 mL/kg
    D. 15 mL/lb.
    E. 45 mL/lb.
    (1:158)

5. Which of the following have been described as complications of airway suctioning?
   I.   Tracheitis
   II. Decreased intracranial pressure
   III. Atelectasis
   IV. Cor pulmonale
      A.   I and III
      B.   II and III
      C.   II, III, and IV
      D.   I, II, and III
      E.   I, II, and IV
   (1:267–268) (2:526–527 and 754–755)

6. Which of the following methods is (are) recommended to reduce the severity of mucosal damage that may complicate airway suctioning?
   I.   Use of catheters with multiple side holes
   II. Not jabbing catheter up and down
   III. Limiting magnitude subatmospheric pressure
   IV. Limiting attempts to a Q shift basis
      A.   I, II, and IV
      B.   I only
      C.   II and III
      D.   I, II, and III
      E.   I and IV
   (1:269) (2:524–527)

7. Which of the following bronchodilators should not be mixed with sodium bicarbonate solutions?
   A.   Terbutaline
   B.   Metaproterenol
   C.   Isoetharine
   D.   A and C are correct.
   E.   All of the above
   (25:Chap 8, pp 3–4) (40)

8. Which of the following catheters is designed to facilitate suctioning of the left mainstem bronchus?
   A.   Whistle tip
   B.   Ring tip
   C.   Coudé
   D.   Multiple side hole tip
   E.   McGill
   (1:269)

9. Which of the following is the *maximum* allowable suction catheter size for use on a patient with a 5-mm I.D. endotracheal tube?
   A.   6 French
   B.   8 French
   C.   10 French
   D.   12 French
   E.   14 French
   (2:524–527)

10. Which two of the following lung segments are the most common sites of retained secretions among hospitalized patients?
    I.   Superior basal
    II. Anterior basal
    III. Lateral basal
    IV. Posterior basal
    V.   Medial basal
       A. I and III
       B. I and IV
       C. II and III
       D. III and IV
       E. III and V
    (1:198-200)

11. Which of the following are side effects of metaproterenol therapy that the respiratory therapy practitioner should be aware of?
    I.   Short duration of action
    II. Tachyarrhythmias
    III. Tremor and nervousness
    IV. Excessive vasopressor activity
       A. II and III
       B. I and III
       C. II, III, and IV
       D. I, II, III, and IV
       E. II and IV
    (2:470-484)

12. Which of the following may be considered contraindications to postural drainage techniques?
    I.   Recent food consumption
    II. Putrid lung abscess
    III. Undrained empyema
    IV. Intracranial hypertension
    V.   Mucosal edema
       A. I and III
       B. II, III, and IV
       C. I, III, and IV
       D. I and V
       E. I, III, and V
    (7:206) (1:202)

13. Prone, a pillow under the patient's abdomen, and the bed flat describes the position for draining:
    A. Basal lobes, apical segment
    B. Basal lobes, posterior segment
    C. Basal lobes, lateral segment
    D. Basal lobes, anterior segments
    E. A and C are correct.
    (7:212)

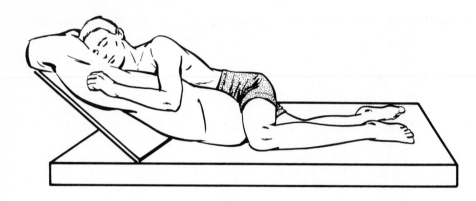

Figure IV-35.

14. The above diagram shows a patient lying on his right side with head at a 30° angle and chest and abdomen at a 45° angle. In this position, which segment will drain?
    A. Upper lobe, posterior segment on the left
    B. Upper lobe, apical segment on the right
    C. Upper lobe, anterior segment on the left
    D. Upper lobe, posterior segment on the right
    E. Upper lobe, apical segment on the left
    (7:211)

15. Which of the following statements about the prone position is (are) true?
    I.   Its use may improve oxygenation.
    II. It should never be used on patients in intensive care units.
    III. It may assist in draining secretions from dependent lung zones.
        A. I and III
        B. II and III
        C. I only
        D. I and II
        E. II only
    (1:198–201) (7:206–210)

16. In patients with extrinsic asthma, cromolyn sodium has been shown to:
    I.   Reduce the frequency of allergic asthmatic episodes
    II. Reduce the need for systemic corticosteroids
    III. Treat acute bronchospasm
        A. I and III
        B. II and III
        C. I and II
        D. II only
        E. I, II, and III
    (2:488–489)

17. Which of the following bronchodilators might the respiratory therapy practitioner recommend for use by asthmatics because of a long duration of action?
    I. Isoproterenol
    II. Metaproterenol
    III. Terbutaline
    IV. Isoetharine
    A. I only
    B. II and III
    C. II, III, and IV
    D. II and IV
    E. I and III
    (2:476–477)

18. Which of the following statements regarding the bronchospasm that may accompany administration of acetylcysteine is (are) true?
    I. It may be preventable through concurrent administration of a bronchodilator.
    II. It is the least important of acetylcysteine's side effects.
    III. It is caused by its sympatholytic activity.
    A. I only
    B. II and III
    C. I, II, and III
    D. I and II
    E. II only
    (2:464) (1:221)

19. A respiratory therapy practitioner positions a patient on his back, one-quarter turn to the left side with the foot of the bed elevated 12 inches. The pulmonary segment being drained is:
    A. Right middle lobe
    B. Anterior segment, right basal lobe
    C. Medial segment, right basal lobe
    D. Lateral segment, right basal lobe
    E. Posterior segment, right basal lobe
    (7:209)

20. The physician wants his patient to receive 0.40 cc metaproterenol diluted with 2.5 cc normal saline (N.S.). The respiratory therapy practitioner in charge of this patient's home care program would have the patient use which of the following household measurements?
    A. Four drops metaproterenol and one teaspoon N.S.
    B. Six drops metaproterenol and one-half teaspoon N.S.
    C. Four drops metaproterenol and one-half teaspoon N.S.
    D. Six drops metaproterenol and one-third tablespoon N.S.
    E. B and D are correct.
    (53) (54)

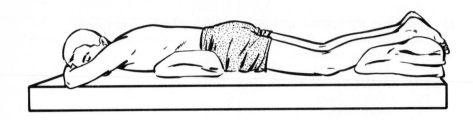

Figure IV-36.

21. The above diagram shows the patient in a prone position with a pillow under the abdomen and ankles. In this position, what segment will drain?
    A. Upper lobe, apical segments bilaterally
    B. Upper lobe, anterior segments bilaterally
    C. Lingula, superior lobe, on the left
    D. Lower lobe, apical segment bilaterally
    E. Lower lobe, posterior-basal segment bilaterally
    (7:213)

22. Which of the following are recommended methods for determining the location of pulmonary infiltrates for purposes of drainage?
    I.   Patient historical data
    II. Bedside physical examination
    III. Analysis of pulmonary angiography
    IV. Chest roentgenograms
    V.   Arterial blood gas analysis
        A. I and III
        B. II and IV
        C. III and V
        D. II and V
        E. I and IV
    (2:682)

23. The respiratory therapy practitioner is asked to perform chest physical therapy on a patient with multiple lung abscesses. On reviewing chest films and other pertinent data, the practitioner notes the presence of consolidation throughout both lung fields apically and basally. The practitioner should drain these segments in which order?
    A. Basal segments first, then middle segments, and apical segments last
    B. Right lung field first, left lung field last
    C. Apical segments first, then middle segments, and basal segments last
    D. Apical segments first, then basal segments, and middle segments last
    E. Basal segments first, then apical segments, and middle segments last
    (2:682)

24. In which of the following conditions is chest physical therapy usually considered an essential part of the therapeutic regimen?
   I.   Cystic fibrosis
   II. Adult respiratory distress syndrome
   III. Myasthenia gravis
   IV. Lung abscess
   V.   Bronchiolitis
      A. II and IV
      B. I and IV
      C. III and IV
      D. I and II
      E. II and III
   (13:117–122) (11:71–73) (1:202)

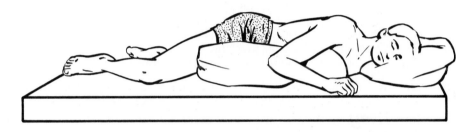

Figure IV-37.

25. The above diagram shows the patient lying on his left side with the right leg ahead of the left. In this position, which segment will drain?
   A. Upper lobe, anterior segment on the right
   B. Lower lobe, posterior-basal segment on the right
   C. Upper lobe, apical-posterior segment on the left
   D. Upper lobe, posterior segment on the right
   E. Lingula, superior segment
      (7:210)

26. Recommended levels of subatmospheric suctioning pressure in adult and pediatric populations include:
   I.   Adult: 100–180 mm Hg
   II. Pediatric: 60–80 mm Hg
   III. Adult: 80–160 mm Hg
   IV. Pediatric: 60–120 mm Hg
   V.   Adult: 80–120 mm Hg
   VI. Pediatric: 40–120 mm Hg
      A. II and III
      B. I and II
      C. II and V
      D. I and VI
      E. V and VI
   (56) (1:269)

27. Which of the following statements regarding racemic epinephrine is (are) true?
    I.   It may be indicated in the treatment of croup.
    II. It may be indicated in the treatment of adult respiratory distress syndrome.
    III. It possesses a strong decongestant action.
    IV. It is a more potent bronchodilator than isoproterenol.
        A. II and III
        B. I and III
        C. I and IV
        D. III and IV
        E. I only
    (2:473)

28. Select the false statement about metaproterenol.
    A. Central nervous system side effects may be noted.
    B. It is completely free of β_1 side effects.
    C. Duration of action is relatively long.
    D. Oral preparations are available.
    E. It is useful in relieving acute bronchospasm.
    (2:476–477)

Answer Key

1. E	7. E	13. A	19. A	25. D
2. B	8. C	14. A	20. B	26. C
3. C	9. C	15. A	21. D	27. B
4. A	10. B	16. C	22. B	28. B
5. A	11. A	17. B	23. C	
6. D	12. C	18. A	24. B	

E. Ensure Ventilation

Questions in this category are designed to assess the candidate's ability to conduct therapeutic procedures that will help the patient achieve adequate, spontaneous, and artificial ventilation. A major goal of this content category is to assess the candidate's understanding of the physiologic basis, indications, contraindications, and hazards of intermittent positive pressure breathing (IPPB) therapy and continuous mechanical ventilatory therapy.

Entry Level Pretest

According to the NBRC, 5% of the questions on the Entry Level Examination are from the ensure ventilation content category. In addition, the Composite Examination Matrix (see reference 80) states that questions in this category assess the candidate's ability to perform the following related tasks on an entry level:

1. Instruct and monitor techniques of incentive spirometry
2. Initiate and adjust IPPB therapy
3. Initiate and adjust continuous mechanical ventilation to maintain adequate alveolar ventilation
4. Initiate and adjust IMV and SIMV to maintain adequate alveolar ventilation.

The following self-study questions were developed from the NBRC Composite Examination Matrix:

1. The respiratory therapy practitioner is asked to initiate mechanical ventilation on a woman who is 5 feet, 3 inches tall and weighs 220 pounds. Select the appropriate delivered tidal volume for this patient.
   A.   300 mL
   B.   400 mL
   C.   600 mL
   D.   1000 mL
   E.   1200 mL
      (25:Chap 15, p 2)

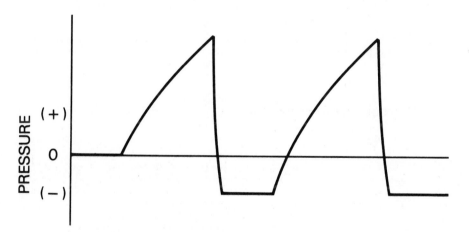

Figure IV-38.

2. The above pressure waveform is best described by which of the following terms?
   A.   ZEEP
   B.   PEEP
   C.   NEEP

D.   EPAP
E.   ZPAP
    (70:517)

3. Which of the following are true regarding the hyperventilation
    that can complicate IPPB therapy?
    I.   Symptoms include dizziness and tingling of extremities.
    II.   It is a rare side effect.
    III. It can usually be prevented through proper patient instruc-
          tion.
    IV.   It is never a serious hazard.
        A.   I, III, and IV
        B.   II and IV
        C.   I, II, and III
        D.   I and III
        E.   I, II, and IV
    (2:571) (1:189–190)

4. The physician's order for IPPB should *not* specify which one of the
    following?
    A. FIo_2
    B.   Ventilator flow rate
    C.   Ventilator sensitivity
    D.   Drugs to be administered
    E.   B and C are correct.
    (2:578)

5. Which of the following is invariably considered to be an absolute
    contraindication for IPPB therapy?
    A.   Active tuberculosis
    B.   Hemoptysis
    C.   Untreated tension pneumothorax
    D.   Pulmonary emphysema
    E.   Postoperative atelectasis
    (1:192)

6. Which of the following statements regarding the use of expiratory
    retard maneuvers used in conjunction with IPPB therapy is (are)
    true?
    I.   A clinical goal is to prevent airtrapping.
    II.   It is believed to decrease expiratory airway resistance.
    III. It may result in a decrease in venous return.
        A.   I and III
        B.   II and III
        C.   I, II, and III
        D.   I and II
        E.   I only
    (54:224)

7. Which of the following are established clinical goals of IPPB therapy?
   I.   Deliver aerosolized medication
   II. Improve bronchial hygiene
   III. Provide long-term improvement in arterial blood gas abnormalities
   IV. Prevent the need for intubation and mechanical ventilation
      A. II and IV
      B. I and IV
      C. I, II, and IV
      D. II and III
      E. I, II, III, and IV
    (2:555–567) (1:186–188)

8. The primary use of sustained maximal inspiratory therapy (incentive spirometry) is to:
   A. Treat atelectasis
   B. Mobilize secretions
   C. Decrease the work of breathing
   D. Prevent atelectasis
   E. Maintain normal blood gases
    (1:196)

9. When used for the administration of continuous ventilatory support, pressure-cycled ventilators may have which of the following disadvantages?
   I.   Volume delivery may be unreliable.
   II. Precise FIo_2 administration may require equipment modification.
   III. They are generally more expensive than volume-cycled ventilators.
   IV. They cannot be adapted to include exhaled tidal volume monitors.
      A. I and II
      B. I and IV
      C. II, III, and IV
      D. I, II, and IV
      E. II only
    (2:589–591)

10. Which of the following I:E ratios would be most preferable for a patient with neurologic trauma who is receiving continuous ventilatory support?
   A. 2:1
   B. 1:1
   C. 1:1.5
   D. 1:2
   E. 1:3
    (2:753–754)

11. Hand-held, unpressurized nebulizers are an effective and efficient means of administering adrenergic bronchodilators. Their use over that of positive pressure devices (IPPB) may be encouraged in all but which one of the following cases?
     A. Patients with intrinsic asthma
     B. Patients with abdominal distention
     C. Patients with severely diminished pulmonary reserves
     D. Patients who have had thoracic surgery
     E. Patients who have received IPPB in previous hospitalization
     (1:187–188)

12. The volume of anatomic deadspace in a healthy 100-kg adult is believed to be:
     A. 100 mL
     B. 220 mL
     C. 150 mL
     D. 250 mL
     E. 300 mL
     (5:73)

13. Which of the following is *not* an example of pulmonary baro-trauma that may result from the administration of continuous ventilatory support?
     A. Subcutaneous emphysema
     B. Tension pneumothorax
     C. Pulmonary interstitial edema
     D. Cardiovascular depression
     E. Mediastinal emphysema
     (1:386–388)

14. Which of the following are recognized as hazards of IPPB therapy?
     I.   Cerebral hypotension
     II.   Oxygen-induced hypoventilation
     III. Pulmonary barotrauma
     IV.   Bacterial cross-contamination
     V.   Fluid overload
          A. I, III, and IV
          B. II and III
          C. I, II, IV, and V
          D. II, III, and IV
          E. II, III, IV, and V
     (1:182 and 189–191)

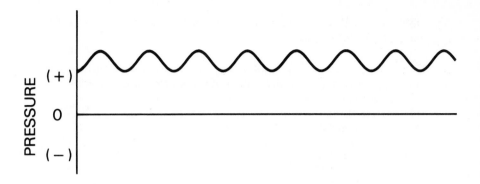

Figure IV-39.

15. The above pressure waveform is most accurately described by
     which of the following terms?
     A. NEEP
     B. ZEEP
     C. PEEP
     D. CPAP
     E. EPAP
     (79:518)

Answer Key

1. C	4. E	7. C	10. E	13. D
2. C	5. C	8. D	11. C	14. D
3. D	6. C	9. A	12. B	15. D

Advanced Practitioner Pretest

According to the NBRC, 7% of the questions on the Advanced Practitioner Examination are from the ensure ventilation category. In addition, the Composite Examination Matrix (see reference 80) states that
questions in this category assess the candidate's ability to perform the
following related tasks on an advanced practitioner level:

1. Select the appropriate mechanical ventilator
2. Initiate and adjust continuous mechanical ventilation to provide
    adequate alveolar ventilation
3. Initiate and adjust IMV and SIMV to achieve adequate alveolar
    ventilation

The following self-study questions were developed from the NBRC Composite Examination Matrix:

1. Rapid reduction in Pa_{CO_2} following initiation of continuous ventilatory support may result in which of the following disorders?
    I.   Convulsions
    II. Arrhythmias
    III. Iatrogenic alkalosis
        A. II and III
        B. I, II, and III
        C. I and III
        D. I and II
        E. II only
    (7:167)

2. Which of the following disorders/conditions is (are) known to lead to increases in physiologic deadspace?
    I.   Acute decreases in cardiac output
    II. Use of positive pressure ventilation
    III. Pulmonary emphysema
        A. I and III
        B. II and III
        C. I and II
        D. I, II, and III
        E. II only
    (5:186)

3. Which of the following methods has (have) been recommended to minimize the cardiovascular side effects of positive pressure ventilation?
    I.   Use of IMV and SIMV
    II. Maintenance of inverse I:E ratios
    III. Trendelenburg positioning
    IV. Appropriate volume expansion
        A. I, II , and IV
        B. II, III, and IV
        C. II and IV
        D. I only
        E. I and IV
    (1:334–335) (2:602–603) (7:166)

4. Which of the following statements is (are) true about the use of mechanical deadspace?
    I.   It is used to correct alveolar hyperventilation.
    II. It acts by decreasing minute alveolar ventilation.
    III. Its use in conjunction with IMV is recommended.
    IV. It will not affect ventilator tubing compliance.
        A. II and III
        B. II and IV
        C. I only

    D. I, II, III, and IV
    E. I, II, and III
  (1:351–352) (39:22–23) (50)

5. Which of the following are reported advantages of IMV?
    I. Weaning may be enhanced.
    II. Carbon dioxide homeostasis may be facilitated.
    III. Cardiovascular depression may be minimized.
    IV. It allows for use of much lower FIo_2s.
      A. II and IV
      B. II, III, and IV
      C. I, II, and IV
      D. I, II, and III
      E. I and III
  (2:599–601) (1:339–341)

6. Which of the following statements regarding ventilator external circuit compliance is (are) true?
    I. Compliance may decrease as humidifier water volume decreases.
    II. Values less than 1.0 cc/cm H_2O are often advisable in neonatal circuits.
    III. Values are generally improved by the use of thick-walled tubing.
      A. I and III
      B. II and III
      C. III only
      D. II only
      E. I only
  (4:12–13) (50) (43) (39:22–23)

7. Which of the following is (are) most likely to occur when negative end-expiratory pressure (NEEP) is applied to the patient's airways during expiration?
    I. Decrease in venous return
    II. Reduction in small airway caliber
    III. Increase in intracranial pressure
    IV. Decrease in intrathoracic pressure
      A. II and IV
      B. II and III
      C. II only
      D. I and III
      E. I, II, aı.d III
  (2:592)

8. Most modern volume ventilators are capable of producing a ventilatory pattern that incorporates an end inspiratory pause. Which of the following statements regarding the clinical use of this technique is (are) true?
    I. It may improve V/Q relationships.
    II. It may alter I:E ratios.

III.   It must be used with caution to prevent cardiovascular depression.
IV.   It should not be used on patients with abnormal pulmonary compliance.
    A.   I and II
    B.   II and IV
    C.   I, II, and III
    D.   II, III, and IV
    E.   II only
   (1:358–359) (24:290–291)

9. All of the following modalities have been advocated as means of preventing postoperative atelectasis. Which of these will most likely lead to increases in the mean intrathoracic pressure?
   I.   IPPB
   II.   Incentive spirometry
   III. CO_2 rebreathing techniques
   IV.   Use of blow bottles
    A.   I and IV
    B.   IV only
    C.   I, II, and IV
    D.   I and II
    E.   I and III
   (1:193–196 and 321–325) (2:539–541 and 557–559)

10. Which of the following has (have) been implicated in the formation of positive water balance in mechanically ventilated patients?
   I.   Decreased levels of antidiuretic hormone
   II.   Increased levels of antidiuretic hormone
   III.   Abnormal renal perfusion
    A.   I and III
    B.   II only
    C.   I and II
    D.   I only
    E.   II and III
   (7:167) (1:389) (31:30–31)

11. Mechanical hyperventilation may be used therapeutically to:
   I.   Decrease intracranial pressure
   II.   Prevent patient "fighting" of the ventilator
   III.   Aid the management of chronic metabolic acidosis
   IV.   Reduce the urine output
    A.   I, III, and IV
    B.   I and IV
    C.   II and IV
    D.   I, II, and III
    E.   II, III, and IV
   (2:753) (25:Chap 15, p 12) (1:338–339)

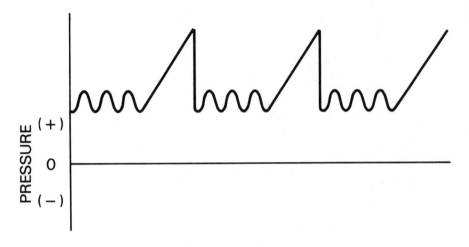

Figure IV-40.

12. The above pressure waveform may be most accurately described by which of the following terms?
     A. CPAP
     B. PEEP
     C. IMV with PEEP
     D. EPAP
     E. NEEP
        (70:518)

13. Which of the following would generally be considered indications for continuous mechanical ventilation for the newborn?
     I.   Prolonged apnea
     II. Pa_{O_2} of 40 mm Hg on 50% oxygen
     III. Pa_{O_2} of 40 mm Hg on 12 cm H_2O CPAP and 80% oxygen
     IV. Pa_{CO_2} of 60 mm Hg on 30% oxygen

          A. II, III, and IV
          B. I and IV
          C. I, III, and IV
          D. I, II, and III
          E. I, II, III, and IV
        (29:205–210)

14. Which of the following will most likely result when a 5% carbon dioxide and 95% oxygen mixture is administered to a 35-year-old postoperative patient?
     I.   Cerebral vasoconstriction
     II.   Hyperpnea
     III. Arterial hypocarbia
     IV.   Increased tidal volume

    A. II and IV
    B. III and IV
    C. III only
    D. I and III
    E. I, II, and IV
    (3:298)

15. Fluid retention is a reported side effect of continuous mechanical ventilation. This phenomenon may lead to which of the following pulmonary changes?
    I. Widened $P(A-a)_{O_2}$
    II. Increased effective static compliance
    III. Decreased lung volumes
    IV. Decreased V_D/V_T
    A. I and III
    B. II and III
    C. III and IV
    D. II and IV
    E. IV only
    (7:167)

16. Which of the following patient groups has (have) demonstrated an increased incidence of gastrointestinal complications during continuous ventilatory support?
    I. Those receiving systemic corticosteroid therapy
    II. Those with preexisting gastrointestinal disorders
    III. Those receiving prophylactic antacid therapy
    A. II only
    B. I and II
    C. II and III
    D. III only
    E. I and III
    (1:388–389) (7:168–169)

17. Widely accepted physiologic indications for continuous mechanical ventilation include:
    I. Vital capacity less than 10–15 mL/kg
    II. Negative inspiratory force less than 50 cm H_2O
    III. V_D/V_T greater than 0.6
    IV. $P(A-a)_{O_2}$ greater than 200 mm Hg (on 100% O_2)
    V. Pa_{CO_2} greater than 60 mm Hg in patients with chronic obstructive pulmonary disease
    A. I and III
    B. II and III
    C. I, III, and IV
    D. II, IV, and V
    E. I, II, III, and IV
    (7:78) (38:60) (11:231)

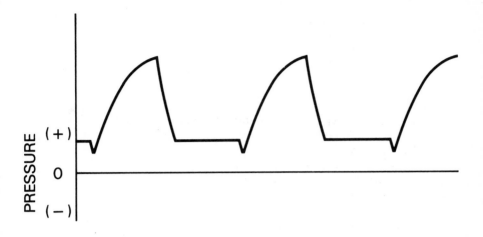

Figure IV-41.

18. The above pressure waveform is most accurately described by which of the following terms?
    A. PEEP with IMV
    B. PEEP with SIMV
    C. PEEP with EPAP
    D. PEEP/assist mode
    E. PEEP with CPAP
    (70:518)

19. Controlling mechanical ventilation through the use of skeletal muscle paralysis is an accepted part of the management of respiratory failure secondary to which of the following disorders?
    A. Drug overdose
    B. Myasthenia gravis
    C. Flail chest
    D. Cardiogenic pulmonary edema
    E. Chronic obstructive pulmonary disease
    (11:214–215) (1:504–505)

20. Which of the following must be known to calculate the physiologic deadspace to tidal volume ratio (V_D/V_T)?
    I.   Minute ventilation
    II.   Anatomic deadspace
    III. Pa_{CO_2}
    IV.   Respiratory rate
    V. $P\bar{E}_{CO_2}$
        A. III and V
        B. I, II, and IV
        C. I, II, III, and IV

D.   III, IV, and V
E.   I, II, III, IV, and V
(5:Chap 8)

Answer Key

1. B	5. D	9. A	13. C	17. A
2. D	6. B	10. E	14. A	18. D
3. E	7. A	11. D	15. A	19. C
4. C	8. C	12. C	16. B	20. A

F.   Ensure Oxygenation

Questions in this category are designed to assess the candidate's ability to conduct therapeutic procedures necessary to achieve adequate arterial and tissue oxygenation. It must be pointed out that the questions on the Advanced Practitioner Examination are concerned with ensuring adequate oxygenation through the use of respiratory waveform manipulation maneuvers such as PEEP and CPAP.

Entry Level Pretest

According to the NBRC, 5% of the questions on the Entry Level Examination are from the ensure oxygenation category. In addition, the Composite Examination Matrix (see reference 80) states that questions in this category assess the candidate's ability to perform the following related tasks on an entry level:

1.   Administer oxygen (on or off the ventilator) to treat hypoxia
2.   Administer PEEP and/or CPAP therapy
3.   Initiate and adjust combinations of IMV, SIMV, and PEEP therapy
4.   Prevent iatrogenic hypoxemia (oxygenate before and after suctioning and equipment changes)
5.   Position the patient to prevent hypoxemia

The following self-study questions were developed from the NBRC Composite Examination Matrix:

1.   In a healthy, resting, adult subject at sea level, the content of oxygen in the arterial blood (Ca_{O_2}) is approximately:
A.   5 vol%
B.   10 vol%

C.   15 vol%
D.   20 vol%
E.   25 vol%
(5:83–84)

2. Which of the following are associated with anatomic shunting?
    I.   Transposition of the great vessels
    II.   Atelectasis and pneumonia
    III. The bronchial and pleural circulations
    IV.   Adult respiratory distress snydrome
       A.   I and IV
       B.   II and IV
       C.   I, II, and IV
       D.   I and III
       E.   II, III, and IV
    (1:189–190)

3. The respiratory therapy practitioner is caring for a patient who has a severe left-sided infiltrate. Positioning the patient on the unaffected side would most likely lead to which of the following?
    I.   Drainage of involved segment
    II.   Worsening Pa_{O_2}
    III. Improvement of V/Q relationships
    IV.   Increasing Pa_{O_2}
       A.   I and II
       B.   II only
       C.   IV only
       D.   I, III, and IV
       E.   I and IV
    (1:88–92) (5:189) (32:213)

4. When the respiratory therapy practitioner is analyzing the oxygen concentration being administered to an infant who is in an Isolette or oxygen hood, he should:
    I.   Analyze as close to the proximal airway as possible
    II.   Ask the nurse to chart the FI_{O_2} for him
    III. Note only the liter flow in his charting
    IV.   Perform analysis at least every day
       A.   I, II, and IV
       B.   I only
       C.   II and III
       D.   I and IV
       E.   I and III
    (13:78–80) (10:Chap 1)

5. Which of the following is the primary physiologic effect of PEEP and CPAP therapy?
    A.   Increase in cardiac output
    B.   Decrease in Pa_{CO_2}
    C.   Increase in anatomic deadspace

D. Increase in functional residual capacity
E. Decrease in urine output
(29:207)

6. Which of the following neonatal disorders are believed to be the result of the toxic effects of oxygen?
    I.   Bronchopulmonary dysplasia
    II.   Infant respiratory distress syndrome
    III. Retrolental fibroplasia
    IV.   Asphyxia neonatorum
       A. II and IV
       B. I and II
       C. I, III, and IV
       D. I, II, and III
       E. I and III
    (29:194–195) (13:81–82)

7. Which of the following conditions is (are) known to cause intra-pulmonary (right-to-left) shunting?
    I.   Sarcoidosis
    II.   Left ventricular failure
    III. Ventricular septal defects
    IV.   Adult respiratory distress syndrome
       A. I, III, and IV
       B. II and IV
       C. II only
       D. III and IV
       E. I only
    (5:188–190)

8. Which of the following statements regarding the administration of helium and oxygen mixtures is (are) true?
    I.   It is usually indicated in the management of acute restrictive disorders.
    II.   Low gas density may decrease the work of breathing.
    III. It should not be used on patients prone to airtrapping.
    IV.   It is of particular benefit when used as a vehicle for medical aerosols.
       A. I and IV
       B. III and IV
       C. I, II, and IV
       D. II only
       E. II and III
    (3:295–298)

9. In which of the following conditions may the administration of hyperbaric oxygen be indicated?
    I.   Carbon monoxide poisoning
    II.   Diaphragmatic hernia
    III. Gas gangrene infections

A. I and II
B. I only
C. III only
D. I and III
E. I, II, and III
(2:395)

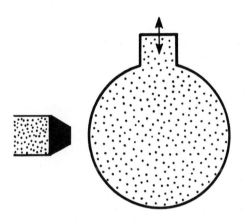

Figure IV-42.

10. The above illustration:
    A. Shows a shunt unit
    B. Shows a deadspace unit
    C. Shows a normal unit
    D. Shows a silent unit
    E. None of the above
    (5:66)

11. The most efficient mechanism the body has to compensate for arterial hypoxemia is:
    A. Pulmonary vasoconstriction
    B. Increased peripheral vascular resistance
    C. Increased cardiac output
    D. Cerebral vasodilation
    E. Increased minute ventilation
    (5:92)

12. The environmental temperature range in which the newborn's oxygen consumption is lowest refers to which of the following?
    A. Thermal neutral zone
    B. Homeothermic zone
    C. Thermoregulatory zone
    D. Hypothermic zone
    E. Internal temperature gradient zone
    (29:97–98)

13. Which of the following are common clinical goals of oxygen therapy?
  I.   To improve alveolar ventilation
  II. To reduce pulmonary workloads
  III. To reduce myocardial workloads
  IV. To increase urine output
    A. II and IV
    B. I and III
    C. II and III
    D. IV only
    E. III and IV
  (1:133–134 and 144–147) (7:119)

14. Which of the following statements regarding oxygen administration is *not* true?
    A. It will frequently decrease cardiopulmonary workloads necessary to maintain a given Pa_{O_2}.
    B. Administration is known to result in hypoventilation.
    C. It cannot correct hypoxemia due to hypoventilation.
    D. It may not be successful in treating hypoxemia due to shunting.
    E. Low concentrations are frequently useful in treating hypoxemia accompanying chronic obstructive pulmonary disease.
      (5:Chap 15) (1:Chap 7) (2:241–242 and 394–395) (32:64–66)

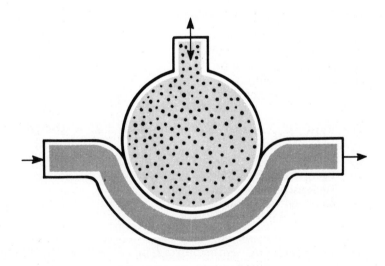

Figure IV-43.

15. The above diagram illustrates:
    A. A shunt unit
    B. A normal alveolar unit

    C. A silent unit
    D. A deadspace unit
    E. None of the above
    (5:66)

16. Which position is associated with the highest Pa_{O_2} among populations with normal lungs?
    A. Supine
    B. Upright (erect)
    C. Low Fowler's
    D. High Fowler's
    E. Prone Trendelenburg
    (2:236)

17. Which of the following will enhance the tendency of oxygen to dissociate from the hemoglobin molecule at the tissue level?
    I. Acidosis
    II. Hypocarbia
    III. Hyperthermia
        A. II and III
        B. I only
        C. I and II
        D. I, II, and III
        E. I and III
    (5:81–88) (3:104–112) (2:237–238)

18. Tissue hypoxia will most frequently lead to which one of the following disorders?
    A. Cardiogenic shock
    B. Lactic acidosis
    C. Hypercapnia
    D. Cor pulmonale
    E. Metabolic alkalosis
    (5:49–51 and 96)

19. In a healthy, resting, adult subject at sea level, the content of oxygen in mixed venous blood ($C\bar{v}_{O_2}$) is approximately:
    A. 5 vol%
    B. 10 vol%
    C. 15 vol%
    D. 20 vol%
    E. 25 vol%
    (3:108)

20. The primary therapeutic goal of PEEP therapy is to:
    A. Improve pulmonary compliance
    B. Decrease pulmonary extravascular water
    C. Increase the oxygen tension of the arterial blood
    D. Improve oxygen tissue transport
    E. Decrease the Q_S/Q_T
    (46) (47)

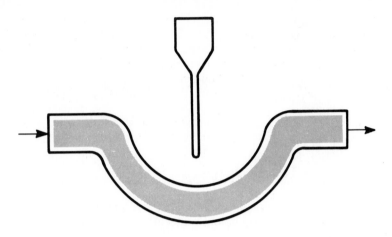

Figure IV-44.

21. The above illustration shows:
     A. A shunt unit
     B. A deadspace unit
     C. A silent unit
     D. A normal unit
     E. None of the above
         (5:66)

22. Hypoxemia due to diffusion defects is associated with which of the
     following conditions?
     A. Chronic bronchitis
     B. Bronchial asthma
     C. Sarcoidosis
     D. Barbiturate overdose
     E. Myasthenia gravis
         (2:241, 394, and 705)

The next two questions refer to the following illustration:

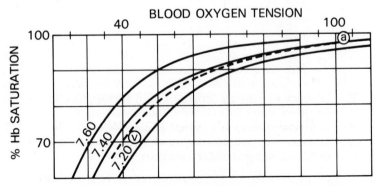

Figure IV-45.

23. In the above illustration, a dashed line is used to represent the change in blood pH that accompanies tissue oxygenation. Which of the following statements regarding this physiologic shift in the oxyhemoglobin dissociation curve is (are) true?
    I.   It is known as the Haldane effect.
    II. It is known to enhance the unloading of oxygen at the tissue level.
    III. It is associated with a decrease in blood P_{50}.
    IV. It represents a decrease in the affinity of hemoglobin for oxygen.
    A. I and III
    B. I, III, and IV
    C. III only
    D. III and IV
    E. II and IV
    (3:127)

24. Which of the following is *least* likely to cause the oxyhemoglobin dissociation curve to shift to the right?
    A. Hyperthermia
    B. Acidosis
    C. Decreased red blood cell 2–3 diphosphoglycerate
    D. Hypercarbia
    E. A and C are correct.
    (3:127)

25. Recognized hazards of PEEP therapy include which of the following?
    I.   Cardiovascular embarrassment
    II. Microatelectasis
    III. Pulmonary barotrauma
    IV. Arterial hypertension
    A. I and III
    B. II and IV
    C. IV only
    D. II and III
    E. I, III, and IV
    (1:373–374) (2:602–603)

26. Which of the following statements regarding pulmonary oxygen toxicity is *not* true?
    A. It is the PI_{O_2}, not the FI_{O_2}, that is causative.
    B. The duration of exposure is a critical factor.
    C. Prevention usually consists of lowering FI_{O_2} to 0.4 as rapidly as possible.
    D. One may safely administer 100% oxygen for up to 96 hours.
    E. It may contribute to adult respiratory distress syndrome.
    (1:147–152) (2:383–393)

27. Which of the following statements represent(s) indications for PEEP therapy?
    I.   Treat refractory hypoxemia

    II.   Enhance ventilator weaning
   III. Allow reductions of FI_{O_2} to nontoxic levels
      A. I only
      B. II and III
      C. I and III
      D. I, II, and III
      E. II only
   (46)

28. Which of the following statements is (are) true regarding indications for CPAP therapy?
     I.   Enhance ventilator weaning
    II.   Treat refractory hypoxemia
   III. Provide more effective alveolar ventilation
   IV. Allow for administration of nontoxic levels of oxygen
      A. I and II
      B. I, II, and IV
      C. II and III
      D. III and IV
      E. IV only
   (1:325 and 384) (29:207–210)

29. Which of the following types of hemoglobin is unable to combine physically with oxygen?
   A. Fetal
   B. Adult
   C. Carboxyhemoglobin
   D. Methemoglobin
   E. C and D are correct.
   (2:239)

30. The peripheral chemoreceptors differ from their central counterparts in which of the following respects?
     I.   They alone are stimulated by hypoxemia.
    II.   They are not stimulated by hypercapnia.
   III. They normally contribute only a fraction of the alveolar ventilation.
   IV. They alone are stimulated by acidosis.
      A. III only
      B. I and III
      C. II and III
      D. I only
      E. I and II
   (2:203)

31. Patients who have longstanding chronic obstructive pulmonary disease are sometimes placed on continuous home oxygen therapy. Which of the following should be present for the patient to derive substantial benefit from this expensive mode of therapy?
   A. Ventilation-perfusion mismatch
   B. Severe pulmonary hypertension
   C. A 40 packs/year smoking history

D.   Hypercarbia
E.   Compensated respiratory acidosis
(11:182–183) (1:489)

32. Which of the following should be monitored immediately after placing a patient on PEEP therapy?
A. Pa_{O_2}
B. FEV_1
C.   Effective static compliance
D. $P(A-a)_{O_2}$
E.   Arterial blood pressure
(6:131)

33. The so-called optimum therapeutic level of PEEP is most accurately defined as that which corresponds to:
A.   The highest Pa_{O_2}
B.   The lowest Q_S/Q_T
C.   The highest functional residual capacity
D.   The highest oxygen tissues transport
E.   The lowest effective static compliance
(46) (47)

Answer Key

1. D	8. D	15. B	22. C	29. D
2. D	9. D	16. B	23. E	30. B
3. D	10. B	17. E	24. C	31. B
4. B	11. C	18. B	25. A	32. E
5. D	12. A	19. C	26. D	33. D
6. E	13. C	20. D	27. C	
7. B	14. C	21. A	28. B	

Advanced Practitioner Pretest

According to the NBRC, 3% of the questions on the Advanced Practitioner Examination are from the ensure oxygenation category. In addition, the Composite Matrix (see reference 80) states that questions in this category assess the candidate's ability to perform the following related tasks on an advanced practitioner level:

1. Initiate and adjust PEEP and CPAP therapy to treat hypoxia
2. Initiate and adjust combinations of IMV, SIMV, and PEEP therapy to treat hypoxia

The following self-study questions were developed from the NBRC Composite Examination Matrix:

1. Which of the following statements regarding CPAP therapy are true?
I.   Physiologic effects are similar to those of PEEP.
II. It is sometimes used as an adjunct to ventilator weaning.

III.   Ability to maintain a normal Paco$_2$ is a contraindication.
IV.   Cardiovascular embarrassment is not a hazard.
    A.   II and IV
    B.   I and IV
    C.   III and IV
    D.   I and II
    E.   I, II, III, and IV
(29:207–210) (13:153) (1:325, 384, and 452–453)

2.   Indications for continuous positive airway pressure (CPAP) therapy in the newborn would include which of the following?
    I.   Pao$_2$ of 40 mm Hg on 35% oxygen
    II.   Paco$_2$ of 80 mm Hg on 21% oxygen
    III.   Pao$_2$ of 40 mm Hg and Paco$_2$ of 50 mm Hg on 80% oxygen
    IV.   Pao$_2$ of 40 mm Hg on 70% oxygen
        A.   I, II, and III
        B.   I and IV
        C.   IV only
        D.   II and IV
        E.   III and IV
(29:205–210)

3.   Which of the following statements is (are) true regarding increases in venous admixture that may result when excessive levels of PEEP are administered?
    I.   They are believed to be the result of increases in cardiac output.
    II.   They may occur if blood flow is redistributed to nonventilated lung units.
    III.   Their occurrence is related to the existence of nonuniformly distributed lung pathology.
        A.   I and III
        B.   II only
        C.   II and III
        D.   III only
        E.   I only
(46:4) (1:374)

4.   Methods of treating hypoxemia that is unresponsive to oxygen administration include which of the following?
    I.   PEEP
    II.   Use of large mechanical tidal volumes
    III.   NEEP
    IV.   Supine positioning
        A.   I and III
        B.   I and II
        C.   II, III, and IV
        D.   II and IV
        E.   I only
(47)

5. Which of the following statements about CPAP therapy is (are) true?
   I.   It is synonymous with the term CPPV.
   II. It will frequently narrow the $P(A-a)_{O_2}$.
   III. It will result in a decreased FRC.
   IV. It is contraindicated in the presence of ventilatory failure.
       A. II and IV
       B. I and IV
       C. II, III, and IV
       D. I and II
       E. II only
   (29:207–210) (1:325 and 384)

6. Which of the following is *least* likely to be a clinical goal of the administration of PEEP therapy?
   A. Improve CO_2 hemostasis
   B. Treat refractory oxygenation failure
   C. Allow administration of nontoxic levels of oxygen
   D. Improve existing pulmonary pathology
   E. Improve V/Q relationships
   (46:2)

7. The most acceptable method of reducing the incidence of pulmonary oxygen toxicity is to:
   A. Administer He/O_2 mixtures instead
   B. Administer megadoses of vitamin E
   C. Administer PEEP and reduce the FI_{O_2} to 40% as rapidly as possible
   D. Place patient on 21% oxygen for 1 hour each shift
   E. Lower FI_{O_2} despite clinical evidence of hypoxia
   (1:147–151) (2:313 and 390–391)

8. The respiratory therapy practitioner is monitoring a 15-year-old patient who is receiving an FI_{O_2} of 0.6 via a T tube setup. The following data are noted at this time:

Respiratory rate	32
Pa_{O_2}	40 mm Hg
Pa_{CO_2}	36 mm Hg
pH	7.38
Base excess	−3.8 mEq/L
Historical data:	Patient is seen 3 days post admission for acute viral pneumonia and has been on continuous mechanical ventilation for 24 hours

   True statements regarding this situation include:
   I.   Refractory oxygenation failure exists.
   II. PEEP would be detrimental.
   III. An FI_{O_2} of 1.0 would increase the Pa_{O_2} dramatically.
   IV. CPAP may be beneficial.

A. I, II, and IV
B. I and IV
C. II, III, and IV
D. I and III
E. II and IV
(1:Chaps 24 and 30 and pp 129, 144, 312, 313, and 321)
(32:63–68 and 114–119)

9. Acute decreases in venous return seen following administration of PEEP or CPAP therapy may result in which of the following?
   I.   Decreased cardiac output
   II.   Depression of the systolic blood pressure
   III. Decreased urine output
   IV.   Increased $P\bar{v}_{O_2}$
      A. I, II, and III
      B. II and III
      C. I, III, and IV
      D. I only
      E. I and III
   (46:4–5) (6:123) (1:373) (25:Chap 4, pp 13–14) (31:31–32)

10. Among patients who are not being monitored with a pulmonary artery (Swan-Ganz) catheter, which of the following would provide the most accurate information regarding the proper level of positive end-expiratory pressure (PEEP)?
   A. Arterial blood pressure
   B. Effective static compliance
   C. Q_S/Q_T
   D. Pa_{CO_2}
   E. Pa_{O_2}
   (46) (47)

11. Which of the following may be seen when PEEP or CPAP is applied to patients in acute oxygenation failure?
   A. Decreases in cardiac output
   B. Increases in static effective compliance
   C. Decreases in intrapulmonary shunting
   D   A and B are correct.
   E. All of the above are correct.
   (46:3) (47)

12. PEEP has been shown to influence the reliability of PWP measurements. To minimize PEEP and airway pressure related artifact, the tip of the catheter is usually placed:
   A. In the apical lung zones
   B. In the abdominal aorta
   C. in the basal lung zones
   D. Adjacent to the pulmonary lymphatics
   E. In the anterior lung zones
   (25:Chap 13, p 23)

13. Which of the following statements about the effect of PEEP on PWP measurements is (are) true?
    I.   It usually results in falsely low values.
    II. The PWP is not affected except when the patient has adult respiratory distress syndrome.
    III. High levels of PEEP may affect reliability of these measurements.
    A. I only
    B. II and III
    C. I and III
    D. III only
    E. I and II
    (46:4) (25:Chap 13, pp 25–26)

14. All of the following are used in assessing the tissue oxygenation status of patients receiving PEEP. Which is believed to be the *least* reliable indicator?
    A. Pa_{O_2}
    B. $P\bar{v}_{O_2}$
    C. $\dot{Q}_T$
    D. $C(a-\bar{v})_{O_2}$
    E. $(\dot{Q}_T)(Ca_{O_2})$
    (1:310) (46:4–5) (47)

15. The respiratory therapist is administering continuous ventilatory support to a 60-year-old patient 48 hours post emergency laparotomy. The patient is on a volume ventilator with an FI_{O_2} of 0.7, 5 cm H_2O PEEP, a tidal volume of 12 cc/kg, and a rate of 15 in the assist mode. The following arterial blood gases are obtained on these settings:

Pa_{O_2}	39 mm Hg
Pa_{CO_2}	42 mm Hg
pH	7.33
HCO_3^-	18 mEq/L
Base excess	−4.6 mEq/L

    Based on the above information, the therapist should recommend which of the following?
    A. Increase FI_{O_2}
    B. Increase respiratory rate
    C. Increase FI_{O_2} and decrease tidal volume
    D. Increase PEEP
    E. Repeat arterial blood gas studies; laboratory error exists!
    (46) (38:Chaps 4 through 6 and p 63) (32:64–66)

16. Indications for CPAP in the newborn include which of the following?
    I.   Hypocarbia and hypoxemia on 70% oxygen via hood
    II. Pa_{CO_2} greater than 60 in the presence of pulmonary atelectasis
    III. Hypoxemia and normocarbia on 30% oxygen
    IV. Prolonged apnea accompanied by hypercarbia

A. I only
B. I and III
C. I and IV
D. II and IV
E. I, II, and III
(29:206–207)

Answer Key

1. D	4. B	7. C	10. B	13. D
2. C	5. A	8. B	11. E	14. A
3. C	6. A	9. A	12. C	15. D
				16. A

G. Assess Patient Response to Therapy

Questions in this category are designed to assess the candidate's ability to evaluate and monitor the patient's response to respiratory care techniques. This is one of the most important and difficult content categories on the NBRC examinations, and fully 20% of the questions on the Advanced Practitioner Examination are drawn from this area. Questions in this category share a similar scenario: a patient is receiving respiratory care. During that therapy, various bedside and/or laboratory diagnostic data are made available to the respiratory therapy practitioner. Based on that data, the practitioner must make an assessment. That is, the practitioner must evaluate the patient's response to the respiratory therapy techniques in question. Typical questions involve the practitioner noting that a hazardous reaction to therapy is taking place. Other questions may involve determining whether hypoxemia is due to low V/Q or shunting.

Entry Level Pretest

According to the NBRC, 5% of the questions on the Entry Level Examination are from this content category. In addition, the Composite Examination Matrix (see reference 80) states that questions in this area are designed to test the candidate's ability to evaluate the following bedside and laboratory data on an entry level to assess patient response to respiratory care procedures:

1. Cardiopulmonary vital signs
2. Cardiac arrhythmias
3. Chest roentgenograms
4. Chest physical data
5. Subjective and objective response to therapy

6.   Cough and sputum evaluation
7. FI_{O_2} and oxygen liter flow
8.   Basic pulmonary function data
9.   Arterial blood gas and acid-base data
10. Subjective and objective response to continuous ventilatory support (take and assess ventilator parameters)
11. Weaning data
12. Endotracheal or tracheostomy tube cuff pressure
13. Effective compliance values
14. V_D/V_T
15. $P(A-a)_{O_2}$

The following are self-study questions from this category:

1.   A satisfactory definition of respiratory insufficiency is:
     A.   Inability to maintain normal arterial blood gases
     B.   Ability to maintain normal arterial blood gases only by increasing cardiopulmonary workloads
     C. Pa_{CO_2} less than 30 mm Hg with a Pa_{O_2} less than 50 mm Hg
     D.   Inability to maintain normal venous blood gases
     E.   B and C are correct.
     (1:299–301) (11:221–222) (49)

2.   Which of the following statements regarding cyanosis is *least* true?
     A.   Patients may be cyanotic but not significantly hypoxic.
     B.   Cyanosis is not usually considered a reliable clinical sign.
     C.   Hypoxia may exist without the presence of cyanosis.
     D.   In general, cyanosis is considered a sign of mild hypoxia.
     E.   Patients with cyanide and carbon monoxide poisoning may not exhibit cyanosis.
     (30:127–130) (2:235–242)

3.   Which of the following would be the *least* likely cause of arterial hypercapnia in a 70-kg patient?
     A. V_D/V_T of 0.8
     B.   A minute alveolar ventilation of 2.5 L
     C.   Administration of 60% oxygen to a patient with a baseline Pa_{CO_2} of 75 mm Hg
     D.   Hyperthermia
     E.   Hypothermia
     (7:75)

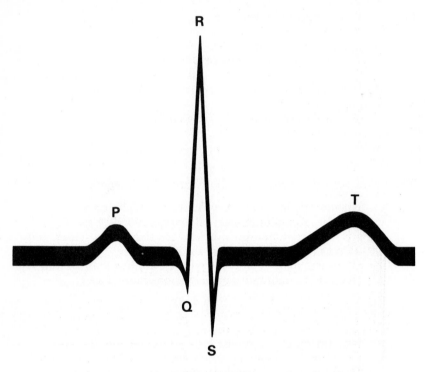

Figure IV-46.

4. The above illustrates a normal cardiac cycle. If there were no uniform ventricular repolarization, which of the following waves would disappear?
   A. P wave
   B. T wave
   C. QRS complex
   D. Q wave
   E. R wave
   (25:Chap 6, p 59)

5. Which of the following would be most helpful in assessing the adequacy of tissue oxygenation?
   A. $\dot{Q}_T$
   B. Pa_{O_2}
   C. $P\bar{v}_{O_2}$
   D. $\dot{Q}_S/\dot{Q}_T$
   E. Arterial pH
   (1:377) (46:5)

6. The presence of which of the following may be used to assess that a 70-kg patient is capable of being weaned from continuous ventilatory support?
   I. $P(A-a)_{O_2}$ less than 600 mm Hg
   II. Vital capacity less than 10 mL to 15 mL/kg

III. V_D/V_T less than 0.8
IV. Resting spontaneous minute volume greater than 15 L/min
V. Pa_{O_2} greater than 70 mm Hg on 40% oxygen
VI. Negative inspiratory force greater than 20 cm to 30 cm H_2O
    A. I, II, V, and VI
    B. V and VI
    C. III, IV, and V
    D. I, III, and V
    E. I, II, III, V, and VI
(7:189) (2:667)

7. The decision to initiate continuous ventilatory support in patients with myasthenia gravis is most frequently made by assessment of which of the following parameters?
    A. Pa_{CO_2}
    B. FEV_1
    C. Vital capacity
    D. V_D/V_T
    E. Q_S/Q_T
(7:363) (2:761)

8. A patient on a volume ventilator is noted to have his plateau pressure increase from 30 cm H_2O to 40 cm H_2O. Which of the following is (are) correct assessments regarding this situation?
    I. The static effective compliance has decreased.
    II. The effective dynamic compliance has increased.
    III. There has been an increase in lung thorax distensibility.
    IV. The airway resistance has increased.
    A. I, II, and IV
    B. I and III
    C. I only
    D. II and III
    E. I and IV
(50) (34:122–126)

9. The respiratory therapy practitioner would not generally consider the PWP elevated until it exceeds:
    A. 9 cm H_2O
    B. 12 mm Hg
    C. 9 mm Hg
    D. 25 cm H_2O
    E. 4 mm Hg
(33:200–204) (1:409)

10. In assessing the overall status of the newborn immediately following delivery, which is the most important clinical sign?
    A. Respirations
    B. Reflex irritability
    C. Muscle tone
    D. Cyanosis
    E. Heart rate
(29:Chap 2) (13:51–55)

11. Which of the following hemodynamic measurements is believed to reflect left ventricular filling pressures (preload) most reliably?
  A.   Central venous pressure
  B.   Pulmonary artery systolic pressure
  C.   Pulmonary wedge pressure
  D. $C(a\text{-}\bar{v})o_2$
  E.   Mean peripheral arterial pressure
     (1:466–469) (2:954–955)

12. The single most important therapeutic effect resulting from the administration of oxygen to a patient with chronic obstructive pulmonary disease who has developed cor pulmonale is:
  A.   Decreased right ventricular workloads
  B.   Decreased left ventricular workloads
  C.   Decreased work of breathing
  D.   Improved renal function
  E.   Increase in Pao_2
     (1:144–147 and 489) (11:Chap 20)

13. Which of the following clinical signs does *not* indicate the presence of respiratory distress in the newborn?
  A.   Nasal flaring
  B.   Expiratory grunting
  C.   Sternal retractions
  D.   Tachypnea
  E.   Loud crying
     (29:184)

14. The clinical diagnosis of ventilatory failure is best assessed by noting which of the following laboratory measurements?
  A. Pao_2
  B. $C(a\text{-}\bar{v})o_2$
  C. $Paco_2$
  D. $FEV_1\%$
  E.   Maximal voluntary ventilation maneuvers
     (49) (5:109)

15. For which of the following should the respiratory care practitioner allow one point when using the Apgar scoring system?
   I.   Absent reflex irritability
  II.   Weak respiratory effort
 III.   Pulse rates less than 100
  IV.   Central or generalized cyanosis
   V.   Some flexion of extremities
     A.   II, III, and V
     B.   I, III, and IV
     C.   II and III
     D.   II, III, IV, and V
     E.   II and V
  (29:Chap 2) (13:51–55)

16. The respiratory therapy practitioner is assessing a patient who has become distressed while receiving continuous ventilatory support.

Bedside examination performed while the patient is being ventilated with a bag-valve unit reveals a dull percussion note on the
left side. Further physical examination reveals a hyperresonant
percussion note on the right side. Under these circumstances, the
cause of this patient's distress may be assessed most rapidly by:
   A.   Obtaining stat arterial blood gases
   B.   Obtaining a portable chest roentgenogram
   C.   Retracting the endotracheal tube slightly
   D.   Paging the physician
   E.   Noting the presence or absence of tactile fremitus
   (32:211–213)

17.   The respiratory therapy practitioner is monitoring a patient in the
      intensive care unit who is being ventilated with a Bourns Bear II
      ventilator. Suddenly the high pressure alarm begins sounding reg-
      ularly. Possible causes include:
        I.   Patient fighting the ventilator
       II.   Mobilization of a large mucus plug
      III.   Tension pneumothorax
       IV.   Kinking of endotracheal tube
            A.   I, II, and III
            B.   II and IV
            C.   I, III, and IV
            D.   I, II, III, and IV
            E.   I, II, and IV
      (32:Chap 12) (60)

18.   The respiratory therapy practitioner is performing a physical
      examination on a patient who has become distressed during con-
      tinuous ventilatory support. Auscultation reveals absent breath
      sounds over the right basal lung field. Percussion yields a flat note
      over the right basal and middle lobes. There is also a noticeable
      tracheal shift to the left. Based on the above information, the most
      probable cause of the patient's distress is:
      A.   Left-sided pneumothorax
      B.   Right-sided hemothorax
      C.   Right mainstem intubation
      D.   Massive right-sided atelectasis
      E.   Herniation of endotracheal tube cuff
      (32:Chap 12)

19.   Which of the following are findings that would indicate slippage of
      an endotracheal tube into the right mainstem bronchus during
      continuous mechanical ventilation?
        I.   Musical inspiratory note
       II.   Hyperresonant percussion note on the right side
      III.   Decrease in effective static compliance
       IV.   Decreased aeration on the left side
            A.   I, II, and IV
            B.   I, II, and III
            C.   II and III

   D.   III and IV
   E.   II, III, and IV
   (32:Chap 12) (34:122–126)

20.   The respiratory therapist is called to the bedside of a patient who is on a Bennett MA-I ventilator because of sounding of a low pressure alarm. On entering the room, the practitioner notes that the ventilator's monitoring bellows spirometer is rising during the inspiratory phase. The practitioner should assess that the most likely cause of the above problem is:
   A.   There is leakage around the endotracheal tube cuff.
   B.   The black spirometer line is disconnected.
   C.   Malfunction of the exhalation valve exists.
   D.   A tension pneumothorax exists.
   E.   The spirometer needs to be changed.
   (32:216–217) (57)

21.   The respiratory therapy practitioner is monitoring a 150-kg patient on a Bourns Bear ventilator. The tidal volume is 1100 mL, the FIo_2 is 0.6, and the patient is receiving 15 cm H_2O PEEP. Suddenly the ventilator inoperative alarm sounds. The practitioner should assess that the *most* probable reason for the above occurrence is:
   A.   Electrical power failure
   B.   Patient has become apneic
   C.   Patient has become disconnected from the ventilator
   D.   Herniation of the endotracheal tube cuff
   E.   A and B are correct.
   (50)

22.   The respiratory therapy practitioner is assessing a patient who has become severely distressed while receiving continuous mechanical ventilation. While the patient is being manually ventilated, the therapist performs a rapid physical examination. Auscultation at this time reveals absent breath sounds over the left apical lung field. The percussion note is dull on the right and hyperresonant on the left. Tracheal shift to the right is also noted. The most likely cause of this patient's distress is:
   A.   Right-sided hemothorax
   B.   Left-sided tension pneumothorax
   C.   Right mainstem intubation
   D.   Ventilator malfunction
   E.   Right-sided tension pneumothorax
   (32:121–213)

23.   A 72-year-old patient with steady state chronic obstructive pulmonary disease is seen in the emergency department after being admitted in respiratory distress. His respirations are labored and he is noted to be cyanotic. Further data collected with the patient breathing room air are as follows:

   pH   7.26
   $Paco_2$ 80 mm Hg

Pa_{O_2}	39 mm Hg
HCO_3^-	38 mEq/L
BP	160/120
Pulse	130
Respiratory rate	35
Minute ventilation	20 L/min

Administration of 40% oxygen to this patient will most likely have which of the following results?
I.   An increase in alveolar ventilation
II. Worsening of respiratory acidosis
III. Blunting of the hypoxic drive
IV. Worsening of cardiovascular vital signs
    A.   I only
    B.   II and IV
    C.   II, III, and IV
    D.   I and III
    E.   II and III
(1:479–480)

Answer Key

1. B	6. B	11. C	16. C	21. C
2. D	7. C	12. A	17. D	22. B
3. E	8. C	13. E	18. B	23. C
4. B	9. B	14. C	19. E	
5. C	10. E	15. A	20. C	

Advanced Practitioner Pretest

According to the NBRC, 20% of the questions on the Advanced Practitioner Examination are from this content category. In addition, the Composite Examination Matrix (see reference 80) states that questions in this category are designed to test the candidate's ability to evaluate the following bedside and laboratory data on an advanced level to assess patient response to respiratory care procedures:

1. Cardiac arrhythmias
2. Advanced pulmonary function data
3. Arterial blood gas and acid-base data
4. Transcutaneous blood gas data
5. Blood chemistry data (i.e., hemoglobin, electrolytes, white blood cell count, eosinophil count)
6. Fluid intake and output
7. Subjective and objective response to mechanical ventilation
8. Endotracheal and tracheostomy tube cuff pressure
9. Central and peripheral vascular pressure and waveform data (i.e., CVP, PWP, pulmonary arterial pressures, peripheral arterial pressures)

10. Cardiac output and other hemodynamic information
11. Exhaled CO_2 tension
12. V_D/V_T
13. $P(A\text{-}a)o_2$
14. Q_S/Q_T
15. $C(a\text{-}\bar{v})o_2$
16. Effective compliance values

The following self-study questions were developed from the NBRC Composite Examination Matrix:

1. Which of the following are known to cause the P_{50} to rise above normal?
   I. Acidosis
   II. Decreased red blood cell 2–3 DPG levels
   III. Carbon monoxide poisoning
   IV. Hypercarbia
      A. I and III
      B. I, II, and IV
      C. I, III, and IV
      D. II and IV
      E. I and IV
   (2:237–239)

2. When a patient who has a large right-to-left intrapulmonary shunt is administered 100% oxygen for 20 minutes, which of the following will apply?
   I. The $P(A\text{-}a)o_2$ will narrow.
   II. The Pao_2 will increase dramatically.
   III. The Q_S/Q_T will increase.
   IV. Nitrogen washout will occur.
      A. I and IV
      B. II and IV
      C. III and IV
      D. IV only
      E. I only
   (5:Chap 19)

3. Which of the following statements regarding perfusion in excess of ventilation $\dot{V}/\dot{Q}$ abnormalities (low $\dot{V}/\dot{Q}$) is *not* true?
   A. It is a common cause of hypoxemia.
   B. It is associated with a normal $P(A\text{-}a)o_2$.
   C. It is associated with an uneven distribution of ventilation.
   D. It will often respond dramatically to low concentrations of oxygen.
   E. It is associated with chronic obstructive pulmonary disease.
   (5:Chap 15, pp 90–91) (2:241–242 and 394–395)

4. A patient is seen in the intensive care unit. Following administration of 100% oxygen, a $P(A\text{-}a)o_2$ of 500 is noted. In the respira-

tory therapy practitioner's assessment, the *least* likely cause(s) is (are):
I.   Physiologic shunting
II. Decreased cardiac output
III. Low $\dot{V}/\dot{Q}$
IV. Diffusion defect
    A. I and IV
    B. II only
    C. I and II
    D. II and III
    E. III and IV
(5:Chaps 19 and 20, pp 92–94 and 232–235) (2:394–395)

5. A 17-year-old girl is brought to the emergency department after having ingested an unknown quantity of Thorazine® at home. Stat blood gas analysis reveals a Pa_{O_2} of 45 mm Hg, a Pa_{CO_2} of 80 mm Hg, and a pH of 7.21. Based on the above data, the respiratory therapy practitioner would determine that administration of 40% oxygen to this patient:
I.   Will likely result in further respiratory depression
II. Will succeed in correcting the hypoxemia
III. Will result in dramatic widening of the $P(A-a)_{O_2}$
    A. I and II
    B. II and III
    C. III only
    D. I only
    E. II only
(2:241–242 and 394–395)

6. A 37-year-old, 70-kg patient is seen in the intensive care unit following a splenectomy. The following data are gathered at this time, with the patient receiving an FI_{O_2} of 0.7 via a T tube setup:

Pa_{O_2}	40 mm Hg
Pa_{CO_2}	40 mm Hg
pH	7.33
Base excess	−3.9 mEq/L
Temperature	37°C
Tidal volume	560 cc
Respiratory rate	44/min

Based on these data, which of the following assessments are true?
I.   The patient's hypoxemia is due to a diffusion deficit.
II. The patient's V_D/V_T is probably elevated.
III. Refractory hypoxemia exists.
IV. The patient is hyperventilating.
    A. II, III, and IV
    B. II and IV
    C. I and II
    D. II and III

E.   I, II, and III
(5:129) (2:394–395) (38:60)

7. Cyanosis is *least* likely to occur despite a significant degree of hypoxemia in which of the following patients?
    I.   Those who are polycythemic
    II. Those with high cardiac output
    III. Those with low cardiac output
    IV. Those who are anemic
        A.   I and III
        B.   II and III
        C.   I and IV
        D.   I only
        E.   II and IV
    (30:129–130)

8. In the absence of cardiac output monitoring capabilities, which of the following would best allow the respiratory practitioner to assess a normothermic patient's tissue oxygen transport?
    A.   Effective static compliance
    B. Pa_{O_2}
    C. Q_S/Q_T
    D. $P(A-a)_{O_2}$
    E. $C(a-\bar{v})_{O_2}$
    (46) (47)

9. Which of the following statements regarding the arterial minus venous oxygen content difference, $C(a-\bar{v})_{O_2}$, is (are) true?
    I.   It is generally unaffected by changes in cardiac output.
    II. Accurate measurement requires placement of a pulmonary artery catheter.
    III. A value of 7.2 vol% generally indicates presence of excellent cardiovascular reserves.
    IV. The normal value for a healthy resting subject is approximately 5.0 vol%.
        A.   I and IV
        B.   IV only
        C.   II and IV
        D.   I, III, and IV
        E.   II and III
    (5:Chap 20)

10. All five of the following patients are intubated and are receiving 100% oxygen via a volume ventilator in the control mode. In addition, each one has a Pa_{O_2} of 50 mm Hg and an oxygen consumption ($\dot{V}_{O_2}$) of 250 mL O_2/min. Based on this and the following information, which patient will have the largest physiologic shunt ($\dot{Q}_S/\dot{Q}_T$)?
    A.   Patient A has a $C(a-\bar{v})_{O_2}$ of 2.5 vol%.
    B.   Patient B has a $C(a-\bar{v})_{O_2}$ of 3.5 vol%.
    C.   Patient C has a $C(a-\bar{v})_{O_2}$ of 5.0 vol%.

D. Patient D has a $C(a-\bar{v})o_2$ of 6.0 vol%.
E. Patient E has a $C(a-\bar{v})o_2$ of 8.0 vol%.
(46:3)

11. Five patients with identical physiologic shunt fractions ($\dot{Q}s/\dot{Q}_T$) of 20% are seen in the intensive care unit. They all have varying $C(a-\bar{v})o_2$ values as listed below. Assuming that their oxygen consumptions ($\dot{V}o_2$) are all 300 mL/min, which one of the following is likely to have the lowest Pao_2?
A. Patient A: 2.5 vol%
B. Patient B: 3.5 vol%
C. Patient C: 4.5 vol%
D. Patient D: 6.0 vol%
E. Patient E: 8.0 vol%
(5:233)

12. Assuming a steady state oxygen consumption, as a patient's cardiac output falls, which of the following most likely will take place?
I.   An increase in $C(a-\bar{v})o_2$
II. An increase in Pao_2
III. A decrease in $P\bar{v}o_2$
A. I and III
B. II and III
C. III only
D. I and II
E. I only
(46:4–5) (47) (1:419–420) (5:Chap 19 and p 232)

13. A 70-kg patient is seen in the intensive care unit. The respiratory therapy practitioner is asked to assess this patient's pulmonary status. In so doing the following data are collected:

BP	160/120
Pulse	135/min
V_T	750 cc
Respiratory rate	40/min
Temperature	37.4°C

Assuming this patient's V_D/V_T is normal, which of the following would most likely represent this patient's current $Paco_2$?
A. 15–25 mm Hg
B. 25–35 mm Hg
C. 35–45 mm Hg
D. 45–55 mm Hg
E. 55–65 mm Hg
(1:308–309)

14. The respiratory therapy practitioner is monitoring a patient who is receiving continuous ventilatory support via a volume ventilator. At this time he notes that the pulmonary wedge pressure is 27

mm Hg. Which of the following is *least* likely to be responsible for this abnormality?

A. Aortic stenosis
B. Mitral valvular disease
C. Left ventricular failure
D. Hypervolemia
E. Adult respiratory distress syndrome
   (41) (58) (32:Chap 5) (33:203–205) (25:Chap 15, p 17)

15. The respiratory therapy practitioner is monitoring a 60-kg patient who is intubated and is receiving positive pressure ventilation with an FI_{O_2} of 0.6 and a corrected V_T of 700 mL via a Bennett 7200 ventilator. Pertinent data collected with the tidal volume held constant are as follows:

	1:00 PM	2:00 PM
Peak Pressure	48 cm H_2O	61 cm H_2O
Plateau Pressure	26 cm H_2O	47 cm H_2O
PEEP	5 cm H_2O	10 cm H_2O
Inspiratory Flow Rate	40 L/min	65 L/min

True statements regarding the above include:
   I. There is a decrease in pulmonary compliance.
   II. There is an increase in airway resistance.
   III. There is a decrease in airway resistance.
   IV. There is an increase in pulmonary elastance.
   A. II and IV
   B. I, III, and IV
   C. I and III
   D. I and II
   E. I, II, and IV
   (50) (34:122–126)

16. The respiratory therapy practitioner is monitoring a patient who is receiving continuous ventilatory support via a Bennett MA-II ventilator. Over the span of one hour, the peak pressure is noted to increase from 32 cm H_2O to 49 cm H_2O. Concurrently, the plateau pressure remains constant and unchanged. Noting that there have been no changes in tidal volume or flow rate, which of the following conditions are most likely responsible for the recorded changes?
   I. Cardiogenic pulmonary edema
   II. Bronchospasm
   III. Leak in the ventilator circuit
   IV. Upper airway obstruction
   V. Tension pneumothorax
   A. I, II, and IV
   B. II and IV
   C. II and III
   D. I, IV, and V

E. I, II, and III
    (57) (50) (34:122–126) (2:627–631)

17. Which of the following statements regarding the central venous pressure is (are) true?
   I.   It is measured in the right ventricle.
   II. It assesses right ventricular filling pressures.
   III. It may not accurately reflect left ventricular functions.
   IV. Normal value is 15 mm Hg to 25 mm Hg.
     A. II and III
     B. II only
     C. II, III, and IV
     D. III and IV
     E. I, II, and III
    (1:406–409) (2:954–955)

18. Which of the following hemodynamic parameters may be determined through the use of a properly functioning four-channel pulmonary artery catheter?
   I.   Pulmonary arterial pressures
   II. Cardiac output
   III. $S\bar{v}_{O_2}$
   IV. Central venous pressure
   V. Pulmonary wedge pressure
     A. I, II, IV, and V
     B. II, III, IV, and V
     C. I, III, IV, and V
     D. I, III, and IV
     E. I, II, III, IV, and V
    (2:954–955) (1:406–409)

19. Which of the following complications are known to be related to the use of pulmonary artery catheters?
   I.   Subcutaneous emphysema
   II. Cerebral thromboembolus
   III. Pulmonary venous rupture
   IV. Pulmonary infarction
     A. I and IV
     B. I, III, and IV
     C. I, II, III, and IV
     D. I, II, and IV
     E. II and III
    (2:955) (1:407–408)

20. The respiratory therapy practitioner is monitoring a mechanically ventilated patient in the intensive care unit. The patient's PWP has just increased rapidly from 10 mm Hg to 32 mm Hg. Which of the following is the most likely cause?
     A. Right ventricular failure
     B. Left ventricular failure
     C. Adult respiratory distress syndrome
     D. Septic shock

E.   Renal failure
   (1:431–436) (2:726)

21. A P$\bar{v}_{O_2}$ of 26 mm Hg would indicate the presence of:
   A.   Low Q$_T$
   B.   Arterial hypoxemia
   C.   Increased metabolic demands
   D.   Tissue hypoxia
   E.   Cyanide poisoning
   (1:377) (46:5)

22. The monitoring of end tidal carbon dioxide tensions (P$_{ETCO_2}$) is most frequently used to approximate:
   A.   Ventilation-perfusion disorders
   B.   Physiologic deadspace
   C.   Anatomic deadspace
   D.   Arterial CO$_2$ tensions
   E.   Capillary shunting
   (59:190)

23. A patient with longstanding chronic obstructive pulmonary disease is being managed in the respiratory intensive care unit. Despite all efforts, he is increasingly unable to manage his upper airway secretions. Blood gases drawn just prior to the patient's being placed on a ventilator show a Pa$_{CO_2}$ of 110 mm Hg and a pH of 7.16. Two hours after being placed on the ventilator, he begins to display seizure activity. The respiratory therapy practitioner would assess that the most likely cause of this phenomenon is:
   A.   Increased intracranial pressure
   B.   Rapid reduction in Pa$_{CO_2}$
   C.   Cerebrospinal fluid acidosis
   D.   Central nervous system hypoxia
   E.   Underlying seizure disorder
   (7:167)

24. Which of the following will not cause increases in pulmonary vascular resistance?
   A.   Acidosis
   B.   Hypoxia
   C.   Pulmonary embolic disease
   D.   Tolazoline (Priscoline®) administration
   E.   Polycythemia
   (11:182–183) (18:36–39)

25. All but which one of the following may be present in a patient who is suffering from severe hypovolemia?
   A.   Hypotension
   B.   Hypoxia
   C.   Increased tissue capillary blood flow
   D.   Lactic acidosis
   E.   Oliguria
   (25:Chap 15, p 17) (12:398–399)

26. Which of the following disorders is (are) known to contribute to the development of hypoproteinemia?
    I. Nasogastric feedings
    II. Protein malnutrition
    III. Parenteral alimentation
    IV. Hepatic failure
        A. I and III
        B. II and IV
        C. III and IV
        D. IV only
        E. III only
    (25:Chap 15, p 17)

27. A 60-year-old patient with adult respiratory distress syndrome is inadvertently administered an excessive amount of lactated Ringer's solution while receiving continuous ventilatory support. This will most likely result in which of the following?
    I. A decrease in the PWP
    II. A decrease in static effective compliance
    III. An increase in the $P(A-a)o_2$
    IV. A decrease in the shunt fraction (Q_S/Q_T)
        A. I and II
        B. I and III
        C. II and III
        D. I and IV
        E. III and IV
    (34:122–126) (1:399 and 410) (25:Chap 15, p 17) (38:Chap 3) (50)

28. A 23-year-old, 70-kg patient is seen in the intensive care unit while receiving volume ventilation with an FIo_2 of 0.7 and 12 cm H_2O PEEP. Based on radiologic and clinical evidence, a diagnosis of pulmonary edema is made. Clinical data obtained at this time are as follows:

Pao_2	63 mm Hg
$P\bar{v}o_2$	33 mm Hg
PWP	28 mm Hg
CVP	15 mm Hg
Oxygen consumption	250 mL/min
$C(a-\bar{v})o_2$	2.5 vol%
Colloidal osmotic pressure	26 mm Hg
Total serum proteins	8.0 g/dL

Based on the above data, the respiratory therapy practitioner is able to assess that the most important contributor to this patient's pulmonary edema is:
A. Left ventricular failure
B. Increased pulmonary vascular resistance
C. Hypervolemia

D.   Hypoproteinemia
E.   Right ventricular failure
   (41) (42) (25:Chap 5, p 17) (1:Chaps 26 through 30)
   (32:Chap 5) (5:Chap 20)

29. The respiratory therapy practitioner is monitoring a 65-kg, 22-year-old patient in the intensive care unit. The patient is seen 24 hours following severe trauma sustained in a motorcycle accident. The following data are noted at this time with the patient receiving 60% oxygen via T tube setup:

Pa_{O_2}	40 mm Hg
Pa_{CO_2}	50 mm Hg
P_B	760 mm Hg
$C(a-\bar{v})_{O_2}$	2.5 vol%
Oxygen consumption	250 mL/min

Which of the following assessments regarding the above information is (are) true?
   I.   The $P(A-a)_{O_2}$ is 200 mm Hg.
   II. CPAP is indicated at this time.
   III. This patient's cardiovascular reserves appear to be excellent.
   IV. Continuous ventilatory support is indicated at this time.
      A.   I, III, and IV
      B.   IV only
      C.   II and III
      D.   III and IV
      E.   I and IV
   (5:Chaps 19 and 20, pp 92–94 and 232–235) (2:394–395)
   (38:38–42) (50)

30. A 75-year-old, 50-kg man from a nursing home is admitted in cardiorespiratory failure. He is placed on a volume ventilator, and an FI_{O_2} of 0.6 with 15 mm H_2O PEEP is required to maintain a Pa_{O_2} greater than 50 mm Hg. A radiologic diagnosis of interstitial and alveolar edema is made. The following information is subsequently gathered:

Pa_{O_2}	55 mm Hg
$S\bar{v}_{O_2}$	55%
$C(a-\bar{v})_{O_2}$	3.5 vol%
PWP	15 mm Hg
CVP	10 mm Hg
Colloidal osmotic pressure	12 mm Hg
Total serum proteins	3.0 g/dL
Oxygen consumption	250 mL/min
Cardiac output	7.1 L/min
P.A. systolic	38 mm Hg
P.A. diastolic	21 mm Hg

Based on this information, the respiratory therapy practitioner's assessment reveals which of the following as being the most important contributor to the patient's pulmonary edema?
A. Left ventricular failure
B. Hypoproteinemia
C. Right ventricular failure
D. Pulmonary hypertension
E. Hypovolemia
(41) (25:Chap 15, p 17) (42) (1:397–398; Chaps 26 through 30)

31. In which of the following patient groups will the central venous pressure frequently *not* reflect left ventricular function?
   I. Those with increased pulmonary vascular resistance
   II. All patients
   III. Those with myocardial infarction
      A. I and II
      B. II only
      C. I and III
      D. III only
      E. I only
   (1:406–409) (2:955) (32:Chap 5)

32. The quantity of oxygen being consumed per minute can be determined by which of the following formulas?
   A. $\dfrac{Cc'_{O_2} - Ca_{O_2}}{Q_T}$
   B. $(Q_T)(Ca_{O_2})$
   C. $(Q_T)[C(a\text{-}\bar{v})_{O_2}]$
   D. $(Ca_{O_2} - Cv_{O_2})(Q_S/Q_T)$
   E. $(Q_T) \div [C(a\text{-}\bar{v})_{O_2}]$
   (5:232–235)

33. The respiratory therapy practitioner is monitoring a 53-year-old, 60-kg patient in the intensive care unit. Clinical information gathered and reported at the time is as follows:

Patient's age	53 years
Body weight	62 kg
V_T	490 mL
Respiratory rate	36/min
Pa_{O_2}	72 mm Hg
FI_{O_2}	0.28
Pulse	110
BP	140/100
Pa_{CO_2}	43 mm Hg

Based on the above data, select the most correct assessment.
A. The patient's hypoxemia is due to shunting.
B. The patient is hyperventilating.
C. Further oxygen administration will result in respiratory depression.

D.   It is likely the patient's V_D/V_T is elevated.
E.   Hypopnea exists.
    (1:308–309)

34. While performing endotracheal suctioning on a 1500-g newborn, the respiratory therapy practitioner notes that the pulse has dropped from 175 to 90. This problem:
    I.   May be caused by vagal stimulation
    II.   May be prevented through administration of parasympathomimetics
    III. Is uncommon in neonatal units
    IV.   May be caused by hypoxia
        A.   III only
        B.   I and III
        C.   II, III, and IV
        D.   I and IV
        E.   I, II, III, and IV
    (2:527)

35. Which of the following parameters must be measured to calculate the intrapulmonary shunt?
    I. Ca_{O_2}
    II. Pa_{CO_2}
    III. $P(A-a)_{O_2}$
    IV. $C\bar{v}_{O_2}$
    V. $P\bar{v}_{O_2}$
    VI. $\dot{Q}_T$
        A.   I, IV, V, and VI
        B.   I, III, and IV
        C.   I, III, and V
        D.   I, II, III, and VI
        E.   I, II, IV, V, and VI
    (5:224)

36. The respiratory therapy practitioner is monitoring a patient who has a noncolloidal serum osmotic pressure of 340 mOsmol/L. This value is consistent with:
    I.   Pyschogenic polydipsia
    II.   Increased antidiuretic hormone secretion
    III. Fresh water drowning
    IV.   Uncontrolled diabetes mellitus
    V.   Hypernatremia
        A.   I and II
        B.   II, III, and IV
        C.   I, II, III, IV, and V
        D.   IV and V
        E.   III and IV
    (94:Chap 2) (7:Chap 14)

37. The respiratory therapy practitioner is monitoring a patient who has a noncolloidal serum osmotic pressure of 240 mOsmol/L. The above is consistent with:
   I.   Hyponatremia
   II. Salt water drowning
   III. Decreased antidiuretic hormone secretion
   IV. Psychogenic polydipsia
      A. I, III, and IV
      B. I and II
      C. I and III
      D. II, III, and IV
      E. IV only
   (94:Chap 2) (7:Chap 14)

38. The respiratory therapy practitioner is monitoring a patient who has a serum osmolality of 290 mOsmol/L. This value is consistent with:
      A. Hypoproteinemia
      B. Normal serum osmolality
      C. Hyperosmolality
      D. Hyponatremia
      E. Hypokalemia
   (94:Chap 2) (7:Chap 14)

39. The respiratory therapy practitioner is monitoring a patient who has a total protein concentration of 4.0 g/dL. This value is most consistent with:
   I.   Hyperproteinemia
   II. Protein malnutrition
   III. Serum hyperosmolality
   IV. Adult respiratory distress syndrome
      A. I and IV
      B. IV only
      C. II and III
      D. II and IV
      E. II only
   (94:Chap 2) (7:Chap 14)

40. The respiratory therapy practitioner is monitoring a serum sodium level of 142 mEq/L and a serum potassium level of 6.4 mEq/L. These values are consistent with:
   I.   Hypokalemia
   II. Diuretic administration
   III. Normal sodium levels
   IV. Cushing's syndrome
      A. I only
      B. III only
      C. III and IV
      D. II, III, and IV
      E. I and III
   (94:Chap 2) (7:Chap 14)

Answer Key

1. E	9. C	17. A	25. C	33. D
2. C	10. A	18. E	26. B	34. D
3. B	11. E	19. A	27. C	35. B
4. E	12. A	20. B	28. C	36. D
5. E	13. A	21. D	29. D	37. A
6. D	14. E	22. D	30. B	38. B
7. E	15. B	23. B	31. C	39. E
8. E	16. B	24. D	32. C	40. B

H. Modify Therapy

Questions in this category are designed to assess the candidate's ability to make necessary modifications in therapeutic procedures based on patient response. This content category is a logical extension of the previous one in which the practitioner was asked to assess the patient's response to therapy. Now, having made his or her assessment, the respiratory therapy practitioner must modify therapy to achieve a more optimal therapeutic response. Obviously, there are many modifications in therapy that the therapist cannot make alone and that require a physician's order. That is the subject of the next NBRC content category.

Entry Level Pretest

According to the NBRC, 5% of the questions on the Entry Level Examination are from the modify therapy content category. In addition, the Composite Examination Matrix (see reference 80) states that questions in this category assess the candidate's ability to properly and safely modify all respiratory therapy techniques on a basic level.

The following self-study questions were developed from specific competencies listed in the NBRC Composite Examination Matrix:

1. A 69-year-old man with advanced chronic obstructive pulmonary disease is admitted to the emergency department in respiratory distress and considerable confusion. The patient's baseline $Paco_2$ is known to be in excess of 60 mm Hg. The physician wants the respiratory therapy practitioner to place the patient on low concentration oxygen and then draw a blood gas sample. Which of the following would be the *least* advisable means for the respiratory therapy practitioner to administer O_2 to this patient?
    A.   One liter via nasal cannula
    B.   24% air entrainment mask
    C.   Two liters via nasal cannula
    D.   28% air entrainment mask
    E.   Three liters via nasal cannula
    (49) (7:84)

2. The respiratory therapy practitioner is administering 0.5 mL metaproterenol with 2.0 mL normal saline to a 22-year-old asthmatic via hand-held nebulizer. During the treatment, the patient complains of nervousness and anxiety. At this time, the therapist observes that the patient's extremities are extremely tense and are shaking uncontrollably. The therapist should:
   A. Stop therapy and notify the physician
   B. Realize this is a cardiovascular side effect and chart it as such
   C. Stop therapy and administer only half the bronchodilator dose next time
   D. Wait until the patient calms down and then resume therapy
   E. Stop therapy and chart the results
   (2:477 and 580)

3. The respiratory therapy practitioner is helping transport an apneic patient to the radiology department for a CAT scan. The patient has a tracheostomy tube in place and is being ventilated with a pressure-cycled ventilator. As the patient's transport cart is being pushed onto the elevator, the patient coughs violently, causing the tracheal tube to fall down into the elevator shaft. What action should the respiratory therapy practitioner take at this time?
   A. Run to the nearest nurses' station and call your medical director
   B. Ventilate the patient in any way possible
   C. Have an aide get a sterile tube
   D. Obtain a manual resuscitation unit as rapidly as possible
   E. Begin external cardiac compressions on the patient
   (1:276)

4. During the administration of IPPB, the respiratory therapy practitioner observes his patient cough up sputum containing a moderate amount of fresh blood. The therapist should:
   A. Discontinue therapy and chart the results
   B. Discontinue therapy and notify the physician
   C. Page the physician and inform him that hemoptysis is a contraindication to IPPB
   D. Continue therapy if the patient will agree to it
   E. Wait 5 minutes and then continue therapy
   (2:580) (1:191)

5. While administering IPPB to a patient with advanced emphysema, the respiratory therapy practitioner observes that the patient is unable to exhale completely following assisted ventilations. The proper therapeutic modification would be to:
   A. Review therapeutic instructions with patient
   B. Increase flow rate
   C. Employ expiratory retard device
   D. Decrease cycling pressure
   E. Increase ventilator sensitivity
   (1:360–363) (70:516)

6. While administering IPPB the respiratory therapist notes that the patient's respiratory rate is 25 breaths per minute. Which of the following is the proper therapeutic modification?
    A. Make no modification
    B. Decrease the flow rate
    C. Decrease the sensitivity
    D. Instruct the patient to pause between each breath
    E. Increase the cycling pressure
    (75)

7. The respiratory therapist finds that due to the thickness and tenacity of tracheobronchial secretions, only scant amounts can be aspirated through a patient's orotracheal tube. Which of the following therapeutic modifications may facilitate removal of this patient's secretions?
    I.   Instilling 5 mL to 10 mL of distilled H_2O
    II.   Flexing the patient's head and neck during attempts
    III. Increasing suctioning pressure to 140 mm Hg
    IV.   Using postural drainage techniques prior to attempts
        A. I and IV
        B. II and IV
        C. III and IV
        D. I and II
        E. I and III
    (2:523–526)

8. A patient is receiving 40% oxygen via heated aerosol mask following triple vein/coronary artery bypass graft. She is progressing well, and solid foods are ordered as tolerated. To prevent hypoxia the respiratory therapy practitioner would place his/her patient on _____ liters via nasal cannula while eating.
    A. 2
    B. 3
    C. 4
    D. 5
    E. 6
    (1:141)

9. The respiratory therapy practitioner finds a patient who has a long history of chronic obstructive pulmonary disease who is apparently asleep. At this time, the therapist notes that the patient is being administered 6 L oxygen via cannula. The therapist should immediately:
    A. Remove nasal oxygen
    B. Begin to ventilate
    C. Establish unresponsiveness
    D. Establish an airway
    E. Get a stat arterial blood sample
    (37:12–13) (7:85)

10. A patient on a volume ventilator becomes acutely distressed. The high pressure alarm is sounding with each breath, and fluctua-

tions in the patient's arterial blood pressure are noted. Which of the following is the most appropriate therapeutic modification at this time?

A. Raise the pressure limit to 80 cm H_2O and check the ventilator for malfunctions
B. Have a colleague manually ventilate the patient while checking the ventilator circuit for leaks
C. Manually ventilate the patient while a colleague performs a physical examination
D. Recommend insertion of a chest tube
E. Page the physician stat
   (32:209)

11. A respiratory therapist is administering IPPB to a patient who is 3 days post left upper lobectomy. Suddenly the patient complains of sharp chest pains. Rapid physical examination reveals that the left lung field is hyperresonant to percussion and that the trachea has shifted to the right. Which of the following therapeutic modifications must the practitioner make at this time?

A. Terminate therapy and chart the above information
B. Terminate therapy and have a nurse notify the physician
C. Terminate therapy and insert a chest tube
D. Terminate therapy, call for help, and administer supplemental oxygen
E. Terminate therapy and page your supervisor
   (1:191) (37)

12. A patient is receiving continuous flow IMV via a Bennett MA-I ventilator with a 5-L reservoir bag in the system. The mandatory rate is 6 and the patient is not receiving PEEP therapy. During the patient's spontaneous respirations, the therapist notes that the system pressure manometer reads −8 cm H_2O. Based on the above information, the therapist should perform which of the following corrective actions?

A. Increase the continuous flow rate
B. Increase the sensitivity as well as the continuous flow rate
C. Decrease the sensitivity
D. Use a smaller reservoir bag system
E. Decrease the continuous flow rate
   (71) (57)

13. The arterial blood gases of a patient who is on continuous mechanical ventilation are consistent with respiratory alkalosis. Which of the following is the *least* appropriate corrective action?

A. Switch to IMV
B. Decrease tidal volume
C. Sedate patient
D. Wait for metabolic compensation to occur
E. Decrease respiratory rate
   (2:599–601) (1:349–352)

14. The respiratory therapist is administering 2.0 mL of 20%
acetylcysteine and 2.0 cc distilled water via a Bird Mark 7 ventilator to a patient with tenacious secretions. During the therapy the
patient becomes acutely dyspneic. Audible wheezes are noted
throughout both lung fields. The most appropriate action for the
respiratory practitioner to take at this time is to:
   A. Wait 5 minutes and perform nasotracheal suctioning
   B. Discontinue therapy and notify the physician
   C. Reduce acetylcysteine dosage and continue therapy
   D. Wait until dyspnea subsides and resume therapy
   E. Add 0.5 mL isoproterenol to the medication cup and con-
       tinue therapy
       (2:577–581)

15. The respiratory therapist receives an order to administer 1.0 mL
metaproterenol with 2.0 cc normal saline to a 65-year-old patient
with severe chronic obstructive pulmonary disease. Believing the
bronchodilator dosage might be in error, the practitioner contacts
the physician who states that the order is correct as written.
Under these circumstances, the practitioner should:
   A. Refuse to administer this dosage of isoproterenol
   B. Ask the physician to administer this drug himself
   C. Administer the therapy as ordered and notify the physician
       immediately should the patient experience side effects
   D. Administer therapy as ordered but increase nebulizer flow so
       that less drug deposition will occur
   E. Report this incident immediately to the medical director
       (2:577)

16. The physician orders 0.3 cc metaproterenol diluted to a 1:4 ratio
with one-half normal saline and administered every 2 hours to an
asthmatic patient. During the second treatment, the pulse is noted
to rise from 100 to 135. Based on this information, the respiratory
therapy practitioner should:
   A. Administer 0.25 cc isoproterenol next treatment
   B. Stop therapy and notify the nurse
   C. Stop therapy and notify the physician
   D. Wait until the pulse returns to baseline and resume therapy
   E. Stop therapy and chart observations
       (2:573 and 579–580)

17. The respiratory therapist receives an order to administer 24%
oxygen via nasal catheter to a severely dyspneic patient with
chronic obstructive pulmonary disease. There are no nasal cathe-
ters available and the physician cannot be reached for comment.
Which of the following therapeutic modifications should the prac-
titioner take at this time?
   A. Administer 24% oxygen via air entrainment mask
   B. Administer 1 L oxygen via nasal cannula
   C. Do nothing until the physician gives new orders
   D. Administer emergency IPPB therapy

E.   Administer 28% oxygen via air entrainment mask
(1:138–142)

18. The respiratory therapy practitioner is administering IPPB to a
patient with a Bennett PR-II. Suddenly the ventilator begins to
cycle on very rapidly. Which of the following therapeutic modifi-
cations should the practitioner make at this time?
I.   Check the ventilator sensitivity
II.   Instruct the patient not to pause so long between breaths
III.   Check the ventilator rate control
IV.   Stop therapy and change ventilators
A.   II and IV
B.   I only
C.   I and III
D.   I and IV
E.   IV only
(4:Chaps 9 and 10) (57) (68)

19. During the administration of IPPB with a Bird Mark 7 ventilator
to an alert patient, the respiratory therapy practitioner notes that
the inspiratory phase has become abruptly short. The most appro-
priate therapeutic modification would be to:
A.   Instruct the patient to follow instructions more carefully
B.   Check for an obstruction in the inspiratory mainline
C.   Check for a disconnected exhalation line
D.   Decrease the cycling pressure
E.   Check the expiratory flow for apnea control
(2:589–597) (68)

20. IPPB is being administered to a patient via a Bird ventilator. The
therapist notices that the system pressure gauge reads −10 cm
H_2O just prior to initiation of the inspiratory phase. The practitioner should make which of the following therapeutic modifications?
A.   Increase the flow rate setting
B.   Check for leaks in the high pressure line
C.   Adjust the pressure magnet and clutch assembly
D.   Increase ventilator sensitivity
E.   Instruct the patient not to expire too vigorously
(4:249–253) (68)

21. The respiratory therapist is administering IPPB to a postoperative
patient via mouthpiece. During the treatment, the patient is
unable to cycle the ventilator off. The most appropriate action(s)
would be:
I.   Adjust the sensitivity control
II.   Check for a leak in the system
III.   Check exhalation valve function
IV.   Decrease the cycling pressure to 10 cm H_2O
A.   II and III
B.   I and III
C.   I and II

D.   III and IV
E.   II only
(70:646–647) (2:589–591) (69)

22. The respiratory therapy practitioner is administering oxygen via a
partial rebreathing mask. Noting that the reserve bag collapses
completely during inspiration, the practitioner should:
A.   Replace the one-way valve between the mask and reservoir
bag
B.   Tape the ambient entrainment valve shut
C.   Get a blood gas analysis stat
D.   Increase the oxygen flow rate
E.   Have the patient sedated to decrease minute ventilation
(70:468)

23. The respiratory therapy practitioner is to administer oxygen therapy to a patient via simple oxygen mask. After attaching the
device, he notices that the humidifier's safety valve repeatedly
pops off. The practitioner should make which of the following
modifications?
A.   Replace the mask with a new one
B.   Tape the valve shut
C.   Leave well enough alone and get a blood gas sample
D.   Realize the oxygen tubing is obstructed and correct the
problem
E.   Page the nursing supervisor
(69)

24. The respiratory therapy practitioner is administering IPPB to an
alert patient via a Bennett PR-II ventilator. During the inspiratory phase, the system pressure gauge does not rise above atmospheric pressure and the patient must occlude the mouthpiece to
cycle the ventilator off. Which of the following therapeutic modifications corrects the above problem?
A.   Increasing the sensitivity
B.   Increasing the flow rate
C.   Adding terminal flow
D.   Administering therapy via sealed mouthpiece
E.   Decreasing the sensitivity
(2:589–591) (57)

25. IPPB is being administered to an alert 50-kg patient with 0.5 cc
isoetharine 1 day post orthopaedic surgery. With a cycling pressure of 27 cm H_2O, volumes of approximately 3000 cc are being
administered at a rate of 8 per minute. Several minutes into the
treatment the patient complains of lightheadedness and tingling of
her extremities. Which of the following actions should the respiratory therapy practitioner perform at this time?
A.   Stop the treatment and notify the physician
B.   Stop the treatment and decrease bronchodilator dosage
C.   Tell the patient to pause between each breath
D.   Lower the cycling pressure

E. Have the patient rest for several minutes and then resume
    therapy with settings unchanged
    (2:570–573)

Answer Key

1. E	6. D	11. D	16. C	21. A
2. A	7. A	12. A	17. A	22. D
3. B	8. D	13. D	18. C	23. D
4. B	9. C	14. B	19. B	24. B
5. C	10. C	15. C	20. D	25. D

Advanced Practitioner Pretest

According to the NBRC, 7% of the questions on the Advanced Practitioner Examination are from the modify therapy content category. In
addition, the Composite Examination Matrix (see reference 80) states
that questions in this category assess the candidate's ability to properly
and safely modify all respiratory therapy techniques on an advanced
level.

The following self-study questions were developed from specific competencies listed in the NBRC Composite Examination Matrix:

1. The respiratory therapist notes that even with proper hyperinfla-
    tion and hyperoxygenation, a 1650-g newborn repeatedly experi-
    ences bradycardia shortly after initiation of tracheal suctioning
    through a 3.5-mm endotracheal tube. Which of the following
    therapeutic modifications would be *least* helpful in preventing this
    side effect?
    A. Use of pulmonary drainage techniques
    B. Lavage with physiologic saline to thin secretions
    C. Administration of sympatholytics prior to therapy
    D. Use of smaller size suction catheter
    E. Exercising extreme care not to overstimulate upper airway
        tissues
        (1:267–270) (56:284) (2:525–527)

2. Which of the following pediatric patients should the respiratory
    therapy practitioner monitor with great caution because of the
    danger of oxygen-induced hypoventilation?
    I.   Those with infant respiratory distress syndrome
    II.   Those with bronchiolitis
    III. Those with cystic fibrosis
    IV.   Those with patent ductus arteriosus
    V.   Those with bronchial asthma
        A. III only
        B. II and III
        C. III and IV
        D. I, II, and V

E.   I, II, III, IV, and V
(29:176 and 178) (13:121)

3. The high pressure alarm of a Bennett MA-I ventilator is sounding with each breath and the patient is acutely distressed. The respiratory therapist begins manually hyperinflating while a colleague performs a rapid chest physical examination. The practitioner notes that each manual breath takes a great deal of effort and is accompanied by a musical inspiratory note. Severely diminished aeration is noted bilaterally, and tracheal shift is not noted. Which of the following corrective actions should the respiratory therapist perform at this time?
A.   Recommend insertion of a chest tube
B.   Retract the airway slightly
C.   Change the airway
D.   Deflate the tracheal tube cuff
E.   Inflate the tracheal tube cuff
(1:275) (32:211)

4. The respiratory therapy practitioner is asked to place a 90-year-old patient on a Bennett 7200 ventilator with an FI_{O_2} of 0.4 following orthopaedic surgery. The following arterial blood gas study was reported on the above FI_{O_2} with the alert patient in the assist/control mode:

Pa_{O_2}	59 mm Hg
Pa_{CO_2}	40 mm Hg
pH	7.43
Base excess	−0.4 mEq/L

Which of the following therapeutic modifications should the respiratory therapy practitioner make at this time?
A.   Increase the FI_{O_2} to 0.6
B.   Place the patient on 5 cm H_2O PEEP
C.   Increase the minute ventilation
D.   Place the patient on IMV
E.   No setting changes are indicated
(5:130 and Chap 12)

5. The respiratory therapy practitioner is caring for a patient with myasthenia gravis who is receiving continuous ventilatory support via a Bennett 7200 ventilator. Because of excessive parasympathetic activity, the volume of secretions above the tracheal tube cuff is usually considerable. Which of the following is the *least* acceptable method of managing these secretions?
A.   Instruct the patient to suction his pharynx on a p.r.n. basis
B.   Suction below the cuff, above the cuff, then deflate the cuff and manually sign the patient to help expel any remaining secretions
C.   Recommend the administration of parasympatholytics
D.   Deflate the endotracheal tube cuff prior to suctioning the trachea

E. Use appropriate drainage techniques
    (73) (78) (103:200–202)

6. The respiratory therapy practitioner is given an order to increase
    the end expiratory pressure of a patient on a Bourns Bear II venti-
    lator from 0 cm H_2O to 10 cm H_2O. Assuming this was the only
    change ordered, which of the following ventilator controls and
    alarms will have to be reset?
    A. High pressure and low exhaled tidal volume alarms
    B. High pressure and low pressure alarms
    C. High pressure, low pressure, and apnea alarms
    D. High pressure and ventilator inoperative alarms
    E. High pressure, low pressure, and low exhaled tidal volume
        alarms
    (60)

7. A 20-year-old, apneic, 100-kg patient with considerable neuro-
    logic trauma sustained in a suicide attempt is brought to the
    emergency department and immediately placed on a volume ven-
    tilator in the control mode. The following data were collected half
    an hour later with an FI_{O_2} of 0.4:

Pa_{O_2}	52 mm Hg
Pa_{CO_2}	30 mm Hg
pH	7.50
HCO_3^-	20 mEq/L
Base excess	−1.4 mEq/L
V_T	900 mL
Respiratory rate	24
Peak flow rate	50 L/min

Which of the following modifications should the respiratory therapy practitioner make at this time?
    A. Decrease the tidal volume and add 5 cm H_2O PEEP
    B. Decrease the respiratory rate and increase the FI_{O_2}
    C. Increase the flow rate and increase the FI_{O_2}
    D. Add 200 cc mechanical deadspace and increase the FI_{O_2}
    E. Increase the flow rate and add 10 cm H_2O PEEP
    (72) (1:500–501) (25:Chap 15, p 11)

8. The physician asks the respiratory therapy practitioner to begin
    weaning a 50-kg patient who has a vital capacity of 440 mL and a
    negative inspiratory force of 14 cm H_2O. The patient is currently
    on a volume ventilator in the assist/control mode. His blood gases
    on an FI_{O_2} of 0.4 are as follows:

Pa_{O_2}	78 mm Hg
Pa_{CO_2}	34 mm Hg
pH	7.49
HCO_3^-	27.3 mEq/L

The most appropriate modification would be to:

A.   Switch the patient to SIMV with a mandatory rate of 5
B.   Place the patient on a T tube setup with an FIo_2 of 0.4
C.   Switch the patient to SIMV with a mandatory rate of 12
D.   Place the patient on a T tube setup with an FIo_2 of 0.5
E.   Place the patient on 70% oxygen via heated aerosol mask
     (66) (2:670)

9.   The neonatologist asks the respiratory therapy practitioner to increase the level of PEEP to raise a 850-g newborn's mean airway pressure from 10 cm H_2O to 12 cm H_2O. Subsequently, the therapist observes the esophageal pressure (P_{ESO}) has not changed from previous values. Regarding the above information, the most appropriate therapeutic modification would be which of the following?

A.   Decrease the PEEP
B.   Increase the PEEP
C.   Make no modification at this time
D.   Decrease the ventilator rate
E.   Implement high-frequency ventilation
     (9:291)

10. The physician writes an order asking the respiratory therapist to make whatever ventilator changes are necessary to keep a 1200-g newborn's arterial blood gases within normal limits. The most recent results show a Pao_2 of 42 mm Hg and a $Paco_2$ of 40 mm Hg on an FIo_2 of 0.7. Which of the following therapeutic modifications is most appropriate at this time?

A.   Increase the PEEP
B.   Increase the FIo_2
C.   Increase the ventilator rate
D.   Get another blood gas sample
E.   Increase the pressure limit
     (29:217)

11. Following traumatic nasotracheal intubation, the respiratory therapist notes that a patient is bleeding profusely from upper airway soft tissues. The proper action for the respiratory therapy practitioner to take at this time is to:

A.   Page the physician and recommend orotracheal intubation
B.   Apply 1:100 epinephrine topically to achieve hemostasis
C.   Deflate the cuff periodically and carefully suction blood and secretions
D.   Replace the airway with a foam cuff type tube
E.   Notify the physician, keep the cuff inflated, and suction the pharynx as needed
     (73) (78) (80)

12. Shortly after the initiation of control mode continuous ventilatory support, an 80-kg patient's systolic blood pressure is noted to drop 20 mm Hg during every mechanical breath. The patient is receiving a tidal volume of 800 mL with a flow rate of 40 L/min

and at a rate of 26 L/min. Which of the following is the most appropriate action for the respiratory therapist to take at this time?
A. Administer 100 mL 5% albumin
B. Decrease the tidal volume
C. Increase the peak flow rate
D. Recommend further sedation of the patient
E. Decrease the peak flow rate
    (1:303–304 and 415) (72)

13. The respiratory therapy practitioner is administering continuous ventilatory support to an apneic 70-kg patient. The following information is charted with the patient receiving a tidal volume of 600 cc, an FI_{O_2} of 0.5, and a respiratory rate of 14:

Pa_{O_2}	156 mm Hg
Pa_{CO_2}	52 mm Hg
pH	7.33
HCO_3^-	26 mEq/L

Which of the following therapeutic modifications should the practitioner make at this time?
A. Decrease the FI_{O_2} and increase the tidal volume
B. Increase the respiratory rate
C. Increase the tidal volume to 800 cc
D. Add mechanical deadspace and lower the FI_{O_2}
E. Decrease the FI_{O_2} and decrease the respiratory rate
    (49)

14. During tracheal suctioning of a 30-year-old patient, the onset of bigeminal and multifocal premature ventricular contractions is noted on the cardiac monitor. The patient's color becomes ashen and he complains of dizziness. At this time, the respiratory therapy practitioner should take which of the following actions?
A. Lower the suctioning pressure and resume therapy
B. Page the physician stat
C. Stop therapy, call for assistance, and ensure ventilation and oxygenation by whatever means possible
D. Let the patient rest and then continue suctioning
E. Ask a nurse practitioner to interpret the rhythm strip
    (2:270) (25:Chap 6, pp 18–21)

15. A spontaneously breathing 55-year-old patient with noncardiogenic pulmonary edema is intubated and placed on a Bennett MA-I ventilator with an FI_{O_2} of 0.6 and 5 cm H_2O PEEP. Twenty minutes later the following blood gas and acid-base data are charted:

Pa_{O_2}	40 mm Hg
Pa_{CO_2}	36 mm Hg
pH	7.40

$$HCO_3^- \qquad 24.0 \text{ mEq/L}$$

Base excess -1.1 mEq/L

Based on the above information, which of the following ventilator modifications needs to be made at this time?

A. Leave settings unchanged
B. Increase FIo_2 to 0.7
C. Decrease ventilator sensitivity
D. Increase PEEP to 10 cm H_2O
E. Decrease minute ventilation
   (5:130) (49)

16. Which of the following modifications could the respiratory therapy practitioner use as a method to reduce condensation of water in the ventilatory circuit of a newborn who is on a Baby Bird ventilator?

A. Using a disposable circuit
B. Decreasing the proximal airway temperature to 32°C
C. Placing the ventilatory tubing inside the Isolette
D. Using a thick-walled, narrow-bore tubing
E. Using corregated tubing
   (29:220)

17. One hour after being placed on a volume ventilator, an apprehensive 68-year-old patient with chronic obstructive pulmonary disease is experiencing ventricular arrhythmias and generalized seizures. Arterial blood gas analysis at this time in the assist/control mode with an FIo_2 of 0.4 reveals a Pao_2 of 62 mm Hg, a $Paco_2$ of 42 mm Hg, a pH of 7.65, and an HCO_3^- of 34 mEq/L. Which of the following is the correct modification of this patient's respiratory therapy?

A. Add 400 cc mechanical deadspace and pharmacologically paralyze
B. Adjust ventilator to allow $Paco_2$ to return to baseline values
C. Increase the backup rate and administer acetazolamide (Diamox®) to control metabolic alkalosis
D. Place patient on 5 cm H_2O PEEP and pharmacologically paralyze
E. Leave settings unchanged and monitor cardiac output
   (2:599–600) (7:167)

18. The respiratory therapist is performing nasotracheal suctioning on a patient in the intensive care unit. Looking at the cardiac monitor, the therapist notes the onset of ventricular tachycardia. Which of the following is the most acceptable sequence of actions?

A. Stop therapy and notify the physician at once
B. Leave the catheter in place and administer 6 to 10 L oxygen through it
C. Call for help, establish an airway, and ensure ventilation with supplemental oxygen
D. Place patient on nasal oxygen and wait for arrhythmia to subside

E. Lower suctioning pressure and resume therapy
(1:270) (25:Chap 6, pp 20–21)

Answer Key

1. C	5. D	9. C	13. A	17. B
2. A	6. B	10. A	14. C	18. C
3. D	7. C	11. E	15. D	
4. E	8. C	12. C	16. C	

I. Recommend Modifications in Therapy

Questions in this category are designed to assess the candidate's ability to recommend modifications in the respiratory care plan based on the patient's response to respiratory therapy. It is important to note that this content category is an extension of the previous two. In category G the practitioner was asked to assess the patient's response to the various respiratory techniques. In category H the practitioner was asked to modify respiratory therapy based on his/her previous assessment. As noted previously, there are many modifications that cannot be made without a physician's written order. This is the nature of this particular content category. Here the practitioner must act as a consultant to the physician, recommending modifications in therapy that are necessary.

The importance of this content category is underscored by the fact that 22% of the questions on the Advanced Practitioner Examination are taken from this area. Questions from this category are arguably the most difficult on the NBRC examinations, for not only must the practitioner be able to assess what is wrong with the patient, but he or she must also know specifically what type of therapeutic modality is indicated in the treatment of the patient's disorder.

Entry Level Pretest

According to the NBRC, 4% of the questions on the Entry Level Examination are from this category. In addition, the Composite Examination Matrix (see reference 80) states that questions from this category assess the candidate's ability to recommend on an entry level modifications in all respiratory care techniques to appropriate medical personnel.

The following self-study questions were developed from specific competencies listed in the NBRC Composite Examination Matrix:

1. Which of the following aerosolized medications would the respiratory therapist be *least* likely to recommend for patients with croup or postextubation laryngeal edema?
A. Racemic epinephrine
B. Corticosteroids

C. Isoproterenol
D. Cool, aqueous electrolyte solutions
E. Phenylephrine
(2:473)

2. For which of the following patients could the respiratory therapy practitioner recommend the use of pressure-cycled ventilators as a means of providing continuous ventilatory support?
A. Those with chronic obstructive pulmonary disease
B. Those with adult respiratory distress syndrome
C. Those with neuromuscular disorders who require long-term ventilatory support
D. Those with pulmonary fibrotic disorders
E. None of the above
(2:589–591) (32:116–117)

3. For patients with which of the following conditions would the respiratory therapy practitioner *not* recommend postural drainage techniques?
A. Bronchiectasis
B. Empyema
C. Lung abscess
D. Cystic fibrosis
E. Chronic bronchitis
(1:202)

4. The respiratory therapy practitioner is monitoring a 65-kg patient with acute neuromuscular disease. Bedside pulmonary function tests reveal the following:

Respiratory rate	44
Vital capacity	430 mL
Negative inspiratory force	12 cm H_2O

Based on the above information, which of the following is the most appropriate recommendation?
A. Administer high concentration oxygen
B. Do a before and after bronchodilator study
C. Administer continuous ventilatory support
D. Administer CPAP
E. Obtain stat chest film and repeat blood gas study
(1:302–305) (11:222–230) (7:362–365)

5. Which of the following could the respiratory therapy practitioner recommend as a means of correcting hypocarbia in a patient who is being mechanically ventilated?
A. Decrease inspiratory flow rate
B. Administer sodium bicarbonate
C. Add mechanical deadspace
D. Administer PEEP
E. Perform elective tracheotomy
(1:351–352)

6. The respiratory therapy practitioner is instructed to place his or her patient on the level of PEEP that corresponds to the best cardiovascular function. In so doing the following data are collected on various levels of PEEP:

Level of PEEP	Sa_{O_2}	$S\bar{v}_{O_2}$
0	70%	43%
3	72%	46%
6	76%	51%
9	82%	59%
12	84%	63%
15	86%	56%
18	87%	52%

The level of PEEP the therapist should recommend is:
A. 6 cm H_2O
B. 9 cm H_2O
C. 12 cm H_2O
D. 15 cm H_2O
E. 18 cm H_2O
(46:2–5) (47)

7. Which of the following methods would the respiratory therapy practitioner be *least* likely to recommend to help stabilize the chest wall of a patient with flail chest who also requires continuous ventilatory support?
A. Pharmacologic paralysis and controlled mechanical ventilation
B. IMV with PEEP
C. PEEP
D. NEEP
E. Assisted ventilation with large tidal volumes
(64) (1:504–505)

8. In general, the respiratory therapy practitioner would *not* recommend atropine for bronchodilator therapy in which of the following patients?
  I. Those subject to tachyarrhythmias
 II. Those who do not respond to sympathomimetic bronchodilators
III. Those with thickened and tenacious secretions
  A. II and III
  B. II only
  C. I and III
  D. I and II
  E. I only
(2:490) (53:134–136)

9. Which of the following bronchodilators should the respiratory therapy practitioner recommend for use in a patient who has suffered a recent myocardial infarction?
A. Atropine
B. Isoproterenol

C. Epinephrine
D. Metaproterenol
E. Racemic epinephrine
   (25:Chap 3, p 9)

10. Within minutes following extubation, a 45-year-old patient is noted to develop moderate inspiratory stridor. The patient is alert and otherwise in no distress. Which of the following recommendations would be appropriate for the respiratory therapist to make at this time?
   I.   Perform emergency intubation stat
   II. Administer a continuous cool aerosol
   III. Administer aerosolized decongestants and/or corticosteroids
   IV. Be prepared to reintubate
       A. I and III
       B. II and IV
       C. I only
       D. II, III, and IV
       E. IV only
   (1:282–285)

11. A physician's order reads: "IPPB every 2 hours with 0.5 mL isoetharine and 4 cc of 4.2% $NaHCO_3$." The most appropriate recommendation for the respiratory therapy practitioner to make would be:
   A. Inform the physician that bicarbonate solutions cannot be aerosolized
   B. Ask the physician to use metaproterenol instead of isoetharine
   C. Inform the physician that sympathomimetics lose effectiveness in an alkaline medium
   D. Recommend that acetylcysteine be administered instead
   E. Administer therapy as ordered
   (25:Chap 8, pp 3–4) (40)

12. A respiratory therapy practitioner is monitoring a patient who is receiving PEEP therapy. The physician wants the practitioner's help in determining the optimal level of this modality. The practitioner should recommend monitoring which of the following parameters to help determine this dosage?
   A. Pa_{O_2}
   B. $\dot{Q}_S/\dot{Q}_T$
   C. Arterial blood pressure
   D. Effective static compliance
   E. Effective dynamic compliance
   (46:5) (47) (31:21)

13. Which of the following therapeutic modalities would the respiratory therapy practitioner recommend for a comatose neurotrauma victim who has a respiratory rate of 33, a negative inspiratory

force of 30 cm H_2O, a Pa_{CO_2} of 45 mm Hg, and a P_{O_2} of 60 mm Hg while receiving 8 L oxygen via simple oxygen mask?
A. IPPB every 2 hours with isoetharine
B. Oxygen therapy via nonrebreathing mask
C. CPAP therapy
D. Continuous mechanical ventilation
E. 50% oxygen via T tube
(38:60)

14. Which of the following methods of oxygen administration would the respiratory therapy practitioner be *least* likely to recommend for a hypoxemic, low birth weight newborn?
A. Oxygen catheter
B. Oxygen hood
C. Nasal CPAP prongs
D. Isolette
E. Endotracheal tube
(13:78–88)

15. A 39-year-old, 50-kg woman is brought to the emergency department following barbiturate overdose. She is comatose and her eyes are fully dilated. The following laboratory data are collected immediately after admission:

FI_{O_2}	0.21
pH	7.19
Pa_{O_2}	53 mm Hg
Pa_{CO_2}	74 mm Hg
HCO_3^-	26.2 mEq/L
Base excess	−3.0 mEq/L

Which of the following is the most appropriate recommendation regarding this patient?
A. Place on 3 L oxygen via nasal cannula and administer IPPB
B. Intubate and place on assist/control with a V_T of 500, a backup rate of 8, and an FI_{O_2} of 1.0
C. Intubate and place on a Bennett PR-II ventilator with a cycling pressure of 20 cm H_2O
D. Intubate and place on assist/control with a V_T of 600, a backup rate of 15, and an FI_{O_2} of 0.3
E. Intubate and place on assist/control with a V_T of 1000, a backup rate of 20, and an FI_{O_2} of 0.25
(1:Chap 22) (38:Chap 6) (58) (2:394–395)

16. An alert, 17-year-old patient is scheduled for surgery to repair tendon and ligament damage sustained in a football game. As part of a routine preoperative workup, the following data are gathered:

Pa_{O_2}	43 mm Hg
Pa_{CO_2}	47 mm Hg
pH	7.35

FIo_2	0.21
Respiratory rate	12
Pulse	45
BP	110/60
Temperature	37.4°C

Which of the following should the respiratory therapy practitioner recommend regarding the above data?
A. An electrocardiogram
B. Administration of 6 L oxygen via nasal cannula
C. Repeating the arterial blood gas studies
D. Intubation and continuous mechanical ventilation
E. Postponing the surgery
   (5:155 and Chap 12)

17. A physician's order reads: "Administer 4 L oxygen via hood." The patient is a 2100-g newborn who was born approximately 1 month preterm. The respiratory therapy practitioner should:
A. Administer therapy as ordered
B. Obtain a chest roentgenogram
C. Ask the physician to specify a concentration of oxygen
D. Refuse to administer therapy
E. Suggest nasal prongs instead
   (13:153)

18. The respiratory therapy practitioner receives an order to administer IPPB every 2 hours to a 33-year-old patient who is recovering from upper abdominal surgery performed approximately 16 hours earlier. During the treatment, the patient consistently achieves tidal volumes in excess of 2.4 L, with a cycling pressure of 15 cm H_2O. Further investigation reveals that the patient's spontaneous vital capacity is 25 cc/kg. Based on this information, which of the following is the most appropriate recommendation?
A. All respiratory therapy should be discontinued
B. Aerosol therapy followed by postural drainage
C. Sustained maximal inspiratory therapy (incentive spirometry) every hour while awake
D. Blow bottles every other day four times a day
E. Metaproterenol, 0.5 cc, via hand-held nebulizer
   (1:194–195) (3:883–885)

19. An order is received to administer incentive spirometry to an 84-year-old woman who is recovering from hip surgery performed 18 hours previously. However, even after thorough instructions, the therapist finds that the patient is unable to accomplish a proper sustained inspiratory maneuver. Further investigation reveals this patient's vital capacity is 15 cc/kg. Based on the above information, which of the following is the most appropriate recommendation?
A. Intubation and administration of CPAP therapy is indicated.
B. Respiratory therapy should be discontinued.

C. Postural drainage and percussion is indicated.
D. IPPB should be administered instead of incentive spirometry.
E. Therapy as ordered should be continued.
   (1:194–195) (2:883–885)

20. A 25-year-old patient with advanced cystic fibrosis is brought to the emergency department by her parents. She is cyanotic and distressed but is able to protect her airway. She is placed on 3 L oxygen via nasal cannula, and an intravenous line is started. Twenty minutes later arterial blood is analyzed, revealing:

Pa_{O_2}	40 mm Hg
Pa_{CO_2}	90 mm Hg
pH	7.12
Base excess	+8 mEq/L
HCO_3^-	30 mEq/L
Hb concentration	18.9 g/dL

Following consideration of this information, the respiratory therapy practitioner should recommend:
A. Decreasing the liter flow to 1 L/min
B. Placing patient on a 35% air entrainment mask
C. Initiation of continuous mechanical ventilation with an FI_{O_2} of 0.35
D. Placing the patient on 4 L oxygen via nasal cannula
E. Obtaining another arterial blood gas sample because laboratory error exists
   (49) (38:64–66) (63:102–121) (32:92–96) (2:1010)

21. Which of the following should the respiratory therapy practitioner recommend as the *most* effective means of administering therapeutic aerosols with a very high density to the tracheobronchial tree?
A. Nondisposable all-purpose nebulizer
B. Disposable pneumatic all-purpose nebulizer
C. Ultrasonic nebulizer
D. Hydronamic type nebulizer
E. Spinning disk type nebulizer
   (1:172 and 179)

22. Which of the following means of oxygen administration would the respiratory therapy practitioner recommend for a patient who has a carboxyhemoglobin concentration of 30%?
A. Nonrebreathing mask
B. Partial rebreathing mask
C. Simple oxygen mask
D. Nasal cannula
E. Nasal catheter
   (1:497–498)

23. The physician wants the respiratory therapy practitioner to place the patient on the level of PEEP that corresponds to the best effec-

tive static compliance. With the corrected tital volume held constant, the following data are accumulated:

Level of PEEP	Plateau Pressure
0 cm H_2O	48 cm H_2O
3 cm H_2O	50 cm H_2O
6 cm H_2O	52 cm H_2O
9 cm H_2O	51 cm H_2O
12 cm H_2O	51 cm H_2O
15 cm H_2O	52 cm H_2O
18 cm H_2O	58 cm H_2O
21 cm H_2O	66 cm H_2O

Which of the following levels of PEEP should the respiratory therapist recommend?
A.   9 cm H_2O
B.   12 cm H_2O
C.   15 cm H_2O
D.   18 cm H_2O
E.   21 cm H_2O
   (47) (50) (1:375)

24.   Which of the following should the respiratory therapy practitioner *not* recommend to help facilitate the weaning of a patient from supportive ventilation?
A.   Deflation of the tracheal tube cuff during the procedure
B.   Not suctioning the patient during weaning attempts
C.   Using an FIo_2 10% higher than on the ventilator
D.   Positioning the patient in a sitting or semirecumbent position
E.   Monitoring of an electrocardiogram during the process
   (2:668–670)

25.   A patient with a history of chronic obstructive pulmonary disease is brought to the emergency department after several days of increasing respiratory distress. After a baseline arterial sample is drawn, oxygen is administered via nasal cannula at a flow rate of 2 L/min. Pertinent arterial blood gas data are revealed below:

	Room Air	2 L Oxygen
Pao_2	35 mm Hg	45 mm Hg
$Paco_2$	75 mm Hg	70 mm Hg
pH	7.24	7.31
HCO_3	33 mEq/L	36 mEq/L

Based on the above clinical data, the respiratory therapy practitioner should recommend which of the following changes in this patient's therapy?
A.   Increase the oxygen flow to 5 L/min
B.   Intubate and place on assist/control with an FIo_2 of 0.35
C.   Place on a 28% air entrainment mask
D.   Increase oxygen flow to 3 L/min

   E.   Place patient on IMV with an FI_{O_2} of 0.4
        (49) (38:64–66) (63:101–121) (32:92) (1:Chaps 7 and 32)
        (5:180–183)

26. A respiratory therapy practitioner receives an order to use pos-
     tural drainage techniques on a patient who underwent surgery 24
     hours previously to repair a cerebral aneurysm. On reviewing the
     patient's chest roentgenogram the practitioner notes the presence
     of considerable infiltrates in the right lateral and posterior basal
     segments. The most appropriate course of action for the respira-
     tory therapy practitioner to take would be to:
   A.   Drain the affected segments as best as possible while a nurse
        monitors the patient's arterial blood pressure
   B.   Inform the physician that postural drainage is in fact contra-
        indicated for this patient
   C.   Refuse to perform the therapy as ordered
   D.   Drain the affected segments using accepted drainage posi-
        tions
   E.   Inform the physician of possible hazards and ask for further
        orders
        (1:202) (7:205–207) (76)

Answer Key

1. C	6. C	11. C	16. C	21. C
2. E	7. D	12. D	17. C	22. A
3. B	8. C	13. D	18. C	23. C
4. C	9. D	14. A	19. D	24. B
5. C	10. D	15. D	20. C	25. D
				26. E

Advanced Practitioner Pretest

   According to the NBRC, 22% of the questions on the Advanced Practitioner Examination are from the recommend modifications in therapy
content category. In addition, the Composite Examination Matrix (see
reference 80) states that questions from this category assess the candidate's ability to recommend modifications in all respiratory care techniques on an advanced level to appropriate medical personnel.
   The following self-study questions were developed from the competencies listed in the NBRC Composite Examination Matrix:

1.   After 9 days on continuous ventilatory support in the assist/con-
     trol mode, a 53-year-old patient regains consciousness. Because
     of an improving clinical picture, the respiratory therapy practi-
     tioner is asked to gather the following data for weaning purposes:

Weight	75 kg
Pa_{O_2}	96 mm Hg
Pa_{CO_2}	29 mm Hg

FIo$_2$	0.4
pH	7.48
Vital capacity	13 cc/kg
Negative inspiratory force	21 cc/kg
Resting spontaneous minute volume	16 L/min

Based on the above data, which of the following would be the most appropriate recommendation?
A. Place on IMV with an FIo$_2$ of 0.7
B. Add 200 cc deadspace and get an arterial sample
C. Place on IMV with an FIo$_2$ of 0.4
D. Place on T tube with an FIo$_2$ of 0.6
E. Place on T tube with an FIo$_2$ of 0.5
    (2:670) (66)

2. The respiratory therapy practitioner is administering IPPB to a patient in the cardiac care unit when he notes the following rhythm on a cardiac monitor:

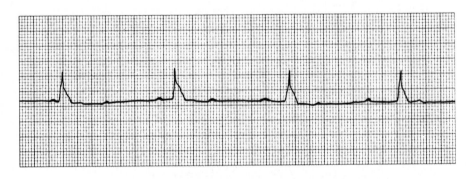

Figure IV-47.

Which of the following therapeutic modalities should the therapist recommend at this time?
A. Lidocaine
B. Morphine
C. Pacemaker
D. Sodium bicarbonate
E. Epinephrine
    (25:Chap 6, p 27)

3. The respiratory therapist is asked to help correct a neonatal condition in which the Pao$_2$ is 45 mm Hg while breathing 35% oxygen via Isolette. At the same time, a pH of 7.42 and a Paco$_2$ of 40 mm Hg are noted. Which of the following is to be recommended?
A. Administer 60% oxygen via Isolette
B. Administer 50% oxygen via hood
C. Intubate and place on 4 cm H$_2$O CPAP with an FIo$_2$ of 0.5

D. Administer 100% oxygen via hood
E. Initiate continuous ventilatory support with an FIo_2 of 0.7
    (29:206 and 209) (13:78–88)

4. A comatose 37-year-old patient is admitted to the emergency
    department following a suicide attempt involving ingestion of an
    unknown quantity of secobarbital (Seconal®). The following data
    are obtained at this time with the patient breathing room air:

Pao_2	35 mm Hg
$Paco_2$	78 mm Hg
pH	7.11
Base excess	−6.8 mEq/L

    Based on the above data, which of the following would the respi-
    ratory therapy practitioner *not* recommend as part of this patient's
    management?
    A. Continuous ventilatory support
    B. Naloxone (Narcan®)
    C. Supplemental oxygen
    D. Emergency airway
    E. Cardiovascular support
        (53:231–232) (7:369–376) (2:394–395)

5. Cardiopulmonary resuscitation is in progress for a 60-year-old
    patient in the cardiac care unit. The monitor shows a fine ventric-
    ular fibrillation. Two initial attempts at defibrillation with 250
    watts/sec are unsuccessful in treating this arrhythmia. Which of
    the following should the advanced respiratory therapy practitioner
    not recommend at this time?
    A. Emergency intubation
    B. Ventilation with 100% oxygen
    C. $NaHCO_3$ administration
    D. Epinephrine administration
    E. Additional attempts at defibrillation with 400 watts/sec
        (25:Chap 2, pp 5–7)

6. A 63-year-old asthmatic who has developed adult respiratory dis-
    tress syndrome and Gram-negative hypotensive shock is placed on
    volume ventilation with an FIo_2 of 0.6 and 8 cm H_2O PEEP. Sub-
    sequently the decision is made to paralyze the patient pharmaco-
    logically and control her ventilation. Which one of the following
    drugs should the therapist recommend to accomplish this goal?
    A. Succinylcholine
    B. Pancuronium bromide (Pavulon®)
    C. Curare
    D. Neostigmine
    E. Sodium pentothal
        (53:365–369)

7. An 18-year-old, 40-kg woman is seen in the intensive care unit 2
    days after being found comatose by friends at home. She is on a
    volume ventilator in the assist/control mode with an FIo_2 of 0.4.

Because she has regained consciousness and is fighting the ventilator, the physician asks the respiratory therapist to collect appropriate weaning data. The following information is charted at this time:

Pa_{O_2}	88 mm Hg
Pa_{CO_2}	24 mm Hg
Vital capacity	1760 mL
Negative inspiratory force	58 cm H_2O
pH	7.56

The respiratory therapist would most likely be correct in recommending which of the following?
A. Placing the patient on a T tube system with an FI_{O_2} of 0.5
B. Sedating the patient to prevent her from fighting the ventilator
C. Placing the patient on IMV with an FI_{O_2} of 0.4
D. Adding 200 cc mechanical deadspace and obtaining a blood gas analysis
E. Extubating the patient and placing her on a 50% heated aerosol mask
   (1:339–341, 381, and 384) (2:599–601 and 670) (62) (66)

8. The respiratory therapy practitioner is monitoring a hemodynamically stable 1200-g (32-week gestation) newborn who is being ventilated by a time-cycled controller in the continuous flow IMV mode. Umbilical arterial blood gases on an FI_{O_2} of 0.9, a mandatory rate of 20, 3 cm H_2O PEEP, and an 1:E ratio of 1:3 are as follows:

Pa_{O_2}	40 mm Hg
Pa_{CO_2}	65 mm Hg
pH	7.20
Base excess	−5.1 mEq/L
HCO_3^-	15.6 mEq/L

Based on the above information, which of the following should the respiratory therapy practitioner recommend?
A. Increase the PEEP and use an 1:E ratio of 1:4
B. Increase the PEEP and the FI_{O_2}
C. Increase the PEEP and the IMV rate
D. Increase the FI_{O_2} and use inverse 1:E ratios
E. Increase the IMV rate and raise the FI_{O_2} to 1.0
   (29:206–212)

9. Which of the following size (I.D.) endotracheal tubes should the respiratory therapy practitioner recommend for an average-size patient who is 8 years old?
A. 4.0 mm
B. 6.0 mm
C. 7.5 mm

D. 8.0 mm
E. 9.0 mm
   (25:Chap 17, p 3)

10. A 70-year-old patient with a long history of bronchitis and emphysema is brought to the emergency department because of respiratory distress and increasing confusion. Blood gas analysis results obtained 30 minutes after being placed on 3 L oxygen via nasal cannula are as follows:

Pa_{O_2}	88 mm Hg
Pa_{CO_2}	75 mm Hg
pH	7.34
HCO_3^-	38 mEq/L
Pulse	100
Blood pressure	130/90

Based on the above data, what would be the most appropriate recommendation for the respiratory therapy practitioner to make at this time?
A. Place on 5 cm H_2O mask CPAP
B. Do not change present therapy
C. Decrease oxygen flow to 2 L/min
D. Intubate and place on assist/control with an FI_{O_2} of 0.4
E. Increase oxygen flow to 4 L/min
   (49) (38:64–66) (63:102–121) (32:92–96)

11. A 30-year-old patient received a vagotomy and partial pyloroplasty 8 days previously. Three days postoperatively, he became septic and was taken back to the operating room to repair a perforated ileum. Since that time he has been on a volume ventilator with high levels of PEEP and FI_{O_2}s of 0.7 or greater. Because of the danger of oxygen toxicity, the pulmonary physician makes the decision to raise the patient's PEEP to 28 cm H_2O and at the same time lower his FI_{O_2} to 0.5. Concurrent and pertinent information is noted below:

	20 cm H_2O PEEP	28 cm H_2O PEEP
Pa_{O_2}	46 mm Hg	46 mm Hg
$S\bar{v}_{O_2}$	57%	47%
$C(a-\bar{v})_{O_2}$	3.5 vol%	5.8 vol%
Qs/Q_T	34%	28%
FI_{O_2}	0.7	0.5
PWP (on ventilator)	6 mm Hg	9 mm Hg
Oxygen consumption	250 mL/min	250 mL/min

Further orders are to leave the FI_{O_2} at the 0.5 level despite any cardiovascular depression noted at 28 cm H_2O PEEP. At this

time, which of the following should the advanced respiratory therapy practitioner recommend to treat this patient's hypoxia?
A.   Lower the PEEP to 15 cm H_2O
B.   Raise the PEEP to 30 cm H_2O
C.   Induce hypothermia to lower metabolic demands
D.   Expand intravascular volume
E.   Apply inflation hold of 0.5 second
   (46) (49) (47)

12. A 12-year-old boy sustains trauma including a long-bone fracture and is admitted to the emergency department in shock. After appropriate fluid resuscitation, he is hemodynamically stable. The chest roentgenogram on admission is unremarkable. Twelve hours later the following data are obtained while the patient is receiving an FIo_2 of 0.6 via T tube setup:

Pao_2	40 mm Hg
$Paco_2$	27 mm Hg
pH	7.42
HCO_3^-	12 mEq/L
Base excess	−7.4 mEq/L

Based on the above information, which of the following is the most appropriate recommendation?
A.   A stat chest roentgenogram
B.   Place on 5 cm CPAP with an FIo_2 of 0.5
C.   Place on controlled mechanical ventilation with an FIo_2 of 1.0
D.   Place on assist/control with 8 cm H_2O PEEP and an FIo_2 of 0.7
E.   Place on assist/control with an FIo_2 of 0.9
   (49:2) (32:64–66 and 117–118) (38:Chaps 4 through 6 and 63)

13. A 1650-g (33-week gestation) newborn is seen in the nursery 5 hours after an uneventful delivery. The following is noted with the patient breathing room air:

Respiratory rate	75
Pulse	195
Blood pressure	65/35
Expiratory grunt	Audible with stethoscope
Sternal retractions	Some noted
Color	Peripheral cyanosis

Which of the following should the respiratory therapy practitioner recommend at this time?
A.   Intubate and place on 2 cm H_2O CPAP
B.   Place patient on 4 cm H_2O nasal CPAP
C.   Place on 60% oxygen via hood
D.   Place on 40% oxygen via Isolette
E.   Intubate and place on IMV
   (29:206–212)

14. The intern is unable to pass an oral endotracheal tube despite repeated attempts. In desperation, he asks someone to give him the antidote for the succinylcholine he has administered to facilitate tracheal intubation. The respiratory therapist should promptly hand him:
    A. Neostigmine
    B. Pancuronium bromide (Pavulon)
    C. Edrophonium chloride (Tensilon®)
    D. Pyridostigmine bromide (Mestinon®)
    E. A bag-valve-mask unit
    (53:371)

15. A 20-year-old, 60-kg patient is seen in the emergency department during a severe asthma attack. The following information is noted at that time with the patient receiving 3 L oxygen via nasal cannula:

Pa_{O_2}	60 mm Hg
Pa_{CO_2}	40 mm Hg
pH	7.34
HCO_3^-	20 mEq/L
Vital capacity	20 cc/kg

    Regarding the above information, which is the correct recommendation?
    A. The patient should be given intramuscular and aerosolized sympathomimetics and admitted to a medical ward immediately.
    B. The patient should be intubated and transferred to the intensive care unit.
    C. Isoetharine should be administered via IPPB and the patient sent home.
    D. Appropriate bronchodilator and oxygen therapy should be administered and the patient transferred to the intensive care unit.
    E. A before and after bronchodilator study using isoproterenol should be performed stat.
    (32:Chap 8)

16. Which of the following antimicrobial agents should the respiratory therapist recommend for a patient who has coccidioidomycosis?
    A. Polymixin B
    B. Amphotericin B
    C. Penicillin G
    D. d-tubocurarine
    E. Amikacin
    (2:491)

17. Administration of which of the following therapeutic modalities would be *least* beneficial in decreasing the venous return of a patient who has developed acute cardiogenic pulmonary edema?
    A. IPPB

B.   Phenylephrine hydrochloride
C.   Morphine sulfate
D.   Rotating tourniquets
E.   Furosemide
     (1:Chap 27) (53:123-124)

18. A 43-year-old patient is admitted to the progressive care unit with a diagnosis of acute bronchial asthma. On admission, he is ordered "IPPB every 2 to 3 hours while awake and p.r.n. at night with 0.5 cc isoetharine." Because of the complaint that this therapy is not providing significant benefit, his physician asks the respiratory therapy practitioner to recommend methods to evaluate therapeutic effectiveness. Which of the following will provide the physician with the information he needs when the patient is monitored both before and after therapy?
     I. $\dfrac{FEV_1}{FVC}\%$
     II.   Pulse
     III. Forced vital capacity
     IV.   Blood pressure
     V.   Chest physical findings
           A.   I, IV, and V
           B.   I, II, and IV
           C.   II, III, and IV
           D.   I only
           E.   I, III, and V
     (13:278-280) (1:189 and 231)

19. Which of the following delivered energy settings should the respiratory therapy practitioner recommend for initial attempts at defibrillation when performed on adult patients?
     A.   200-300 watts/sec
     B.   300-400 watts/sec
     C.   400 or greater watts/sec
     D.   1-4 watts/sec/kg
     E.   100-200 watts/sec
     (25:Chap 7, p 4)

20. The physician wants the respiratory therapist to monitor appropriate hemodynamic data and place a severely hypoxic patient on the optimal level of PEEP. The following data are collected at this time:

Level of PEEP (cm H_2O)	Sa_{O_2}	Cardiac Index [(Q_T) (Body Surface Area)]
0	73%	2.9 L/m²
5	78%	3.2 L/m²
10	84%	3.4 L/m²
15	86%	3.0 L/m²
20	88%	2.6 L/m²

Based on the above information, what is the most appropriate
level of PEEP?
A.   0 cm H_2O
B.   5 cm H_2O
C.   10 cm H_2O
D.   15 cm H_2O
E.   20 cm H_2O
   (47) (46)

21. Which of the following would be the most appropriate antibiotic
     for home treatment of pulmonary infections in patients with
     chronic obstructive pulmonary disease caused by Gram-positive
     bacteria?
     A.   Polymixin B
     B.   Amphotericin B
     C.   Amikacin
     D.   Ampicillin
     E.   Gentamicin
        (11:93)

22. Which of the following should the respiratory therapist *not* recom-
     mend as part of the home care plan for a patient with chronic
     bronchitis who also has cor pulmonale?
     A.   Chest physical therapy
     B.   Oxygen therapy
     C.   Aerosol therapy
     D.   IPPB therapy
     E.   High sodium diet
        (38:65)

23. The respiratory therapy practitioner would be *least* likely to rec-
     ommend initiation of continuous ventilatory support as part of the
     treatment of severe chronic obstructive pulmonary disease in
     which one of the following instances?
     A.   Patient inability to protect airway
     B.   Inability to keep pH above 7.20
     C.   On noting mild increases in $Paco_2$ following oxygen admini-
          stration
     D.   Rapid deterioration of sensorium
     E.   Sudden onset of hypotension or arrhythmias
        (49) (38:64–66) (63:102–121) (32:92–96) (1:Chap 7, p 32)

24. The respiratory therapy practitioner is monitoring a hemodynam-
     ically stable 1100-g newborn who is being ventilated with a con-
     ventional time-cycled controller in the continuous flow IMV
     mode. Umbilical arterial blood gases on an FIo_2 of 0.7 and 4 cm
     H_2O PEEP, a mandatory rate of 15, and an I:E of 1:3.5 are as
     follows:

Pao_2	41 mm Hg
$Paco_2$	38 mm Hg
pH	7.32

Base excess   −4.8
HCO_3^- 15.9 mEq/L

Based on the above information, which of the following is the most appropriate recommendation?
A. Increase the PEEP to 6 cm H_2O
B. Increase the FIo_2 to 1.0 and decrease mandatory rate
C. Decrease the PEEP and increase the mandatory rate
D. Place on high-frequency jet ventilation
E. Place on 18 cm H_2O CPAP with an FIo_2 of 1.0
(29:206–212)

25. Which of the following drugs should the respiratory therapy practitioner recommend for topical administration to help control the bleeding that frequently occurs during attempts at nasotracheal intubation?
A. Dexamethasone
B. Isoproterenol
C. Lidocaine
D. Epinephrine
E. Benzocaine
(53:117–119)

26. A 43-year-old patient is seen in the intensive care unit while on 10 cm H_2O PEEP with an FIo_2 of 0.8. Because of severe hypoxemia, the level of PEEP is raised to 15 cm H_2O. The pertinent data are presented below:

	10 cm H_2O PEEP	15 cm H_2O PEEP
Pao_2	45 mm Hg	45 mm Hg
$S\bar{v}o_2$	55%	46%
PWP (on ventilator)	10 mm Hg	13 mm Hg
Qs/Q_T	26%	20%
$C(a-\bar{v})o_2$	3.4 vol%	6.5 vol%

Based on the above information, which of the following should the respiratory therapy practitioner recommend at this time?
A. Increase the PEEP to 18 cm H_2O
B. Leave the PEEP at 15 cm H_2O
C. Lower the PEEP to 5 cm H_2O
D. Lower the PEEP to 12 cm H_2O and increase cardiac output
E. Leave the PEEP at 15 cm H_2O and increase the FIo_2 to 1.0
(46) (1:Chap 27, pp 415–416) (38:Chaps 4 through 6, p 63) (32:64–66) (65)

27. After 96 hours of continuous mechanical ventilation, a 29-year-old woman who aspirated gastric contents during an emergency cesarean section has begun to stabilize. She is presently receiving 15 cm H_2O PEEP with an FIo_2 of 0.7 via a Bennett MA-I ventilator in the IMV mode. The following blood gas data are obtained at this time:

Pao_2 134 mm Hg
$Paco_2$ 37 mm Hg

$$pH \qquad 7.44$$
$$HCO_3^- \qquad 26.1 \text{ mEq/L}$$

Which of the following should the respiratory therapy practitioner recommend at this time?

A. Decrease the FIo_2 to 0.6
B. Decrease the IMV rate
C. Decrease the FIo_2 to 0.4
D. Decrease the PEEP to 12 cm H_2O
E. Decrease the PEEP to 6 cm H_2O
    (46)

28. Following a gunshot wound to the head, a 16-year-old patient develops adult respiratory distress syndrome and requires continuous ventilatory support, PEEP, and high concentrations of oxygen. Six days later the patient is still comatose. A resolving radiologic picture and improving effective static compliance are indications for the following blood gas study drawn with an FIo_2 of 0.4 and 10 cm H_2O PEEP:

Pao_2	148 mm Hg
$Paco_2$	35 mm Hg
pH	7.46
HCO_3^-	24.8 mEq/L
Ventilator mode	Assist/control

Which of the following should the respiratory therapist recommend at this time?

A. Place on SIMV
B. Decrease the backup rate
C. Decrease the PEEP to 6 cm H_2O
D. Decrease the FIo_2 to 0.3
E. Place patient on 5 cm H_2O CPAP with an FIo_2 of 0.55
    (46)

29. The respiratory therapy practitioner is performing tracheal suctioning on a patient in the intensive care unit when he notes the following rhythm on the cardiac monitor:

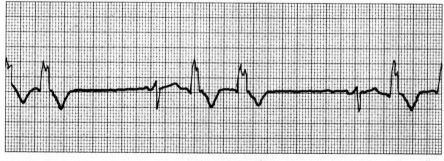

Figure IV-48.

Which of the following therapeutic modalities should the practitioner recommend at this time?
A. Epinephrine
B. Defibrillation with 360 joules (watts/sec)
C. Lidocaine
D. Intubation and ventilation with high concentrations of oxygen
E. Atropine sulfate
    (25:Chap 8, p 103)

30. A severely distressed patient is removed from a Bennett 7200 ventilator and ventilated manually while a physical examination is performed. Dullness to percussion is noted over the right lung field and hyperresonance is present on the left. Additionally, the trachea and the apical pulse are noted to be shifted to the right at this time. Based on the above information, the respiratory therapy practitioner should:
A. Insert a chest tube
B. Advance the endotracheal tube slightly
C. Recommend insertion of a chest tube
D. Recommend reinsertion of the endotracheal tube
E. Have a nurse perform chest physical assessment
    (32:212–213) (80)

31. Which of the following should the respiratory therapist recommend on the basis of noting that a patient has a Pa_{CO_2} of 40 mm Hg and a $P\bar{E}_{CO_2}$ of 30 mm Hg?
A. Continuous ventilatory support
B. Incentive spirometry
C. No therapy is indicated
D. Oxygen therapy
E. Further pulmonary function testing is necessary
    (5:76–78)

32. A patient is seen in the cardiac care unit while receiving continuous mechanical ventilation. Pertinent clinical data are presented below:

Pa_{O_2}	84 mm Hg
Pa_{CO_2}	40 mm Hg
pH	7.54
Base excess	+8.6 mEq/L
Na^+	145 mEq/L
Cl^-	74 mEq/L
K^+	2.9 mEq/L
Total CO_2	34 mEq/L

Which of the following should the respiratory therapist recommend to treat the above acid-base abnormality?
A. Add mechanical deadspace
B. Administer NH_4Cl

C. Administer acetazolamide
D. Administer KCl
E. Decrease minute alveolar ventilation
(32:63) (5:Chap 12, p 130)

33. For which of the following newborns would the respiratory therapy practitioner be *most* likely to recommend the use of nasal CPAP prongs?
A. Those with a cleft palate
B. Those with bilateral choanol artresia
C. Those who weight less than 1200 grams
D. Those who weigh more than 1200 grams
E. Those who are micrognathic and macroglossic
(29:209)

34. A 14-year-old is brought to the emergency department following an automobile accident. The paramedics say that the patient's legs were on fire when they arrived. He is comatose, cyanotic, and is noted to have very weak respiratory efforts. Carotid pulses are palpable, and a blood pressure of 60/20 is obtained. Gross observation reveals extensive thoracic and abdominal trauma from which there is considerable bleeding. Based on the above information, which of the following must be performed first in order to save the patient's life?
A. Control hemorrhage immediately
B. Administer 50 mEq $NaHCO_3$ stat
C. Establish an airway
D. Check pupil response to light
E. Begin external cardiac compressions
(25:Chap 4) (32:83–84)

35. A 32-year-old man is brought to the emergency department in a coma. The following blood gas results are noted at this time with the patient breathing room air:

Pa_{O_2}	104 mm Hg
Pa_{CO_2}	18 mm Hg
pH	7.09
Base excess	−18 mEq/L
HCO_3^-	4 mEq/L

Based on the above data, which of the following is (are) appropriate therapeutic recommendations?
I. Intubate and place on 10 cm H_2O CPAP
II. Monitor vital signs
III. Place on 8 L O_2 via simple oxygen mask
IV. Intubate and place on 5 cm H_2O PEEP
V. Place an oropharyngeal airway
    A. I and II
    B. II and IV
    C. III only
    D. II and V

E.   II and III
(5:195) (59) (38:60)

36. The respiratory therapy practitioner is asked to help set up a home care plan for a patient who is to be discharged with a permanent tracheostomy. Because the patient sustained a midcervical spinal column transection, some diaphragmatic function remains. This is evidenced by a vital capacity of 8 cc/kg. Based on the above information, which of the following would be the *least* appropriate therapeutic recommendation?
A.   Teaching the patient to suction himself
B.   Teaching the patient's family pulmonary drainage techniques
C.   Placing a cuffed, fenestrated tracheostomy tube
D.   Instructing the patient in breathing retraining techniques
E.   Instructing the patient in incentive spirometry
(2:505–506 and 759–760) (1:195)

37. Which of the following would be the *most* appropriate antibiotic for the respiratory therapy practitioner to recommend for a patient who has developed a pneumonia caused by the microorganism *Pseudomonas aeruginosa?*
A.   Kanamycin
B.   Ampicillin
C.   Erythromycin
D.   Tobramycin
E.   Chloramphenicol
(2:492) (11:69)

38. A 33-year-old patient is seen in the intensive care unit following extensive abdominal surgery. The patient is intubated and is receiving an FIo_2 of 0.8 via T tube. The results of arterial blood gas analysis are as follows:

Pao_2	40 mm Hg
$Paco_2$	50 mm Hg
pH	7.25
Base excess	−5 mEq/L
HCO_3^-	18 mEq/L

Based on the above information, which of the following is the most appropriate therapeutic recommendation?
A.   Increase the FIo_2 to 1.0
B.   Place on assist/control with an FIo_2 of 0.6
C.   Place on 10 cm H_2O CPAP with an FIo_2 of 1.0
D.   Place on assist/control with 10 cm H_2O PEEP and an FIo_2 of 0.3
E.   None of the above
(46) (49) (38:Chaps 4 through 6)

39. Which of the following methods is (are) recommended to improve cardiac performance?
    I.   Administering negative inotropic agents
    II. Optimizing venous return
    III. Optimizing left ventricular afterload
        A. I and III
        B. II only
        C. II and III
        D. III only
        E. I and II
    (1:Chap 27 and pp 433–436)

40. Tissue hypoxia is evidenced in a patient receiving continuous ventilatory support when the $S\bar{v}_{O_2}$ is noted to drop to 45%. Which of the following could the therapist recommend to correct this disorder?
    I.   Increasing Ca_{O_2}
    II. Optimizing the P_{50}
    III. Increasing the cardiac output
    IV. Decreasing tissue capillary blood flow
        A. I, II, and IV
        B. I, II, and III
        C. II and III
        D. II and IV
        E. I only
    (58) (65) (38:Chap 6)

41. A 72-year-old patient with a long history of chronic obstructive pulmonary disease is brought to the emergency department following several days of increasing respiratory distress. Arterial blood gas analysis is performed on room air and 2 L nasal oxygen. These data appear below:

	Room Air	2 L Oxygen
Pa_{O_2}	35 mm Hg	45 mm Hg
Pa_{CO_2}	75 mm Hg	78 mm Hg
pH	7.21	7.30
HCO_3^-	31 mEq/L	38 mEq/L
Base excess	+6 mEq/L	+13 mEq/L

Based on the above data, which is the most appropriate therapeutic recommendation?
    A. Place on a 28% air entrainment mask
    B. Intubate and support ventilation with an FI_{O_2} of 0.3
    C. No change in therapy is indicated
    D. Increase oxygen liter flow to 3 L/min
    E. Intubate and support ventilation with an FI_{O_2} of 0.5
    (49) (38:64–66) (32:92–96)

42. Which of the following could the respiratory therapy practitioner safely recommend for emergency treatment of acute congestive heart failure?
    I.   100% oxygen administration
    II. Norepinephrine administration

III. Lasix® administration
IV. KCl administration
    A. I and III
    B. II and III
    C. I and IV
    D. I, III, and IV
    E. III only
    (25:Chap 3, pp 26-28)

43. The respiratory therapy practitioner is monitoring a patient who has the following serum laboratory values:

Sodium	125 mEq/L
Chloride	85 mEq/L
Potassium	5.0 mEq/L
Total osmolality	255 mOsmol/L

Which of the following should the respiratory therapy practitioner recommend at this time?
A. KCl
B. NaCl
C. 15 g albumin
D. 5% dextrose in water
E. Lasix
    (94:Chap 2) (7:Chap 14)

44. The respiratory therapy practitioner is monitoring a patient who has the following serum laboratory values:

Sodium	140 mEq/L
Chloride	105 mEq/L
Potassium	5.0 mEq/L
Blood sugar	400 mg%

Based on the above information, which of the following is the most appropriate recommendation?
A. Mannitol administration
B. KCl
C. 10% dextrose with 0.9% NaCl
D. Insulin administration
E. Total parenteral alimentation
    (94:Chap 2) (7:Chap 14)

45. The respiratory therapy practitioner is monitoring a patient who has the following serum laboratory values:

Sodium	130 mEq/L
Chloride	90 mEq/L
Potassium	2.5 mEq/L
Blood urea nitrogen	5.0 mg/L
Creatinine	1.0 mg/dL

Blood sugar   50 mg/dL
Total serum proteins   5.0 g/dL

Based on the above information, which of the following would be *least* appropriate for parenteral administration?
A. NaCl
B. KCl
C. 5% dextrose
D. Albumin
E. Lasix
(94:Chap 2) (7:Chap 14)

46. The respiratory therapy practitioner would recommend the use of a fenestrated tracheostomy tube for which of the following reasons?
 I.   To prevent aspiration of oropharyngeal secretions
 II. To assist in tracheostomy tube weaning
 III. To provide for better upper airway humidification
 IV. To force the patient to ventilate via upper airway
    A. II and IV
    B. I and IV
    C. I and II
    D. III and IV
    E. IV only
(4:172–173)

47. Tracheostomy buttons may be recommended for all but which one of the following purposes?
A. To wean patients with tracheostomies
B. To maintain stoma patency
C. To provide continuous ventilatory support
D. To ensure a patent suction port
E. To allow for emergency ventilation
(5:174)

48. For which of the following conditions would the respiratory therapy practitioner be most likely to recommend the use of the Rusch Trachoflex tracheostomy tube?
A. To treat status asthmaticus
B. To ensure airway patency in patients with abnormal skin-to-anterior-tracheal-wall distance
C. To evaluate the extent and etiology of tracheal stenosis
D. To allow for more effective patient communication
E. To provide airway patency in patients with tracheal stenosis
(69)

Answer Key

1. C	11. D	21. D	31. C	41. D
2. C	12. D	22. E	32. D	42. A
3. B	13. D	23. C	33. D	43. B
4. B	14. E	24. A	34. C	44. D
5. E	15. D	25. D	35. D	45. E
6. B	16. B	26. D	36. E	46. A
7. A	17. B	27. A	37. D	47. C
8. C	18. E	28. C	38. E	48. B
9. B	19. A	29. C	39. C	
10. C	20. C	30. C	40. B	

J. Initiate Cardiopulmonary Resuscitation (Entry Level Only)

According to the NBRC, this content category is assessed only on the Entry Level Examination. Questions in this category are designed to assess the candidate's ability to initiate, conduct, or modify basic cardiopulmonary and respiratory therapy techniques in an emergency setting.

Entry Level Pretest

According to the NBRC, 5.5% of the questions on the Entry Level Examination are from the initiate cardiopulmonary resuscitation content category. In addition, the Composite Examination Matrix (see reference 80) states that questions in this category assess the candidate's ability to perform the following related tasks:

1. Recognize the need for emergency resuscitation
2. Call for help
3. Initiate, conduct, or modify basic cardiac life support techniques in an emergency setting

The following self-study questions were developed from the NBRC Composite Examination Matrix:

1. The respiratory therapy practitioner is treating a patient who is in a Stryker frame because of trauma involving the cervical spine. During therapy the patient becomes apneic. Which of the following methods should the therapist employ to establish a patent airway?
   A. Place head in "sniffing" position
   B. Flex head slightly
   C. Use a modified jaw thrust maneuver
   D. Hyperextend head and neck
   E. Turn head to the side while applying tracheal pressure
   (37:33)

2. According to the American Heart Association, the condition of pulselessness in an infant victim can best be assessed by palpating which of the following pulses?
    A. Apical
    B. Carotid
    C. Pedal
    D. Femoral
    E. Brachial
       (37:33)

3. All but which one of the following are part of the procedure for relieving upper airway obstruction in the unconscious infant?
    A. Back blows
    B. Stomach thrusts
    C. Tongue-jaw lift
    D. Attempts to ventilate
    E. Calling for help
       (37:31 and 48)

4. Which of the following statements regarding rescue breathing in the infant respiratory arrest victim is (are) true?
    I.   The rate should be 25/min.
    II.   Hyperextension of the head and neck is recommended.
    III. Gastric distention is a known hazard.
          A. I and III
          B. II only
          C. I, II, and III
          D. III only
          E. II and III
       (37:20 and 31-33)

5. The respiratory therapy practitioner finds a patient with advanced chronic obstructive pulmonary disease who has apparently fallen asleep while receiving IPPB. The patient does not respond to being shaken. The therapist should immediately:
    A. Check the patient's FIo_2
    B. Open the airway
    C. Give four quick breaths
    D. Establish breathlessness
    E. Call for help
       (37:12)

6. During the performance of cardiopulmonary resuscitation, which of the following is believed to be a contraindication to external cardiac compressions?
    A. Fracture of three or more ribs
    B. Development of tension pneumothorax
    C. Presence of a carotid pulse
    D. Fracture of the sternum
    E. Presence of constricted pupils
       (37:10 and 24)

7. Which of the following statements regarding external cardiac compression in the adult victim is (are) true?
    I.   The single rescuer rate is 60/min.
    II. The midportion of the sternum should be depressed.
    III. The recommended compression depth is 1½ to 2 inches.
        A. II and III
        B. I, II, and III
        C. I only
        D. I and III
        E. III only
    (37:21-24)

8. According to the American Heart Association, the proper rate for external cardiac compressions in the newborn is:
    A. 60/min
    B. 80/min
    C. 100/min
    D. 120/min
    E. 140/min
    (25:Chap 16, p 6)

9. Because of considerable hazards, which of the following victims should *not* be ventilated with 100% oxygen during the performance of cardiopulmonary resuscitation?
    A. Preterm newborns
    B. Drug overdose victims
    C. Patients with an advanced stage of chronic obstructive pulmonary disease
    D. A and C are correct.
    E. None of the above
    (25:Chap 8, p 2; Chap 16, p 3)

10. Which of the following is most consistent with a diagnosis of partial airway obstruction with poor gas exchange?
    A. Marked sternal and intercostal retractions without air movement
    B. Weak cough, inspiratory stridor, and cyanosis
    C. Inability of rescuer to ventilate after opening the airway
    D. Inspiratory stridor, effective cough, and a complaint of "sore throat"
    E. A and C are correct.
    (37:17 and 27-28)

11. Abdominal thrusts are generally *not* recommended as part of the procedure to relieve complete airway obstruction in which of the following patients?
    I.   Infants
    II. Children
    III. Conscious victims
    IV. Pregnant victims
    V.   Obese victims

A. I and III
B. II and III
C. I, II, and IV
D. II, III, IV, and V
E. I, II, IV, and V
(37:31 and 34)

12. According to the American Heart Association, which of the following is the most effective technique for administering external cardiac compressions to a newborn?
A. Two fingers placed on the lower third of the sternum
B. One finger placed midsternum
C. Two thumbs placed midsternum with the hands encircling the chest
D. Two fingers placed midsternum
E. Two thumbs placed on the lower third of the sternum with the hands encircling the chest
(25:Chap 16, p 6)

13. According to the American Heart Association, during cardiopulmonary resuscitation, properly performed cardiac compressions will result in a carotid artery blood flow that is approximately what percentage of normal?
A. 10–20
B. 15–25
C. 25–35
D. 40–50
E. 70–75
(37:42)

14. The respiratory therapy practitioner has just delivered four quick breaths to an unconscious and apneic adult patient. Now, while carefully palpating the area between the thyroid cartilage and the sternocleidomastoid muscle, he feels a weak but distinct carotid pulse. The practitioner should:
A. Spend another 5 seconds palpating the pulse
B. Begin rescue breathing at a rate of 16/min
C. Begin external cardiac compressions
D. Begin rescue breathing at a rate of 12/min
E. Call for help
(37:19)

15. The respiratory therapy practitioner is assisting in the delivery of a 2000-gram (34-week gestation) newborn. At approximately 1 minute post partum the following vital signs are noted:

Heart rate	40 beats/min
Respirations	Absent
Muscle tone	Flaccid
Reflex irritability	Absent
Color	Central cyanosis

Based on the above information, what is the proper therapeutic recommendation?
A. Suction the· pharynx: dry patient and place under radiant heat warmer
B. Begin external cardiac compression
C. Suction upper airway and ventilate with 100% oxygen via bag-valve-mask unit
D. Hyperoxygenate, intubate, and ventilate with 100% oxygen
E. B and D are correct.
(13:51–55) (15:68–74) (25:Chap 16)

16. Which of the following represents the concentration of oxygen in expired gas during performance of mouth-to-mouth resuscitation?
A. 7–9%
B. 10–12%
C. 13–15%
D. 16–19%
E. 19–21%
(2:915)

Answer Key

1. C	4. D	7. E	10. B	13. C
2. E	5. E	8. C	11. E	14. D
3. B	6. C	9. E	12. C	15. E
				16. D

K. Maintain Records and Communication (Entry Level Only)

According to the NBRC, the maintain records and communication content category is assessed only on the Entry Level Examination. The questions in this category are designed to assess the candidate's ability to maintain proper patient records and communicate effectively relevant information to other members of the health care team. For instance, if the respiratory therapy practitioner were to use terms such as *windpipe* or *stomach* in his or her charting instead of the proper terms, *trachea* and *abdomen,* it would only serve to arouse suspicion as to the competence of that practitioner among other members of the health team.

Entry Level Pretest

According to the NBRC, 1.5% of the questions on the Entry Level Examination are from the maintain records and communication content category. In addition, the Composite Examination Matrix (see reference

80) states that questions in this category assess the candidate's ability to perform the following related tasks:

1. Note and interpret all subjective and objective responses to care procedures
2. Specify therapy administered, including date, time, frequency of therapy, medication administered, and pertinent ventilatory data
3. Communicate pertinent information regarding the patient's clinical status to appropriate members of the health care team
4. Communicate pertinent information relevant to coordinating patient care (scheduling, avoiding conflicts, and proper sequencing of therapies)

The following self-study questions were developed from the NBRC Composite Examination Matrix:

1. Which of the following abbreviations would be *least* likely to be considered acceptable for use in a patient's chart?
   A. q.o.d.
   B. Bronk.
   C. ¼ N.S.
   D. stat
   E. gtts
      (2:1020–1022)

2. A respiratory therapy practitioner has just completed tracheobronchial suctioning of a patient who has multiple lung abscesses. Regarding this procedure, which of the following clinical diagnostic data should be charted as being valid?
   I.   Sputum quantity
   II.   Sputum color
   III. Sputum viscosity
   IV.   Sputum odor
      A. I only
      B. II only
      C. I and III
      D. I, II, III, and IV
      E. I, II, and III
   (2:262) (17:178–179) (7:92)

3. A 24-year-old woman is admitted to the emergency department following an automobile accident in which she suffered multiple abrasions and contusions. She is subsequently transferred to the progressive care unit where 3 L nasal oxygen is ordered along with monitoring of vital signs every 30 minutes. As the respiratory therapy practitioner places this patient on supplemental oxygen, he observes that the patient sleeps when not disturbed but responds briskly and appropriately in response to mild stimuli. Which of the following terms would be the most appropriate for use in charting this patient's level of consciousness?
   A. Drowsy or somnolent
   B. Disoriented to time and place
   C. Deeply comatose

D. Deeply stuporous
E. Comatose
(93)

4. While auscultating the posterior basal segments of a patient who was admitted in congestive heart failure, the respiratory therapy practitioner notes that the patient's expiratory breath sounds are equal in length and intensity to the patient's inspiratory breath sounds. Which of the following terms should the therapist record in the patient's chart to describe these sounds?
   A. Vesicular breath sounds
   B. Amphoric breath sounds
   C. Decreased breath sounds
   D. Normal breath sounds
   E. Bronchovesicular breath sounds
   (2:269–270)

5. Shortly after endotracheal extubation a 48-year-old, postgastrectomy patient is heard making medium-pitched crowing sounds synchronous with labored inspiratory efforts. Which of the following terms should the respiratory care practitioner record in the patient's chart to describe this sound?
   A. Stertorous breathing
   B. Barking cough
   C. Tussive breathing
   D. Stridorous breathing
   E. Labored breathing
   (2:271) (11:236) (1:282–284)

6. Following a cardiac arrest requiring approximately 30 minutes of basic and advanced cardiopulmonary resuscitation, a patient is transported to the cardiac care unit and placed on a Bennett MA-I ventilator. In assessing this patient the respiratory therapy practitioner notes that the patient does not respond at all to painful stimuli. Which of the following should the practitioner record in the chart to describe this patient's sensorium?
   A. Somnolence
   B. Deep coma
   C. Stupor
   D. Light coma
   E. Moderate coma
   (93)

7. Following placement on a Bennett MA-I ventilator, an 82-year-old patient is noted to have significant depressions in her systolic blood pressure that are synchronous with delivered mechanical breaths. Which of the following terms should the respiratory therapy practitioner use to record the above finding in the patient's chart?
   A. Pulsus alternans
   B. Pulsus paradoxus
   C. Pulsus obliternans

    D. Arterial hypotension
    E. Pulsus convulsae
      (7:182)

8. It has been recommended that the respiratory therapy practitioner record all pertinent data regarding any administered therapeutic procedure in the patient's chart. Most respiratory therapy department protocols require the charting of which of the following data with every IPPB treatment?
    I.   Ventilator sensitivity
    II. Occurrence of all adverse effects
    III. Pulse rate
    IV. Auscultatory findings
    V. Ventilator flow rate
    VI. Source gas or delivered FI_{O_2}
      A. I, II, III, V, and VI
      B. II, III, and IV
      C. II, III, IV, and V
      D. II, III, IV, V, and VI
      E. II, III, IV, and VI
      (2:578–580)

Answer Key

1. B   3. A   5. D   7. B
2. D   4. E   6. B   8. E

L. Assist Physician with Special Procedures (Advanced Level Only)

According to the NBRC, the assist physician with special procedures content category is assessed only on the Advanced Practitioner Examination. Questions in this category are designed to assess the candidate's ability to assist the physician with special procedures in a clinical laboratory procedure room or operating room setting.

Advanced Practitioner Pretest

According to the NBRC, 3% of the questions on the Advanced Practitioner Examination are from this category. In addition, the Composite Examination Matrix (see reference 80), states that questions in this category assess the candidate's ability to assist the physician in performing the following special procedures:

1. Bronchoscopy (rigid and flexible fiberoptic)
2. Tracheostomy
3. Thoracocentesis

4. Insertion of chest tubes
5. Invasive cardiovascular monitoring techniques (e.g., insertion of central venous pressure lines, pulmonary artery catheters, arterial lines)

The following self-study questions were developed from the NBRC Composite Examination Matrix:

1. Which of the following is believed to be the most acceptable method of preventing hypoxemia during transnasal fiberoptic bronchoscopy?
   A. Administration of nasal oxygen
   B. Administration of intermittent positive pressure ventilation
   C. Administration of mask oxygen
   D. Inotropic stimulation
   E. Supine positioning
   (104:Chap 8)

2. Which of the following has *not* been associated with the development of tracheal stenosis following tracheal extubation?
   A. Use of high pressure type tube cuffs
   B. High tracheostomy
   C. Low tracheostomy
   D. Excessive removal of tracheal cartilage
   E. Use of excessively angulated tracheostomy tubes
   (36:92)

3. While caring for a patient with a commercial three-compartment pleural evacuation system, the respiratory therapy practitioner notes that bubbling has stopped in the pressure control chamber. Which of the following may be responsible for this?
   I. Excessive levels of wall suction
   II. Absence of a lung leak
   III. Leak somewhere in the system
   IV. Inadequate levels of suction
   V. Evaporation of water in suction control compartment
      A. II, IV, and V
      B. III, IV, and V
      C. I and II
      D. II, III, IV, and V
      E. I and III
   (7:351–357) (32:Chap 7)

4. True statements regarding chest tube removal include:
   I. The procedure should be performed during a forced inspiratory maneuver.
   II. It must be preceded by clinical and radiologic evidence of lung reexpansion.
   III. It is usually not performed during administration of continuous ventilatory support.
      A. I and III
      B. II and III
      C. II only

D. I, II, and III
E. I only
(7:357) (32:Chap 7)

5. All of the following are intraoperative and postoperative complications of tracheotomy. Which is most commonly seen?
A. Hemorrhagic shock
B. Tension pneumothorax
C. Onset of life-threatening arrhythmias
D. Subcutaneous emphysema
E. Respiratory arrest
(36:87–93)

6. Which of the following clinical signs is *least* suggestive of the presence of massive hemothorax?
A. Diminished breath sounds
B. Tracheal shift
C. Rapid, thready pulse
D. Distended neck veins
E. Paradoxical chest wall movement
(7:Chap 18) (32:Chap 7)

7. Which of the following complications is *not* associated with the use of tracheostomy tubes?
A. Pulmonary infection
B. Dysphagia
C. Laryngeal edema
D. Tracheal dilatation
E. Glottic edema
(36:87–90)

8. Which of the following statements is (are) true regarding the technique of elective tracheotomy?
I.   A vertical incision is invariably used.
II.   The trachea is usually incised between the second and third tracheal rings.
III. Hemostasis may be aided by infiltrating the operative site with a dilute epinephrine solution.
A. I only
B. II and III
C. I, II, and III
D. III only
E. I and III
(36:59–66)

9. Which of the following is known to contribute to the development of subcutaneous emphysema following tracheotomy?
A. Use of low pressure tube cuffs
B. Vertical rather than horizontal skin incision
C. Inadequate closure of incision edges postoperatively
D. High tracheostomy
E. Use of overly large tracheostomy tubes
(36:89)

10. Hemorrhagic shock is a potentially lethal postoperative complication of tracheotomy. It is most frequently associated with which of the following?
    A. Incision of miscellaneous jugular anastomoses
    B. Elective performance of procedure
    C. Laceration of the brachiocephalic artery
    D. Erosion of the subclavian vein
    E. Laceration of the left carotid artery
    (36:91)

11. Which of the following statements is (are) true regarding injury to the brachiocephalic (innominate) artery?
    I. It may be precipitated by the use of high pressure tube cuffs.
    II. It is associated with erosion of the anterior tracheal wall.
    III. It frequently results from the performance of a high tracheotomy.
    A. II and III
    B. I and II
    C. II only
    D. I and III
    E. III only
    (36:91)

12. Which of the following would *not* be considered a postoperative complication of tracheotomy?
    I. Hemorrhage
    II. Tracheal stenosis
    III. Pneumothorax
    IV. Air embolism
    V. Tracheomalacia
    A. I, II, and IV
    B. II and V
    C. II only
    D. I and V
    E. III and IV
    (36:88)

13. Vocal cord and laryngeal damage has been noted in patients who have required tracheostomy tubes. This is most frequently associated with which of the following?
    A. Use of high pressure cuffs
    B. High tracheotomy incision
    C. Infection of stomal tissues
    D. Tracheoesophageal fistula
    E. Poor nutritional or immunologic status
    (36:91–93)

14. Which of the following is *not* felt to contribute to the development of brachiocephalic (innominate artery) erosion?
    A. Use of high pressure cuffs
    B. Use of excessively angulated tracheostomy tubes

C. Low tracheostomy
D. Use of tracheostomy tubes that are too short
E. Tracheal tissue infection
   (36:91)

15. In monitoring a patient requiring prolonged mechanical ventilation, the respiratory therapy practitioner notes visible pulsation of the patient's tracheostomy tube. This occurrence:
A. Is of little concern
B. Indicates excessive myocardial workloads
C. May forewarn brachiocephalic (innominate artery) erosion
D. Often accompanies the use of PEEP
E. May indicate a need to adjust the ventilator sensitivity
   (36:91)

16. Which of the following is the most frequent hazard associated with needle biopsy of the lung?
A. Severe hemorrhage
B. Pneumothorax
C. Death
D. Air embolism
E. Anesthesia allergy
   (104:Chap 9)

17. Which of the following are frequently indicated in the treatment of patients with hemothorax?
   I. Platelet administration
   II. Triple-bottle drainage systems
   III. Lasix administration
   IV. Surgical hemostasis
      A. II and IV
      B. III and IV
      C. I and IV
      D. I and II
      E. II and III
   (7:Chap 18) (32:Chap 7)

18. Which of the following statements regarding tension pneumothorax is (are) true?
   I. It cannot be caused by traumatic penetration of the parietal pleura.
   II. Emergency treatment includes insertion of a needle between the second and third ribs.
   III. Single-bottle evacuation systems may be useful.
   IV. It may be caused by rupture of the visceral pleura.
      A. II, III, and IV
      B. II only
      C. I, III, and IV
      D. II and IV
      E. I, II, III, and IV
   (32:Chap 7) (7:344–355)

19. Which of the following statements regarding emergency tracheotomy is (are) true?
    I.   The skin incision should be horizontal rather than vertical.
    II. Preoperative endotracheal intubation should always be performed.
    III. The tracheal incision should ideally be made between the second and third tracheal rings.
    A.   I only
    B.   II and III
    C.   I, II, and III
    D.   I and II
    E.   III only
    (36:66–67)

20. During performance of rigid bronchoscopy, which of the following lung segments tend to be *least* accessible for viewing?
    A.   Right middle lobe, both segments
    B.   Right upper lobe, anterior segment
    C.   Left upper lobe, apical-posterior segment
    D.   Left lower lobe, posterior segment
    E.   Lingula, both segments
    (104:Chap 8)

21. Tracheal intubation with the fiberoptic laryngoscope is frequently recommended in which of the following circumstances?
    A.   Prior to induction of general anesthesia
    B.   Emergency airway placement in the patient with suspected cervical spine fracture
    C.   Management of the severely asphyxiated newborn
    D.   Management of the patient with croup
    E.   To ensure ventilatory support for the patient with neuromuscular disorders
    (36:54)

22. Localized areas of mild to moderate bronchial hemmorhage may frequently be controlled by:
    A.   Proper drainage techniques
    B.   Lavage with 2% Xylocaine
    C.   Careful aspiration
    D.   Lavage with 1% epinephrine
    E.   Lavage with 0.001% epinephrine
    (104:Chap 8)

23. Which of the following statements regarding chest tube placement is (are) true?
    I.   It may be indicated in the treatment of open pneumothorax.
    II. A thoracotomy is performed between the sixth and eighth ribs when air removal is desired.
    III. It should not be performed on an elective basis.
    A.   I only
    B.   II and III
    C.   I and III

    D. II only
    E. I and II
  (7:Chap 18) (32:Chap 7)

24. Bronchoscopy may be used to do all of the following *except:*
    A. Determine the source of hemoptysis
    B. Tracheobronchial toilet
    C. Determine the cause of atelectasis
    D. Transthoracic biopsy
    E. Remove aspirated foreign bodies
    (104:Chap 8)

25. While caring for a patient who has a triple-bottle chest drainage system, the respiratory therapy practitioner notes intermittent bubbling in the underwater seal compartment. Which of the following is most likely responsible for this?
    A. Excessive suction
    B. Leak in the system
    C. Wide fluctuations in intrapleural pressure
    D. Evacuation of pleural gas
    E. Drainage of pleural fluid
    (7:351–357) (32:Chap 7)

26. Which of the following statements regarding triple-bottle chest drainage systems is (are) true?
    I.   They cannot be used for fluid evacuation.
    II. They include a suction control compartment.
    III. They may be used in the treatment of tension pneumothorax.
    A. I and II
    B. II only
    C. I, II, and III
    D. II and III
    E. III only
  (32:Chap 7) (7:351–357)

Answer Key

1. C	6. E	11. B	16. B	21. B
2. C	7. E	12. B	17. A	22. E
3. B	8. B	13. B	18. A	23. A
4. B	9. C	14. D	19. E	24. D
5. D	10. C	15. C	20. C	25. D
				26. D

II

Examination Posttest and Mastery

UNIT I

Entry Level Examination Posttest

The following full-length Entry Level Examination posttest was constructed according to specifications outlined in the current NBRC Composite Examination Matrix (see reference 80). The examination categories and the number of questions the NBRC has allotted to each are listed in the table below. In addition, *the answer key at the end of this test is referenced to the examination matrix so the candidate may further identify his or her weak areas.* For a more thorough discussion of the NBRC Composite Examination Matrix, please refer to the Introduction of this book and to the Examination Category Review and Pretest.

Table 1. Entry Level Examination Content Matrix.

	Examination Category	Number of Questions	Percentage of Questions
I.	Clinical Data	60	30
A.	Review patient records	9	4.5
B.	Collect and evaluate clinical information	21	10.5
C.	Recommend and obtain diagnostic procedures	6	3
D.	Perform and evaluate laboratory procedures	12	6
E.	Assess therapeutic plan	12	6
II.	Equipment	50	25
A.	Select, assemble, check, and correct malfunctions of equipment	42	21
B.	Ensure cleanliness, calibration, and quality control	8	4
III.	Therapeutic Procedures	90	45
A.	Educate patients	3	1.5
B.	Control infection	4	2
C.	Maintain airway	8	4
D.	Mobilize and remove secretions	9	4.5
E.	Ensure ventilation	11	5.5
F.	Ensure oxygenation	11	5.5
G.	Assess patient response to therapy	11	5.5
H.	Modify therapy	10	5
I.	Recommend modifications in therapy	8	4
J.	Initiate cardiopulmonary resuscitation	11	5.5
K.	Maintain records and communication	3	1.5

Examination for Entry Level Respiratory Therapy Practitioners

Time: 3 Hours

Directions: Each of the questions or incomplete statements below is followed by five suggested answers. Select the one that is best in each case and then mark accordingly.

1. The respiratory therapy practitioner is asked to evaluate a distressed patient who is receiving continuous ventilatory support. The patient is on a Bennett MA-I ventilator in the assist/control mode and the respiratory rate is 44/min. The therapist notes that when the patient is temporarily disconnected, the ventilator's orange panel light flashes repeatedly. What is the most appropriate therapeutic modification for the therapist to make at this time?
   A. Decrease the ventilator sensitivity
   B. Have a partner manually ventilate the patient while the therapist replaces the ventilator
   C. Recommend that the patient be sedated
   D. Place the patient on IMV
   E. Increase the ventilator flow rate
   (57) (4:404)

2. If particle size were the only consideration, which of the following aerosol generating devices would be the choice in treatment of postextubation laryngeal edema?
   A. An ultrasonic nebulizer
   B. A hydronamic nebulizer
   C. A sidestream nebulizer
   D. An atomizer
   E. A Cascade humidifier
   (4:122–123)

3. On which of the following ventilators may use of the nebulizer system during the inspiratory phase result in changes in the delivered tidal volume and FI_{O_2}?
   A. Bennett MA-I
   B. Bennett PR-II
   C. Bourns Bear I
   D. Bennett MA-II
   E. Bourns Bear II
   (4:252)

4. The drop in Pa_{O_2} that may accompany administration of isoproterenol has been attributed to:
   I. A B_1 side effect
   II. Increased ventilation to underperfused lung units
   III. Increased perfusion to underventilated lung units
   IV. Pulmonary vasodilatation
   A. I and III
   B. II and III
   C. II and IV
   D. III and IV
   E. IV only
   (2:473)

5. A 39-year-old man presents to the emergency department with fever, respiratory distress, and a cough that is productive of copious quantities of thick, green-tinged sputum. The patient states that he raises several dozen teaspoons of these secretions daily and that he has had recurrent bouts with bronchopneumonia since childhood. Physical examination reveals mild clubbing of digits and a remarkable variety of rhonchi over both lung fields. Based on the above information, which of the following disorders is most likely responsible for this patient's distress?
   A. Bronchogenic carcinoma
   B. Anaerobic lung abscess
   C. Chronic bronchitis
   D. Bronchiectasis
   E. Septic pulmonary infarct
   (11:113–118)

6. The respiratory therapy practitioner is administering IPPB with 0.25 mL isoetharine and 2.0 mL normal saline to a 45-year-old patient who is 2 days post lower abdominal surgery. After several minutes of therapy, the patient complains of lightheadedness and tingling of his extremities. Which of the following actions should the practitioner take at this time?
   A. Discontinue therapy at once and recommend to the physician that IPPB be discontinued
   B. Wait a moment or two and then thoroughly review therapeutic instruction with the patient
   C. Stop therapy at once, notify the physician, and recommend administration of another bronchodilator

D. Wait several minutes then resume therapy without the bronchodilator
E. Decrease ventilator sensitivity
   (1:190) (2:572)

7. For every 10 mm Hg *acute* increase in $Paco_2$ the pH of the blood will drop approximately:
A. 0.5
B. 0.05
C. 0.10
D. 0.15
E. 0.20
   (5:128) (2:246)

8. Which of the following clinical disorders are commonly known to involve or lead to pulmonary edema?
   I.   Left ventricular failure
   II. Hypovolemia
   III. Right ventricular failure
   IV. Adult respiratory distress syndrome
       A. I and IV
       B. I, II, III, and IV
       C. II and IV
       D. III and IV
       E. II and III
   (1:Chap 29)

9. On which of the following ventilators can the inspiratory phase *only* be terminated after a preset pressure has been reached within the ventilator system?
   I.   Bird Mark 7
   II. Bennett PR-II
   III. Bird Mark 8
   IV. Bennett PR-I
       A. I only
       B. II and IV
       C. III and IV
       D. II and III
       E. I and III
   (4:249–260 and 314–324)

10. The respiratory therapy practitioner must wear a gown, mask, and gloves when treating patients who are in which of the following types of isolation?
   I.   Strict
   II. Respiratory
   III. Protective (reverse)
   IV. Enteric
       A. I and III
       B. II and IV
       C. III and IV
       D. I and II

E.   I, III, and IV
(92:29, 39, 45, and 51)

11. An all-purpose jet type nebulizer is being used on a patient in the intensive care unit. Although it is set to deliver 40% oxygen, a properly calibrated analyzer placed at the patient's proximal airway repeatedly reads 46%. Which of the following is (are) the most probably cause(s) for this occurrence?
   I.   Humidity is affecting analyzer accuracy.
   II. There is a leak in the system.
   III. Backpressure is affecting air entrainment valve function.
      A.   II only
      B.   I, II, and III
      C.   III only
      D.   I only
      E.   I and III
   (8:114-115)

12. Which of the following aerosolized bronchodilators is known to be completely free of β_1 activity?
      A.   Isoetharine
      B.   Racemic epinephrine
      C.   Metaproterenol
      D.   Terbutaline
      E.   None of the above
   (2:Chap 20)

13. Which of the following *cannot* be determined through the analysis of pulmonary function data obtained by simple spirometry?
      A. FEF_{50}
      B. $\dfrac{FEV_{1}\%}{FVC}$
      C. $FEF_{200-1200}$
      D.   Expiratory reserve volume
      E.   The average flow rate of the middle 50% of the patient's forced vital capacity
   (16:24-48)

14. A ventilator that is classified as being pressure cycled is generally so termed because:
      A.   The inspiratory phase is initiated after preset conditions of pressure have been achieved.
      B.   The expiratory phase is initiated after preset conditions of flow have been achieved.
      C.   The expiratory phase is initiated after preset conditions of pressure have been achieved.
      D.   The inspiratory phase is terminated after preset conditions of pressure have been achieved.
      E.   C and D are correct.
   (4:218-223)

15. Which of the following is *least* likely to lead to retrolental fibroplasia in the preterm infant?
    A. Perfusion of the retina with Pao_2s greater than 100 mm Hg
    B. Administration of 40% or less oxygen
    C. Intermittent bagging with 100% oxygen
    D. Administration of 100% oxygen directly to the eye itself
    E. Administration of 40% or greater oxygen
    (29:174–177) (13:78–80) (10:178–181)

16. Mild gastric inflation is observed in a cardiac arrest victim who is being ventilated via a manual resuscitator and mask unit. Without interrupting cardiopulmonary resuscitation, the most appropriate action for the respiratory therapy practitioner to take at this time would be to:
    A. Apply pressure to the abdomen during the performance of external cardiac compressions
    B. Reposition the airway
    C. Roll the victim to his side and apply pressure to the upper abdomen
    D. Use two hands to compress the bag-valve unit
    E. Place a pillow under the victim's head
    (37:20 and 34)

17. An increase in the intensity and clarity of spoken voice sounds heard over areas of consolidated lung tissue through a stethoscope best describes:
    A. Vocal fremitus
    B. Egophony
    C. Whispered pectoriloquy
    D. Bronchophony
    E. Bronchovesicular breath sounds
    (95:95)

18. A 68-year-old man is brought to the emergency department in severe distress. An oral history of severe chronic obstructive pulmonary disease is consistent with barrel chest, pursed lipped breathing, and the cyanosis that accompany his presentation. Room air blood gases are as follows:

Pao_2	45 mm Hg
$Paco_2$	75 mm Hg
pH	7.32
HCO_3^-	34 mEq/L
BP	170/120
Pulse	110
Respiratory rate	30

    Administration of 24% oxygen to this patient will most likely have which of the following effects?
    I. Marked increase in minute ventilation
    II. Worsening of cardiovascular vital signs

III.   Improvement in cardiovascular vital signs
IV.   Appreciable relief of hypoxia
   A.   I and IV
   B.   III and IV
   C.   I and II
   D.   I and III
   E.   IV only
   (5:Chap 16)

19.   A patient with bronchogenic carcinoma is receiving continuous flow IMV via a Bennett MA-I ventilator with a 5-L reservoir bag in the system. The patient is noted to become increasingly agitated and distressed for an hour or so prior to his pain medications that are given every 2 hours. During this time the pressure on the manometer is repeatedly noted to fall to −6 cm H_2O during spontaneous breaths. Each time this occurs the ventilator delivers the preset tidal volume of 800 cc. Which of the following modifications should the respiratory practitioner make at this time?
   A.   Make no modifications until more pain medication is ordered
   B.   Decrease the sensitivity and decrease the continuous flow rate
   C.   Increase the sensitivity
   D.   Increase the continuous flow rate
   E.   Increase the continuous flow rate and decrease the sensitivity
   (71) (4:241 and 402) (57)

20.   In which of the following patients might percussion and vibration techniques be contraindicated?
   I.   Those with osteoporosis
   II.   Those with fractured ribs
   III.   Those with resectable lung tumors
   A.   II only
   B.   I only
   C.   I and III
   D.   I, II, and III
   E.   I and II
   (7:Chap 12)

21.   Ventilator weaning attempts are in progress for a 68-year-old patient who is recovering from pneumonia caused by *Klebsiella pneumoniae*. The patient has a history of pulmonary emphysema and has required continuous ventilatory support for the past 5 days. He has been receiving supplemental oxygen via T tube setup for the past hour. Arterial blood gas data gathered during this process appear below:

	After 5 Minutes on T tube	After 30 Minutes on T tube	After 60 Minutes on T tube
FIo_2	0.5	0.5	0.5
Pao_2	62 mm Hg	56 mm Hg	55 mm Hg
$Paco_2$	65 mm Hg	69 mm Hg	74 mm Hg
pH	7.40	7.33	7.20

Based on the above information, what is the correct recommendation?
A.   Extubate at once
B.   Support ventilation at this time
C.   Increase the FIo_2
D.   Obtain an arterial sample
E.   Administer HCO_3^-
   (2:Chap 25) (7:196) (66)

22.   On the Bourns Bear I ventilator, when the tidal volume and respiratory rate are held constant, the I:E ratio then becomes a function of which of the following controls?
A.   I:E ratio control
B.   Expiratory timer
C.   Peak flow control
D.   Assist and sensitivity mechanism
E.   Pressure limit mechanism
   (4:401)

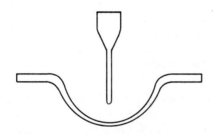

Figure 1.

23.   The above illustration shows:
A.   A normal unit
B.   A shunt unit
C.   A deadspace unit
D.   A silent unit
E.   A and C are correct.
   (5:66)

24.   True statements regarding humidifiers in general include:
   I.   They produce particulate water only.
   II.   They produce water vapor only.
   III. They are incapable of transmitting bacteria.
   IV.   They are incapable of delivering gases at conditions of BTPS.
   A.   II and IV
   B.   II and III
   C.   I and II
   D.   I, II, and III
   E.   II only
   (4:105–109) (2:144)

25. If a properly calibrated galvanic cell type oxygen analyzing device were monitoring a sample of gas that is 100% oxygen at BTPS, the analyzer's meter would most likely read: *saturated*
    A. 100% oxygen
    B. 50% oxygen
    C. Slightly higher than 100% oxygen
    D. Slightly lower than 100% oxygen
    E. 21% oxygen
       (51)

26. A respiratory care practitioner is administering IPPB to a patient who has suffered a recent myocardial infarction. Which of the following signs and symptoms would be most likely to lead the respiratory therapy practitioner to assess that cardiovascular embarrassment is taking place?
    I.   Dyspnea
    II.   Appearance of sonorous rhonchi
    III. Distended neck veins
    IV.   Rapid, thready pulse
          A. I, II, and IV
          B. I, II, and III
          C. I, III, and IV
          D. I only
          E. II and III
       (24:262) (1:190)

27. The respiratory therapy practitioner is asked to select an airway care device for a patient who is to be discharged with a permanent tracheostomy. The physician's order stipulates that the patient stoma is to be used for suctioning purposes only and that he does not anticipate the need for positive pressure ventilation. Which of the following devices might the practitioner select?
    I.   A tracheostomy button
    II.   An Olympic Trach-Talk
    III. A Carlens tube
    IV.   A cuffed Shiley tracheostomy tube with a fenestrated outer cannula
          A. II and III
          B. I only
          C. III and IV
          D. IV only
          E. II and IV
       (2:504-507)

28. The respiratory therapy practitioner is assigned to a neurotrauma patient in the intensive care unit. Gross observation of this patient reveals the fact that he pauses for several seconds at the end of every inspiration. Which of the following terms should the practitioner record in the patient's chart to describe this ventilatory pattern?
    A. Biot's breathing
    B. Hypopnea

C. Apneustic breathing
D. Cluster breathing
E. Ataxic breathing
   (2:751)

29. How long must equipment contaminated by *Mycobacterium tuberculosis* be immersed in a commercial glutaraldehyde solution to ensure that all these organisms have been killed?
A. 12 hours
B. 1 hour
C. 10 to 20 minutes
D. 3 to 10 hours
E. 10 to 20 hours
   (8:195–196)

30. True statements regarding tracheal tube cuff herniation include:
   I. Cuff overinflation may lead to its occurrence.
   II. It is associated with high pressure cuff usage.
   III. It may lead to upper airway obstruction.
   IV. Presence of tracheal shift is diagnostic.
      A. I and II
      B. I and III
      C. II and IV
      D. III and IV
      E. I, III, and IV
   (1:293) (32:211)

31. Which of the following statements regarding disadvantages of the steam autoclaving process is (are) true?
   I. Sterilization is achieved less rapidly than by other means.
   II. It may damage some equipment.
   III. Toxic residues may be left on equipment.
   IV. It is the most expensive means of sterilization.
      A. II only
      B. II and IV
      C. I and III
      D. III only
      E. I and IV
   (2:418–419) (24:335–336) (13:289)

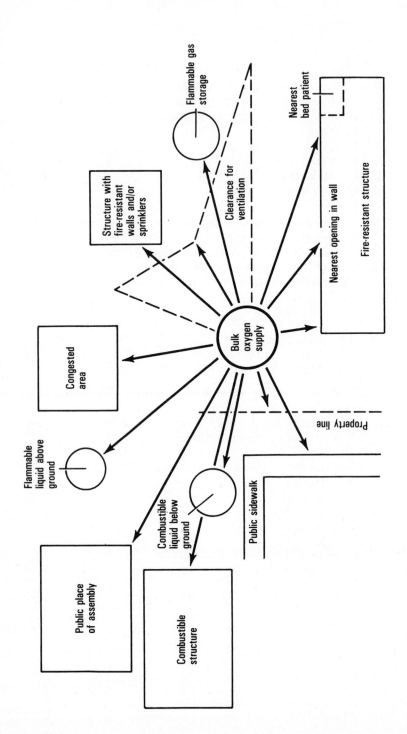

Figure 2.

32. Regarding the above illustration, all of the following are true concerning the distance various objects must be kept from bulk oxygen storage *except:*
    A. 10 feet from the nearest flammable liquid above ground
    B. 50 feet from nearest bed patient
    C. 50 feet from the nearest combustible structure
    D. 5 feet from the property line
    E. 10 feet from a public sidewalk
    (4:46)

33. A 32-year-old woman is brought to the emergency department in a diabetic coma. The following arterial blood gas data were obtained on admission:

FI_{O_2}	0.21
Pa_{O_2}	105 mm Hg
Pa_{CO_2}	19 mm Hg
pH	7.07
HCO_3^-	4 mEq/L
Base excess	-17 mEq/L

    The most correct interpretation of the above results is:
    A. Partially compensated metabolic alkalosis
    B. Partially compensated metabolic acidosis
    C. Partially compensated respiratory acidosis
    D. Fully compensated respiratory acidosis
    E. Fully compensated metabolic acidosis
    (2:1010)

34. Which of the following is *not* part of the normal or resident flora of the upper respiratory tract?
    A. *Candida albicans*
    B. *Hemophilus* species
    C. *Klebsiella* species
    D. Streptococci
    E. Pneumococci
    (11:67) (24:332)

35. Instructions in which of the following techniques would be *least* likely to enhance the deposition of aerosolized medication within the respiratory tract?
    A. End inspiratory breath holding
    B. Mouth breathing
    C. Slow, deep inspirations
    D. Use of accessory muscles during exhalation
    E. Diaphragmatic breathing
    (1:181)

36. Which of the following are believed to be advantages of anesthesia bag type manual resuscitation devices?
    I.   Delivery of any desired concentration of oxygen is possible.
    II. They are truly self-inflating.

III.   Their design allows for "feel" of patient lung mechanics.
IV.   They need not be used by highly trained personnel.
   A.   I and II
   B.   II and III
   C.   I and IV
   D.   III and IV
   E.   I and III
   (8:190) (25:Chap 16, pp 3-4)

37.   In reading the admission note of a patient with severe pulmonary emphysema, the respiratory therapy practitioner would expect the patient's historical data to reveal a chief complaint of:
   A.   Orthopnea
   B.   Dyspnea
   C.   Cough with copious sputum production
   D.   Somnolence
   E.   Sleep apnea
   (11:97)

38.   From which of the following devices may *true* mixed venous blood be obtained under most clinical circumstances?
   A.   Central venous catheter
   B.   Pulmonary venous catheter
   C.   Subclavian catheter
   D.   Pulmonary artery catheter
   E.   A and C are correct.
   (5:231)

39.   Which of the following procedures would be most useful in establishing the existence of a tracheoesophageal fistula in a patient who is receiving continuous ventilatory support?
   A.   Arterial blood gas analysis
   B.   Barium bronchogram
   C.   Methylene blue (dionosil dye) test
   D.   Chest physical examination
   E.   Portable chest roentgenogram
   (31:5 and 9)

40.   The respiratory therapy practitioner is administering IPPB to a patient with a history of chronic obstructive pulmonary disease. After a violent coughing spell, the patient complains of a sudden sharp pain in the left side of his chest. Which of the following modifications should the practitioner make at this time?
   A.   Have the patient transferred to the cardiac care unit for close observation
   B.   Terminate therapy
   C.   Notify the physician and have the patient monitored closely
   D.   Have a Swan-Ganz catheter inserted stat
   E.   B and C are correct.
   (1:191) (2:577-580)

41.   Respiratory therapy equipment constructed from which of the following materials absorbs ethylene oxide readily and consequently

requires the most extended aeration time before it may be safely used?
A. Latex
B. Teflon
C. Polyvinyl chloride
D. Polyethylene
E. Nylon
(24:338)

42. Sympathomimetic bronchodilators are frequently ineffective when administered to:
I. Patients who are severely acidotic
II. Patients with intrinsic asthma
III. Patients with extrinsic asthma
    A. I only
    B. I, II, and III
    C. I and II
    D. II and III
    E. III only
(40)

43. The administration of high concentrations of oxygen (greater than 60%) to patients with adult respiratory distress syndrome would most likely result in which of the following occurrences?
I. Narrowing of the patient's $P(A-a)_{O_2}$
II. Oxygen-induced hypoventilation
III. Little improvement in arterial hypoxemia
IV. Congestive heart failure
    A. I and II
    B. II and IV
    C. III only
    D. III and IV
    E. I and IV
(2:394–395) (46) (32:63–65 and 119)

[handwritten: need PEEP, refractory hypoxemia]

44. The respiratory therapist is asked to place a combative patient on a Bourns Bear I ventilator. The physician asks the practitioner to make sure the ventilator will sound an alarm should the patient become disconnected. Which of the following alarms will the therapist use to accomplish this goal?
I. Exhaled tidal volume
II. Power failure
III. Low source gas pressure
IV. Low inspiratory pressure
V. Apnea
    A. I and IV
    B. II and IV
    C. I, III, and V
    D. II only
    E. I, III, and IV
(1:356–358) (60) (4:477–479)

45. Which of the following is *not* believed to have the same meaning as the term *ventilation-perfusion mismatch?*
    A. Venous admixture
    B. Shunt-like effect
    C. V/Q scatter
    D. Low V/Q
    E. Alveolar hypoventilation
        (5:91 and 185) (2:241 and 394)

46. The hospital's oxygen lines are accidentally connected to a 50-psi nitrous oxide source. Not knowing this, the respiratory therapy practitioner begins mechanically ventilating a comatose patient with what he believes is 100% oxygen. The selection of which of the following ventilators would allow the practitioner to rapidly determine that the wrong source gas was being used?
    A. Bennett MA-I
    B. Bourns Bear II
    C. Bourns Bear I
    D. Ohio CCV
    E. Bennett MA-II
        (51)

47. Which of the following would be the preferred method of maintaining airway patency for a semiconscious patient who is not in respiratory distress?
    A. Oral endotracheal intubation
    B. Nasopharyngeal airway
    C. Oropharyngeal airway
    D. Tracheostomy
    E. Cricothyroidotomy
        (1:237)

48. Excessive delay in the running of a sample of arterial blood may result in which of the following sampling errors?
    I.   High pH
    II.   Low P_{O_2}
    III. Low P_{CO_2}
    IV.   High P_{O_2}
    V.   High P_{CO_2}
        A. II and V
        B. III and IV
        C. I, III, and IV
        D. I, II, and IV
        E. I, II, and III
    (5:158)

49. After delivering four quick breaths to an unconscious and apneic 5-year-old child, the respiratory therapy practitioner is able to palpate a weak carotid pulse. Which is the proper action to take at this time?

A. Begin rescue breathing at a rate of 16/min
B. Begin rescue breathing at a rate of 20/min
C. Begin external cardiac compressions
D. Begin rescue breathing at a rate of 12/min
E. Palpate the femoral pulse
(37:16 and 50)

50. Whenever significant adverse effects occur involving any respiratory therapeutic modality, the respiratory therapy practitioner must immediately terminate the procedure and notify the ordering physician. Which of the following is the *least* appropriate means of communicating this information?
A. Ask the charge nurse to relay the information
B. Ask the shift supervisor to page the physician
C. Page the physician yourself
D. Chart the information and wait for the physician to read it
E. Ask your medical director to relay the information
(96)

51. Which of the following airways should the respiratory therapy practitioner select for an unconscious patient who is breathing spontaneously and adequately?
A. Nasopharyngeal airway
B. Endotracheal tube
C. Tracheostomy tube
D. Oropharyngeal airway
E. Tracheostomy button
(25:Chap 4, p 2) (1:237)

52. Following upper abdominal surgery, the respiratory therapy practitioner finds a 44-year-old male patient completely unwilling to perform deep breathing and coughing exercises. Which of the following are the most appropriate actions under these circumstances?
   I. Synchronize therapy with analgesic administration if possible
  II. Restrain the patient's arms and administer IPPB via mask
 III. Attempt to further instruct the patient
  IV. Support the incision during therapy
        A. I, III, and IV
        B. II and IV
        C. I and IV
        D. I, II, and IV
        E. III and IV
   (2:687–688)

53. The physician wants the respiratory therapy practitioner to place the patient on the level of PEEP that corresponds to the best effec-

tive static compliance. With the corrected tidal volume held constant, the following data are accumulated:

Level of PEEP	Plateau Pressure
0 cm H_2O	48 cm H_2O
3 cm H_2O	50 cm H_2O
6 cm H_2O	52 cm H_2O
9 cm H_2O	51 cm H_2O
12 cm H_2O	51 cm H_2O
15 cm H_2O	52 cm H_2O
18 cm H_2O	58 cm H_2O
21 cm H_2O	62 cm H_2O

Which of the following levels of PEEP should the respiratory therapist recommend?
A.   9 cm H_2O
B.   12 cm H_2O
C.   15 cm H_2O
D.   18 cm H_2O
E.   21 cm H_2O
   (47) (50) (1:375)

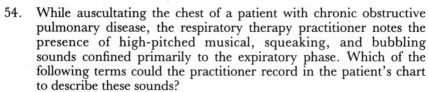

54.   While auscultating the chest of a patient with chronic obstructive pulmonary disease, the respiratory therapy practitioner notes the presence of high-pitched musical, squeaking, and bubbling sounds confined primarily to the expiratory phase. Which of the following terms could the practitioner record in the patient's chart to describe these sounds?
A.   Rales
B.   Wheezes
C.   Pleural friction rub
D.   Sibilant rhonchi
E.   B and D are correct.
   (2:271) (1:103)

55.   All of the following are reportedly reasons why disposable oxygen delivery equipment is desirable. From the standpoint of the respiratory therapy practitioner, which is most significant?
A.   They decrease the cost of sterilization procedures.
B.   They are more cost-effective overall.
C.   Their use allows the therapist to spend more time at the patient's bedside.
D.   They decrease the incidence of cross-contamination.
E.   They do not need to be replaced on a daily basis.
   (2:Chap 7)

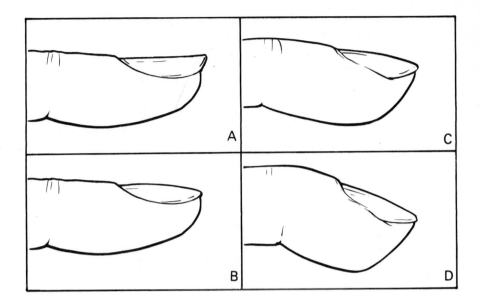

Figure 3.

56. The above diagram shows normal nails in *A* and *B* and clubbed nails in *C* and *D*. All of the following are true about the physical sign of clubbing *except:*
    A. It can often be seen in patients with chronic obstructive pulmonary disease.
    B. It may lead to osteoarthropathy.
    C. It involves soft tissue swelling at the terminal phalanx.
    D. It may be caused by chronic hypoxia.
    E. It is rarely noted in patients with cystic fibrosis.
       (3:190)

57. When an entrainment mask is administering 24% oxygen to a patient, it is entraining how many liters of room air for each liter of driving (source) gas?
    A. 3
    B. 5
    C. 10
    D. 20
    E. 25
       (4:Chap 4) (1:Chap 7)

58. During shift change, it is reported that a patient with a history of chronic obstructive pulmonary disease displayed marked somnolence during his IPPB treatments. Which of the following is the *least* appropriate action for the respiratory therapy practitioner to take at this time?
    A. Check the patient's oxygen therapy orders in his charts
    B. Immediately evaluate the patient to ensure his safety

C.   Check the patient's ventilator to make sure it is not being powered by compressed oxygen
D.   Read the patient chart to see if any other adverse responses to therapy have been noted
E.   Recommend initiation of continuous ventilatory support
     (49) (5:180–183)

59. In a patient with 15 g/dL hemoglobin and a normal cardiac output, cyanosis can be expected to appear first at approximately which of the following oxygen tension levels?
A.   75 mm Hg
B.   65 mm Hg
C.   55 mm Hg
D.   45 mm Hg
E.   35 mm Hg
     (30:129)

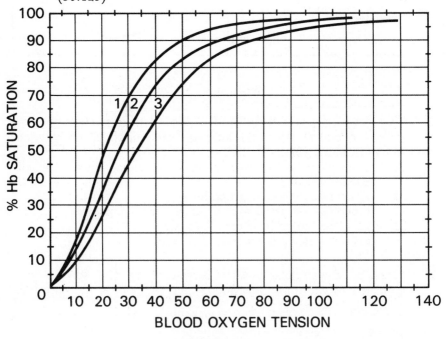

Figure 4.

60. Regarding the above diagram, which of the following statements is *not* true?
A.   The P$_{50}$ is highest in curve number 3.
B.   Curve number 1 displays the highest oxygen affinity.
C.   Curve number 2 represents the normal position of the oxyhemoglobin dissociation curve.
D.   Alkalosis would most likely result in curve number 3.
E.   A decrease in 2-3 DPG would most likely result in curve number 1.
     (3:135)

61. The respiratory therapy practitioner has discovered an unconscious and apneic patient. After calling for help and delivering four quick breaths, the therapist now is attempting to establish pulselessness. According to the American Heart Association, how much time should he or she devote to this effort?
   A. 0–5 seconds
   B. 5–10 seconds
   C. 10–15 seconds
   D. 15–20 seconds
   E. 20–30 seconds
   (37:19)

62. On a pressure-cycled ventilator an increase in lung thorax compliance will most likely result in:
   A. A decrease in delivered volume
   B. An increase in peak airway pressure
   C. Altered machine sensitivity
   D. An increase in the respiratory rate
   E. An increase in delivered volume
   (4:216–248)

63. While inspecting the chest roentgenogram of a dyspneic patient, the respiratory therapy practitioner notes the presence of an extremely thin linear shadow extending along the lateral margin of the right apical and subapical lung area. This is separated from the chest wall by an area of hyperlucency several centimeters wide and approximately 10 cm long. This description is most consistent with:
   A. Alveolar edema
   B. A pleural effusion
   C. Pulmonary emphysema
   D. Mediastinal emphysema
   E. A pneumothorax
   (2:298)

64. A respiratory therapy practitioner is administering continuous ventilatory support to a patient in the coronary care unit using a pressure-cycled ventilator. Suddenly he notices that the inspiratory phase has become extremely short. Which of the following might be responsible for the above occurrence?
   I. The patient's tidal volume may have increased.
   II. The problem may be caused by a leak in the circuit.
   III. The patient may need to be suctioned
   IV. The endotracheal tube may have slipped into the right mainstem bronchus.
   V. A tension pneumothorax may be present.
       A. I, IV, and V
       B. II, III, and V
       C. II, III, IV, and V
       D. I, II, and IV
       E. III, IV, and V
   (4:Chap 8)

65. Which of the following breath sounds are *always* considered abnormal when heard while auscultating the chest?
    I.   Vesicular
    II. Amphoric or cavernous
    III. Bronchial
    IV. Bronchovesicular
        A. II and IV
        B. I and III
        C. III and IV
        D. II only
        E. II and III
    (2:270–271)

66. An average arterial oxygen tension (Pa_{O_2}) for a healthy 60-year-old would be:
    A. 50 mm Hg
    B. 60 mm Hg
    C. 70 mm Hg
    D. 80 mm Hg
    E. 90 mm Hg
       (5:130) (32:63)

67. True statements regarding external cardiac compressions when applied to children include:
    I.   The sternum should be depressed 1 to 1½ inches.
    II. A rate of 100/min should be employed.
    III. The upper portion of the sternum should be depressed.
    IV. The heel of one hand may be used.
        A. I and III
        B. II and IV
        C. III and IV
        D. I and IV
        E. I and II
    (37:33)

68. Which of the following is *not* a recognized hazard of oxygen administration?
    A. Hypoventilation
    B. Absorption atelectasis
    C. Pulmonary edema
    D. Retrolental fibroplasia
    E. Hyperventilation
       (1:147–152) (7:125–127) (32:106–109)

69. Which of the following statements regarding the radial artery is (are) true?
    I.   It is usually accessible among inpatient and outpatient populations.
    II. It generally possesses adequate collateral blood flow.
    III. It is not proximal to nervous or periosteal tissue.
    IV. It is not considered a superficial artery.

      A. I and III
      B. II and IV
      C. I, II, and IV
      D. II only
      E. I and II
      (5:146–150)

70. The respiratory therapy practitioner is reviewing the chart of an extremely obese patient who has been diagnosed as having the classic Pickwickian syndrome. Which of the following findings would the therapist be *least* likely to note in this patient's chart?
    A. Somnolence
    B. Anemia
    C. Hypercapnia
    D. Cor pulmonale
    E. Hypoxemia
        (11:196–199)

71. Gastric inflation is a potential side effect of IPPB therapy. True statements regarding this condition include:
    I.   It may lead to ileus.
    II. It is not common in obtunded patients.
    III. It is more common in patients with nasogastric tubes.
    IV. It may increase the chance of vomiting and aspiration.
          A. II and III
          B. I, II, III, and IV
          C. II, III, and IV
          D. I, III, and IV
          E. III and IV
        (7:168) (54:230)

72. The narrowest portion of the newborn's upper airway is at the level of the:
    A. Trachea
    B. Thyroid cartilage
    C. Oropharynx
    D. Cricoid cartilage
    E. Vocal cords
        (10:85)

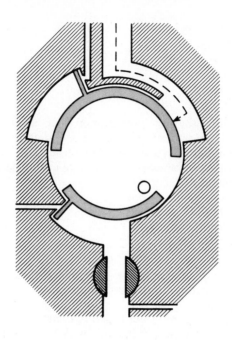

Figure 5.

73. The above illustration shows the Bennett valve in which position?
    I.   Open
    II.   Closed
    III. With the sensitivity control on
    IV.   With peak flow at the minimum setting
        A. I and III
        B. II only
        C. I, III, and IV
        D. I and II
        E. I only
    (3:344)

74. A 35-year-old woman is brought to the emergency department in distress. Historical data include a high fever, shaking, chills, and severe pleuritic chest pain. The patient has a harsh cough that is productive of moderate quantities of rusty-colored sputum. Arterial blood gas analysis reveals hypoxemia and hypocarbia. Based on the above information, which of the following is the most probable cause of this patient's distress?
    A. Gram-negative bacterial pneumonia
    B. Bacterial endocarditis
    C. Bronchiectasis
    D. Pneumococcal pneumonia
    E. Aspiration pneumonitis
    (11:62–64)

75. The breath sounds heard over most of the lung fields in a normal
    subject are termed:
    A. Vesicular
    B. Bronchovesicular
    C. Tracheal
    D. Tubular
    E. Bronchial
        (2:270)

76. When administering oxygen to a premature newborn, umbilical
    arterial oxygen tensions of _____ are usually considered safest.
    A. 20–40 mm Hg
    B. 30–70 mm Hg
    C. 40–80 mm Hg
    D. 80–100 mm Hg
    E. 100–120 mm Hg
        (13:81)

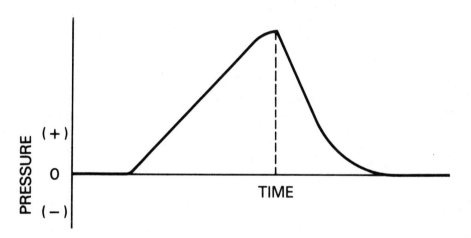

Figure 6.

77. The above pressure waveform is best described by which of the
    following terms?
    A. Assist mode ventilation
    B. Inflation hold
    C. PEEP
    D. Control mode ventilation
    E. Expiratory retard
        (70:517)

78. The administration of excessive doses of oxygen to premature
    newborns is believed to result in the development of which of the
    following disorders?
    I. Retrolental fibroplasia
    II. Alveolar hypoventilation

III. Massive pulmonary hemorrhage
IV. Bronchopulmonary dysplasia
 V. Wilson-Mikitty syndrome
    A. I and III
    B. I and IV
    C. II, IV, and V
    D. I, III, and V
    E. I, II, and IV
  (2:Chap 33)

79. Which of the following physical signs are most typically noted in patients with cor pulmonale?
   I. Rales
  II. Neck vein distention
 III. Mediastinal shift
 IV. Peripheral edema
    A. I and III
    B. III and IV
    C. I and IV
    D. II and III
    E. II and IV
  (17:262)

80. Retrolental fibroplasia:
   I. Will result when the newborn's Pa_{O_2} is greater than 50 mm Hg
  II. Is related to the PI_{O_2}, not the Pa_{O_2}
 III. Is almost invariably seen in the premature newborn
    A. I and III
    B. III only
    C. II only
    D. I, II, and III
    E. I and II
  (13:65 and 81)

81. The deleterious side effects of PEEP on the cardiovascular system are *least* likely to be pronounced in which of the following patients?
    A. Those with normal pulmonary compliance
    B. Those with decreased pulmonary compliance
    C. Those with pulmonary emphysema
    D. Those who are hypovolemic
    E. Those with unstable cardiovascular disease
  (46)

82. A 38-year-old patient is seen in the intensive care unit after being admitted with a severe right-sided infiltrate that occurred as a result of aspiration of gastric contents. Because of severe hypoxemia, this patient is placed on 7 cm H_2O PEEP with an FI_{O_2} of 1.0. Hypoxemia persists, however, despite PEEP therapy and cardiovascular support. The respiratory therapy practitioner

would recommend which of the following positions as being most likely to improve this patient's oxygenation status?
A.   Supine
B.   High Fowler's
C.   Lying on left side
D.   Lying on right side
E.   Low Fowler's
(38:44) (32:216)

83.   Which of the following must be known to calculate the minute alveolar ventilation?
   I.   Respiratory rate
   II.   Anatomic deadspace
   III.   Tidal volume
   IV. Pa_{CO_2}
   V. V_D/V_T
      A.   I, III, and IV
      B.   I, III, IV, and V
      C.   I, II, and III
      D.   I, III, and V
      E.   I, II, III, IV, and V
(5:Chap 8)

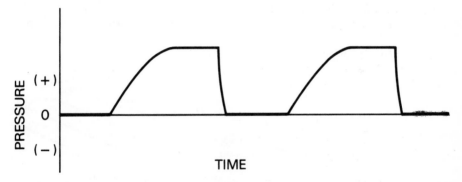

Figure 7.

84.   The above pressure waveform would most likely be generated by which of the following ventilators?
A.   Bennett MA-I
B.   Baby Bird
C.   Bourns Bear-I
D.   Emerson 3P-V
E.   Bird Mark 7
(70:524)

85.   Clubbing of the digits is a physical sign that is known to accompany all of the following disorders *except:*
A.   Bronchogenic carcinoma
B.   Cystic fibrosis

    C.   Infant respiratory distress syndrome
    D.   Chronic bronchitis
    E.   Bronchiectasis
       (17:210–211 and 338)

86. The lung is the most common site of postoperative complications. Which of the following types of surgical procedures is associated with the highest incidence of postoperative pulmonary complications?
    A.   Neurologic
    B.   Lower abdominal
    C.   Orthopaedic
    D.   Upper abdominal
    E.   Thoracic
       (30:37–39)

87. Use of which of the following agents or methods is *not* capable of achieving complete sterilization?
    I.   Alcohols
    II.   Alkaline glutaraldehyde
    III.   Pasteurization
    IV.   Acid glutaraldehyde
        A.   I and III
        B.   III only
        C.   III and IV
        D.   II and IV
        E.   I and II
    (2:418–422)

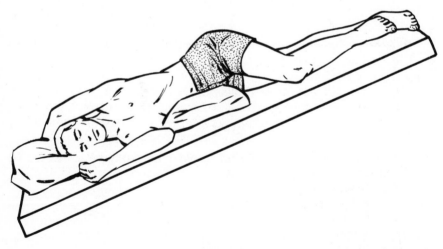

Figure 8.

88. The above illustration shows the patient lying on his right side in Trendelenburg. In this position, which segment will drain?
    A.   Lower lobe, lateral basal segment on the left
    B.   Upper lobe, apical posterior segment on the right

    C.   Lower lobe, posterior basal segment on the right
    D.   Lower lobe, posterior basal segment on the left
    E.   Lower lobe, anterior basal segment on the left
      (7:214)

89. According to the American Heart Association, which of the following are indications for the initiation of basic cardiac life support during the first few minutes of life?
    I.   Apgar score of 4–6
    II. Prolonged periods of apnea
    III. Presence of meconium staining
    IV. Absent cardiac rate
      A. II and IV
      B. III and IV
      C. I and III
      D. II and III
      E. II only
    (25:Chap 16, pp 1–6)

90. Which of the following best describes consolidated lung tissue?
    I.   Porous, well-aerated structure
    II. Relatively poor transmitter of sound
    III. Relatively firm, semisolid structure
    IV. Relatively good transmitter of sound
      A. II only
      B. I and IV
      C. I and II
      D. I and III
      E. III and IV
    (17:195)

91. True statements regarding postextubation edema include:
    I.   Development of respiratory distress shortly after extubation is an unfavorable sign.
    II. Even mildly distressed individuals should be reintubated.
    III. Aerosolization of decongestants and corticosteroids may be helpful.
    IV. Unfavorable response to pharmacologic agents is an indication for immediate tracheotomy.
      A. I and II
      B. II and III
      C. I and III
      D. II, III, and IV
      E. I, II, and III
    (1:282–285)

92. For sterilization to occur, which of the following actions must an agent or method possess?
    I.   Bacteriocidal
    II. Sporicidal
    III. Viricidal

IV. Tuberculocidal
V. Fungicidal
    A. I, II, III, and IV
    B. I, III, IV, and V
    C. II, III, IV, and V
    D. I, II, III, IV, and V
    E. I, II, and IV
  (24:334)

93. Which of the following statements regarding the ratio of compressions to ventilations during basic cardiopulmonary resuscitation (CPR) is (are) true?
  I. During two-rescuer infant CPR it is 5:1.
  II. During one-rescuer adult CPR it is 15:2.
  III. During two-rescuer CPR to children it is 5:2.
    A. I only
    B. I and II
    C. II and III
    D. III only
    E. I, II, and III
  (37:23–24 and 33)

94. For which of the following disorders is cyanosis *least* likely to be a clinical sign?
  A. Neonatal asphyxia
  B. Methemoglobinemia
  C. Carbon monoxide poisoning
  D. Tetralogy of Fallot
  E. Advanced cystic fibrosis
  (17:217–221)

95. Which of the following factors reportedly contribute(s) to the incidence of cuff-related side effects of continuous mechanical ventilation?
  I. Arterial hypertension
  II. Tracheal infection
  III. Use of low pressure cuffs
  IV. Tube movement in the trachea
  V. Prolonged artificial ventilation
    A. II, IV, and V
    B. V only
    C. I, II, and IV
    D. IV and V
    E. I, II, and V
  (1:287–288)

96. During auscultation of the chest, the respiratory therapy practitioner frequently asks the patient to cough. Which of the following chest sounds will most frequently disappear following this maneuver?
  A. Rales
  B. Rhonchi

C. Pleural friction rub
D. Egophony
E. Bronchial breath sounds
   (1:103)

97. Factors that have been held responsible for the extremely high mortality rate among patients developing Gram-negative nosocomial pulmonary infections include:
   I.   Frequent occurrence among immunosuppressed hosts
   II. Concurrent administration of continuous ventilatory support
   III. Use of broad-spectrum antibiotics
   IV. Concurrent development of adult respiratory distress syndrome
      A. I and III
      B. I, III, and IV
      C. I, II, III, and IV
      D. II, III, and IV
      E. II and IV
   (87:438–439) (31:41–42)

98. The respiratory therapy practitioner is asked to help set up a home care program for a quadriplegic patient with a vital capacity of 7 cc/kg. The practitioner notes that the patient is unable to cough effectively. Instruction in which one of the following techniques would be most likely to help improve this patient's cough effort?
   A. Diaphragmatic breathing
   B. Glossopharyngeal ("frog") breathing
   C. Pursed lip breathing
   D. Chest vibration
   E. Segmental chest expansion
   (2:760)

99. Which of the following statements is (are) true regarding the oxygen concentration administered by a Bird Mark 7 ventilator in the air mix mode?
   I.   It will increase as the system pressure increases.
   II. It will decrease as the system pressure increases.
   III. It is not affected by changes in lung compliance.
      A. I and II
      B. II only
      C. I only
      D. I and III
      E. II and III
   (4:258–259)

100. Which of the following would be the emergency airway modality of choice for an unconscious patient on whom attempts at intubation have failed?
   A. Tracheotomy
   B. Oropharyngeal airway

C. Cricothyroidotomy
D. Modified jaw thrust
E. Nasopharyngeal airway
(25:Chap 4, pp 8–9)

101. Patients with refractory hypoxemia accompanied by which of the following presentations are frequently *not* considered good candidates for PEEP therapy?
   I.   Diffuse bibasal pulmonary infiltrates
   II. Unilateral pulmonary infiltrates
   III. Decreased functional residual capacities
   IV. Severely diminished cardiovascular reserves
      A. I and IV
      B. II and III
      C. I and II
      D. III and IV
      E. II and IV
   (46)

102. The respiratory therapy practitioner is teaching a patient the techniques of taking an IPPB treatment. Proper instructions include:
   I.   Exhale through pursed lips only
   II. Initiate inspiration and let the lungs fill and empty passively
   III. Pause for a few seconds between each breath
   IV. Force as much air in and out of the lungs as possible with each breath
      A. II and IV
      B. I and III
      C. III and IV
      D. I and II
      E. II and III
   (2:577–579) (1:189–190)

103. In reviewing a patient's chart, the respiratory therapy practitioner notes that the patient's most recent acid-base study revealed a base deficit of 6.8 mEq/L. This value is most consistent with the presence of:
   A. Alveolar hyperventilation
   B. Metabolic acidosis
   C. Mixed respiratory and metabolic acidosis
   D. Severe respiratory acidosis
   E. Metabolic alkalosis
   (5:101)

104. A 48-year-old man in moderate respiratory distress is brought to the emergency department by his wife. His chief complaint is of progressive numbing and weakness of his extremities that has progressed over the past several days to the point where dyspnea and fatigue are noted on even mild exertion. This was preceded by a severe upper respiratory infection. Based on the above information, the most likely cause of distress is:
   A. Guillain-Barré syndrome

B. Idiopathic thrombocytopenic purpura
C. Myasthenia gravis
D. Chronic obstructive pulmonary emphysema
E. Congestive heart failure
    (11:205–207)

105. Before a pleural effusion may be diagnosed on the basis of physical signs of decreased breath sounds and abnormal percussion note, how much fluid must be present?
A. 0–50 mL
B. 300–500 mL
C. 400–800 mL
D. 50–150 mL
E. 500–1000 mL
    (94:179)

106. The term *pectus excavatum* is most synonymous with which of the following terms?
A. Pigeon chest
B. Barrel chest
C. Funnel chest
D. Bell chest
E. Flail chest
    (95:93)

107. In reviewing the chart of a 20-year-old patient with allergic bronchial asthma, the respiratory therapy practitioner would expect to see evidence of which of the following?
I.   Mucopurulent or mucoid sputum
II. Polycythemia
III. Wheezing on auscultation
IV. Considerable improvement following bronchodilator administration
    A. I, III, and IV
    B. II and III
    C. III only
    D. I and III
    E. I and IV
    (2:707–710) (11:105) (32:157–158)

108. A patient is being given oxygen via a properly fitting 24% air entrainment mask. Which of the following ventilatory patterns will result in the lowest FI_{O_2}?
A. Minute ventilation, 12 L; frequency, 18/min
B. Minute ventilation, 14 L; frequency, 6/min
C. Minute ventilation, 12 L; frequency, 24/min
D. Minute ventilation, 14 L; frequency, 38/min
E. The FI_{O_2} will not vary with the ventilatory pattern.
    (1:136–143)

109. The respiratory therapy practitioner is monitoring a 30-year-old patient who is intubated and receiving an FI_{O_2} of 0.7 via a T tube setup, and acid-base data obtained at that time are as follows:

Pao$_2$	34 mm Hg
Paco$_2$	48 mm Hg
pH	7.32
HCO$_3^-$	19 mEq/L
Base excess	−3.8 mEq/L
Respiratory rate	48/min

Which of the following modifications in therapy should the practitioner recommend at this time?
A. Raise the FIo$_2$ to 1.0
B. Place on 5 cm H$_2$O CPAP with an FIo$_2$ of 0.9
C. Place on assist/control with an FIo$_2$ of 0.8
D. Place on IMV with an FIo$_2$ of 0.8
E. Place on 5 cm H$_2$O PEEP with an FIo$_2$ of 0.8
    (1:384 and 452–453) (38:Chaps 4 through 6, p 63) (32:64–66)
    (46) (49)

110. If during the performance of external cardiac compressions the rescuer's hands inadvertently depress the area over the xiphoid process, which of the following may occur?
A. Lung contusion
B. Laceration of the liver
C. Myocardial contusion
D. Damage to the rescuer's hands
E. Laceration of the ileus
    (37:21)

111. The respiratory therapy practitioner is restocking a crash-cart in the emergency department. In doing so he notices that the intubation roentgenogram contains an endotracheal tube that has the symbol Z-79 but not the letters I.T. Which of the following statements regarding this tube is (are) true?
    I. The tube may not have been implant tested.
    II. The tube probably has a high pressure type cuff.
    III. The tube may be composed of toxic materials.
        A. I and III
        B. II and III
        C. II only
        D. III only
        E. I, II, and III
    (2:517–518)

112. If the respiratory therapy practitioner were to take the external diameter of an endotracheal tube and multiply it by 3.14 (π), he or she would be able to determine which of the following?
A. Proper catheter size for endotracheal suctioning
B. The Forreger size of the tube
C. The French size of the tube
D. The internal diameter of the tube
E. The wall thickness of the tube
    (36:35)

113. In which of the following types of hypoxia is oxygen administration *least* likely to be of benefit?
      A. Hypoxemic
      B. Anemic
      C. Circulatory
      D. Histotoxic
      E. A and C are correct.
      (5:49–50) (7:115–116) (2:241 and 394–395)

114. Which of the following conditions is *least* likely to be associated with the presence of barrel chest?
      A. Infancy
      B. Emphysema
      C. Old age
      D. Middle age
      E. Cystic fibrosis
      (95:93)

115. During the performance of basic cardiopulmonary resuscitation, which of the following is believed to *best* indicate the fact that external cardiac compressions are producing adequate cerebral blood flow?
      A. Improvement in patient's color
      B. Constriction of the pupils in response to light
      C. A palpable carotid pulse
      D. Presence of rib fractures
      E. Presence of a gag reflex
      (37:24)

116. Which of the following types of oxygen analyzers actually measure(s) the partial pressure of oxygen in the monitored gas?
      I.   Paramagnetic devices
      II.   Wheatstone bridge devices
      III. Galvanic cell devices
      IV.   Polarographic devices
           A. II, III, and IV
           B. I and II
           C. II and IV
           D. I only
           E. I, III, and IV
      (51)

117. Which of the following is the *least* likely cause of respiratory alkalosis?
      A. Metabolic alkalosis
      B. Acute hypoxemia
      C. Third-trimester pregnancy
      D. Intracranial hypertension
      E. Fear, pain, and anxiety
      (5:198–208)

118. The respiratory therapy practitioner is asked to continuously monitor the FIo_2 inside an oxygen hood device. Which of the fol-

lowing types of oxygen analyzers would be *most* appropriate for this purpose?
I.   Paramagnetic analyzer
II. Wheatstone bridge type analyzer
III. Galvanic cell type analyzer
IV. Polarographic type analyzer
   A.   I and III
   B.   II and IV
   C.   II and III
   D.   I and II
   E.   III and IV
(51:153–159)

119. Which of the following statements are true regarding the performance of external cardiac compressions to the infant who has suffered a cardiac arrest?
I.   The sternum should be depressed ½ to 1 inch.
II. The rate should be 120/min.
III. The middle of the sternum should be depressed.
IV. The heel of one hand should be used.
   A.   II and III
   B.   I and III
   C.   I and IV
   D.   III and IV
   E.   II, III, and IV
(37:33)

120. The respiratory therapy practitioner can most readily check the accuracy of an oxygen blender device by:
   A.   Checking the air and oxygen lines to lines on the blender on a regular basis
   B.   Checking the flow rate from the blender
   C.   Measuring the patient's arterial oxygen tension every hour
   D.   Employing an oxygen analyzer
   E.   Monitoring the pressure of the bulk oxygen system
(4:142–146)

121. Failure to keep an arterial sample under anaerobic conditions prior to running of the sample is known to result in which of the following errors?
I.   Low pH
II. High P_{O_2}
III. Low Pa_{CO_2}
IV. High P_{CO_2}
V.   Low P_{O_2}
   A.   I, III, and V
   B.   II and IV
   C.   III and V
   D.   II and III
   E.   I, II, and IV
(5:156–157)

122. After performance of a tracheotomy and the insertion of a cuffed tracheal tube, a reasonable estimate of a 50-kg patient's anatomic deadspace would be:
    A. 25 cc
    B. 55 cc
    C. 75 cc
    D. 100 cc
    E. 150 cc
    (20:23) (30:215)

123. Which of the following most correctly describes the term *iatrogenic infection?*
    A. One that results from the use of immunosuppressive agents
    B. One that occurs postoperatively
    C. One that results from the activities of medical or surgical personnel
    D. One that occurs in the hospital
    E. One that occurs from the use of broad-spectrum antibiotics
    (89:686)

124. Which of the following are true statements regarding the color-coding of medical gas cylinders?
    I.   The system was designed by the Compressed Gas Association.
    II. It should be followed *exclusively* in identifying the contents of the cylinder.
    III. If color code and cylinder label information are in conflict, the cylinder should not be used.
    A. I and II
    B. II only
    C. I and III
    D. I only
    E. III only
    (4:37-38)

125. A routine, portable chest roentgenogram generally consists of which of the following projections?
    A. Posteroanterior and lateral views
    B. Posteroanterior views only
    C. Anteroposterior view only
    D. Anteroposterior and lateral views
    E. Oblique and posteroanterior views
    (1:105)

126. True statements regarding the $P(A-a)o_2$ when measured with the patient breathing 100% oxygen include:
    I.   Values greater than 400 mm Hg indicate the presence of oxygenation failure.
    II. Values greater than 400 mm Hg indicate that hypoxemia is probably due to shunting.
    III. Values greater than 100 mm Hg are a contraindication for oxygen therapy.

IV. The normal value for a healthy 20-year-old person is 100 mm Hg.
A. I and II
B. III and IV
C. II and IV
D. III only
E. I and IV
(2:394–395) (5:Chaps 19 and 20, pp 92–94 and 232–235) (38:38–42) (50) (32) (63)

127. The respiratory therapist receives an order to administer sustained maximal inspiratory therapy (incentive spirometry) to a 34-year-old, 100-kg patient who is recovering from a laminectomy performed 4 days previously. The following data are collected by the therapist at the patient's bedside:

BP	120/80
Pulse	88
Respiratory rate	18
Vital capacity	50 cc/kg
Breath sounds	Normal
V_T	750 mL

The therapist should recommend that:
A. Therapy be performed as ordered
B. Therapy be discontinued
C. The patient be discharged from the hospital
D. IPPB be administered instead
E. Aerosol therapy followed by postural drainage and percussion should be administered
(1:173 and 188–189; Chap 14) (2:561–562 and 874–876)

128. Which of the following statements are true regarding wheezing heard while auscultating the chest?
I. It is considered to be a type of rale.
II. It may be described as a musical, whistling, or squeaking sound.
III. It is a frequent finding in patients with congestive heart failure.
IV. It always denotes the presence of asthma.
A. I, II, and III
B. I and II
C. I and III
D. II and IV
E. II and III
(2:271 and 706)

129. Which of the following statements about cromolyn sodium is (are) true?
I. It is not effective against allergic asthma.
II. It is a synthetic corticosteroid.

III. It inhibits the release of slow-reacting substance of anaphy-
        laxis from the mast cell.
IV.   It is a potent bronchodilator.
        A. II and III
        B. III and IV
        C. III only
        D. II, III, and IV
        E. I only
        (2:489) (12:Chap 2)

130. Common effects of mild to moderate hypoxia include all but
        which of the following pathophysiologic actions?
        A. Increased cardiac output
        B. Pulmonary vasoconstriction
        C. Increased arterial blood pressure
        D. Hyperventilation
        E. Decreased cardiac output
        (7:116–118) (30:127–129)

131. A 1340-g male infant is delivered following a 30-week gestation.
        At approximately 1 minute of life, the following vital signs are
        noted:

        Heart rate   110
        Respirations   Absent
        Muscle tone   Flaccid
        Reflex irritability   No response
        Color   Systemic cyanosis

        Based on the above information, which of the following actions
        should the respiratory therapy practitioner recommend at this
        time?
        A. Administer intracardiac epinephrine
        B. Start an intravenous line stat
        C. Intubate and ventilate with 100% oxygen
        D. Continue to monitor closely
        E. Draw an arterial sample stat
        (25:Chap 16, pp 1–6)

132. The respiratory therapy practitioner's therapeutic goal is to mobi-
        lize secretions in a 68-year-old postoperative patient. Which of the
        following modalities would the therapist consider as a last resort?
        A. Aerosol therapy
        B. Instruction in cough technique
        C. Nasotracheal suctioning
        D. Aerosolized mucokinetic agents
        E. Hyperinflation therapy
        (2:525)

133. Which of the following are recommended methods of keeping ven-
        tilator tubing system compliance as low as possible?
        I.   Using thick-walled tubing
        II. Keeping humidifiers filled

III. Keeping gases at BTPS
IV. Using minimal tubing length
    A. I, III, and IV
    B. I, II, and IV
    C. I and IV
    D. II, III, and IV
    E. I, II, III, and IV
    (4:226–230)

134. The respiratory therapy practitioner is administering IPPB therapy to a postoperative patient. About halfway through the therapy, acute dyspnea and tachycardia develop. The patient appears
frightened and complains of sudden anxiety and depression.
Which of the following actions should the practitioner take at this
time?
    A. Console the patient for several minutes and then resume
        therapy
    B. Recommend insertion of a chest tube
    C. Hyperventilate the patient to lower the intracranial pressure
    D. Discontinue therapy and notify the physician
    E. Discontinue IPPB and initiate postural drainage and percus-
        sion techniques
    (1:190) (2:580)

135. Which of the following will likely cause the FIo_2 delivered by an
air entrainment device to decrease significantly?
    I. If the humidity of the driving gas is decreased
    II. If the jet is made smaller
    III. If the jet is made larger
    IV. If the entrainment ports are made smaller
    V. If the entrainment ports are made larger
    A. I and III
    B. II and V
    C. II and IV
    D. III and IV
    E. I and II
    (4:76–78)

136. The respiratory therapy practitioner would be most likely to
employ a nonrebreathing type mask on patients with which one of
the following disorders?
    A. Bronchiectasis
    B. Cystic fibrosis
    C. Anemia
    D. Carbon monoxide poisoning
    E. Ventricular fibrillation
    (4:Chap 3)

137. The respiratory therapy practitioner is operating a Bennett MA-I
ventilator in the control mode with a tidal volume of 650 cc, a
respiratory rate of 14, and a peak inspiratory flow rate of 35 L/
min. If the tidal volume were increased to 1000 cc while maintain-

ing the same I:E ratio and respiratory rate, which of the following would be *least* likely to occur?

A. An increase in inspiratory flow rate
B. An increase in peak pressure
C. Lengthening of the expiratory time
D. No change in the inspiratory time
E. Increase in the volume compressed in the tubing
   (4:216–230 and 233–247)

138. Which of the following is (are) reason(s) why a 10% sodium chloride solution may be preferred for sputum induction purposes?
   I. It is bacteriocidal.
   II. It may increase the volume of pulmonary secretions.
   III. It produces a very small particle size.
   IV. It is believed to be an effective respiratory tract irritant.
      A. I and III
      B. II and IV
      C. III and IV
      D. III only
      E. II and III
   (3:226)

139. If the gas flow through an unheated bubble humidifier is increased from 2 L/min to 6 L/min, which of the following will occur?
   I. The percent body humidity of gases delivered will decrease.
   II. The temperature within the device will increase.
   III. The absolute humidity of the gases will increase.
   IV. The temperature within the unit will decrease.
      A. I and IV
      B. I and II
      C. III and IV
      D. II and IV
      E. I, II, and III
   (8:118–119)

140. In reading his patient's chart prior to IPPB therapy, the therapist notes that the patient had 5+ ankle edema when admitted to the hospital. Which of the following disorders would most likely be responsible for this physical sign?
   A. Bronchial asthma
   B. Adult respiratory distress syndrome
   C. Cor pulmonale
   D. Drug overdose
   E. Neurotrauma
   (11:184)

141. Which of the following abnormalities can usually be treated by increasing alveolar ventilation?
   I. Hypercarbia
   II. Metabolic acidosis
   III. Hypoxia

    IV. Alveolar hypoventilation
    V. Respiratory acidosis
       A. I, II, and V
       B. I, III, and V
       C. II, III, and V
       D. II and III
       E. I, IV, and V
    (5:Chaps 8 and 11) (2:243)

142. Which of the following will enhance the tendency of medical aerosols to "rain out" before entering the patient's smaller airways?
    I. Ninety-degree bends in the delivery tubing
    II. Use of isotonic solutions
    III. Administration with the patient "nose breathing"
    IV. Rapid, shallow patient ventilatory pattern
    V. Administration of aerosol particles greater than 10μ in diameter
       A. I and V
       B. II, III, IV, and V
       C. I, III, IV, and V
       D. I, II, and V
       E. III, IV, and V
    (1:174) (48)

143. For which of the following pulmonary disorders would a hyperresonant percussion note be a common physical finding?
    I. Pleural effusion
    II. Pneumothorax
    III. Emphysema
    IV. Hemothorax
       A. II and III
       B. I, II, and IV
       C. II only
       D. III only
       E. II and IV
    (2:272)

144. Which of the following are advantages associated with the use of high flow oxygen delivery systems?
    I. Changes in ventilatory pattern are less likely to affect the delivered FIo_2.
    II. The temperature and absolute humidity of the inspired gases may be more easily controlled.
    III. The incidence of nosocomial infection is known to be lower with their use.
    IV. Alveolar ventilation tends to increase with their use.
       A. I and II
       B. III and IV
       C. I, II, and III
       D. I, II, and IV
       E. I, II, III, and IV
    (1:132)

145. A 20-year-old woman is admitted to the hospital because of a fractured femur suffered in a hiking accident. Arterial blood gas data
obtained at that time are as follows:

#121

FIo_2	0.21
Pao_2	136 mm Hg
$Paco_2$	18 mm Hg
pH	7.62
Base excess	+0.8 mEq/L

Which of the following is the most likely cause of the above labo-
ratory error?
A. Venous sampling
B. An aerobic sample
C. Too much sodium heparin in sample
D. Delay in running the sample
E. Not enough sodium heparin in sample
   (5:157) (2:1010)

146. Which of the following is the normal value for $\dfrac{FEV_1\%}{FVC}$?
A. Greater than 40%
B. Greater than 60%
C. Greater than 75%
D. Greater than 90%
E. Greater than 95%
   (2:212)

147. Which of the following pulmonary disorders is _not_ associated with
shifts of the mediastinal contents to the unaffected side?
A. Massive atelectasis
B. Pleural effusion
C. Tension pneumothorax
D. Hemothorax
E. Hemopneumothorax
   (17:188) (2:272)

148. In reading a patient's chart, the respiratory therapy practitioner
notes the attending physician's statement that the patient's pri-
mary pathology involves the loss of pulmonary parenchymal elas-
tic recoil. This observation is most consistent with:
A. Chronic bronchitis
B. Emphysema
C. Bronchiectasis
D. Bronchial asthma
E. Adult respiratory distress syndrome
   (11:96)

149. The toxic chemical ethylene chlorohydrin may be formed under
which of the following circumstances?
A. If polyvinyl chloride is left in acid glutaraldehyde solutions
   too long
B. If ethylene oxide gas is ignited

C. If ethylene oxide sterilized items are subsequently steam-autoclaved
D. If ethylene oxide comes in contact with water
E. If previously gamma-irradiated equipment is resterilized with ethylene oxide
    (24:338)

150. When using a Wright respirometer, the respiratory therapy practitioner should be aware that flow rates below which of the following levels can produce inaccurate readings?
A. 3 L/min
B. 30 L/min
C. 10 L/min
D. 15 L/min
E. 20 L/min
    (4:206)

151. An elderly man is brought to the emergency department after being found unconscious. He is febrile and appears extremely malnourished. He is immediately placed on 8 L oxygen via simple oxygen mask, and a sample of arterial blood is drawn and analyzed. These data appear below:

Pa_{O_2}	70 mm Hg
Pa_{CO_2}	27 mm Hg
pH	7.36
HCO_3^-	12 mEq/L
Base excess	−9 mEq/L

Which of the following is the most correct interpretation of the above results?
A. Fully compensated metabolic acidosis
B. Fully compensated respiratory acidosis
C. Acute respiratory alkalosis
D. Acute metabolic acidosis
E. Respiratory alkalosis and metabolic alkalosis
    (2:246) (5:128) (25:Chap 10, pp 2–6)

152. Which of the following bronchodilators is believed to have the shortest duration of action?
A. Isoproterenol
B. Isoetharine
C. Terbutaline
D. Metaproterenol
E. Racemic epinephrine
    (2:473–474)

153. Which of the following is least likely to be responsible for the arterial hypotension that often accompanies states of shock?
A. Hypovolemia
B. Decreased cardiac output
C. Decreased peripheral vascular resistance
D. Left ventricular failure

E.   Increased peripheral vascular resistance
(1:Chap 26)

154.   For which of the following patients could the respiratory therapy
practitioner recommend the use of cromolyn sodium?
A.   An allergic asthmatic during an acute episode
B.   A nonallergic asthmatic during an asthmatic episode
C.   An asthmatic who is in remission
D.   A nonallergic asthmatic who is not receiving bronchodilator
therapy
E.   B and D are correct.
(2:488–489) (32:168)

155.   Which of the following clinical signs would be most likely to
accompany massive unilateral pulmonary atelectasis?
I.   Dull percussion note over the affected area
II.   Tracheal shift to the unaffected side
III.   Vesicular breath sounds over the affected area
IV.   Egophony over the affected area
A.   III only
B.   II and IV
C.   I and IV
D.   III and IV
E.   I and II
(95:95–97) (2:272)

156.   Which of the following tests would most likely be within normal
limits when performed on patients with pulmonary fibrotic lung
disorders?
I. $\dfrac{FEV_1\%}{FVC}$
II.   TLC
III.   FEF $_{200\text{-}1200}$
IV.   FVC
A.   II only
B.   I and IV
C.   II and III
D.   I and III
E.   III and IV
(2:212)

157.   All of the following methods have been recommended to help pre-
vent a patient from fighting a ventilator. Which method report-
edly provides fewest hindrances to the weaning process?
A.   Use of mechanical hyperventilation
B.   Use of analgesics
C.   Use of intermittent mandatory ventilation
D.   Use of paralyzing agents
E.   Use of sedatives and tranquilizers
(1:338–342) (2:598–601 and 664–668)

158. To ensure sterility, equipment must be immersed in heated (60°C) acid glutaraldehyde for how many hours?
   A.   1
   B.   6
   C.   12
   D.   20
   E.   30
   (24:340)

159. Which of the following disorders is *least* likely to be associated with the production of copious amounts of purulent sputum?
   A.   Pulmonary emphysema
   B.   Aspiration pneumonia
   C.   Anaerobic lung abscess
   D.   Bronchiectasis
   E.   Cystic fibrosis
   (2:272)

160. Which of the following features characterize the Bennett PR-I ventilator?
   I.   Volume cycled
   II.   Single circuit
   III.   Flow sensitive
   IV.   Flow adjustable
      A.   I, III, and IV
      B.   II, III, and IV
      C.   I and IV
      D.   II and III
      E.   I, II, III, and IV
   (4:323–324)

161. A P_{50} of _____ would indicate the normal positioning of the oxy-hemoglobin dissociation curve.
   A.   26.5 mm Hg
   B.   25 mm Hg
   C.   40 mm Hg
   D.   97 mm Hg
   E.   29 mm Hg
   (2:238)

162. The physician asks the respiratory therapy practitioner to administer IPPB with 100% oxygen to a patient with acute cardiogenic pulmonary edema. All of the following ventilators are available in the department equipment room. The selection of which one would be *least* desirable?
   A.   Bennett PR-I
   B.   Bird Mark 7
   C.   Bennett AP-5
   D.   Bird Mark 8
   E.   Bennett PR-II
   (4:324)

163. Which of the following formulas would be most useful in helping the respiratory therapy practitioner establish the initial tidal volume for a patient who is to receive continuous ventilatory support?
    A. 15–20 cc/kg
    B. 7–10 cc/kg
    C. 10–15 cc/lb.
    D. 10–12 cc/kg
    E. 15–20 cc/lb.
       (25:Chap 15, p 2) (1:337–338) (24:286)

164. Which of the following statements regarding the esophageal obturator airway is (are) true?
    I.   It is designed to be inserted in the trachea.
    II.   It is equipped with an inflatable cuff.
    III. When inserted properly it allows for relief of gastric distention.
    IV.   It is designed for use by personnel not trained in endotracheal intubation.
       A. I and IV
       B. II and III
       C. II and IV
       D. III and IV
       E. I only
    (4:164–165)

165. The normal range of $P\bar{v}_{O_2}$ for a healthy resting subject is:
    A. 45–50 mm Hg
    B. 25–30 mm Hg
    C. 30–35 mm Hg
    D. 37–43 mm Hg
    E. 50–55 mm Hg
       (5:232)

166. Which of the following is *not* a type of oropharyngeal airway?
    A. Berman
    B. Guedel
    C. Connel
    D. Cole
    E. Safar
       (4:164–165)

167. Which of the following are reported goals of IPPB therapy when used in the management of acute cardiogenic pulmonary edema?
    I.   Relief of dyspnea
    II.   Administration of oxygen
    III. Increase in venous return
    IV.   Administration of mucolytic agents
       A. I, II, III, and IV
       B. II, III, and IV
       C. II and IV
       D. I and II
       E. I + III

E.   I and III
(2:555 and 727–729) (1:435–436)

168. Which of the following common household agents would the
respiratory therapy practitioner recommend to decontaminate
respiratory therapy equipment prescribed for home use?
A.   Common household bleach
B.   Sodium bicarbonate
C.   Acetic acid (vinegar)
D.   Baking soda
E.   Common household cleanser mixed with bleach
(2:452)

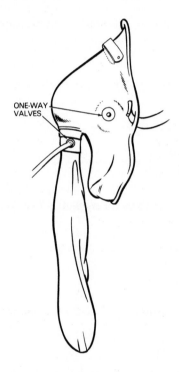

ONE-WAY
VALVES

Figure 9.

169. The above illustration shows:
A.   Simple oxygen mask
B.   Partial rebreathing mask
C.   Nonrebreathing mask
D.   Rebreathing mask
E.   Anesthesia mask
(3:278–283)

170. A 17-year-old girl is brought to the emergency department by her
father after suffering as asthma attack that did not respond to
metered-dose isoetharine at home. The patient's respiratory rate

is 25/min and her pulse is 100. Arterial blood sampled at this time with an FI_{O_2} of 0.21 would most likely reveal:
A. Partially compensated respiratory acidosis with moderate hypoxemia
B. Respiratory alkalosis with moderate hypoxemia
C. Fully compensated metabolic acidosis with mild hypoxemia
D. Respiratory alkalosis with very severe hypoxemia
E. Partially compensated metabolic alkalosis with moderate hypoxemia
(5:201)

171. According to the American Heart Association, irreversible brain damage is usually certain after 10 minutes of pulselessness. Which of the following groups has (have) been known to be exceptions to this rule?
I. Neonatal victims
II. Patients with chronic obstructive pulmonary disease
III. Hypothermic victims
IV. Patients with adult respiratory distress syndrome
A. I, II, and III
B. II, III, and IV
C. I and III
D. III only
E. I, III, and IV
(37:8 and 35)

172. A satisfactory definition of *respiratory failure* is:
A. Inability to maintain normal venous blood gases
B. Inability to sustain internal respiration
C. Inability to sustain external respiration
D. Inability to maintain normal arterial blood gases
E. C and D are correct.
(1:299–301) (11:221–222) (49)

173. The use of which of the following devices would help the respiratory therapy practitioner determine the presence of abnormal concentrations of carboxyhemoglobin?
A. Blood gas analyzer
B. Galvanic cell analyzer
C. CO-oximeter
D. Ear oximeter
E. Tonometer
(5:39)

174. In report, the respiratory therapy practitioner is assigned to a 2100-g newborn who is in an Isolette. On entering the nursery, the practitioner notes that the red flag at the rear of the incubator is in the up position. This most likely indicates:
A. That the Isolette is empty
B. That the patient is in a neutral thermal environment
C. That oxygen should not be administered
D. That that patient's FI_{O_2} is in excess of 40%

E.   That the patient's FIo$_2$ is less than 40%
(4:Chap 3)

175. Which of the following bronchodilators could the respiratory ther-
apist recommend for subcutaneous administration?
A.   Isoetharine
B.   Epinephrine
C.   Terbutaline
D.   Metaproterenol
E.   B and C are correct.
(2:479)

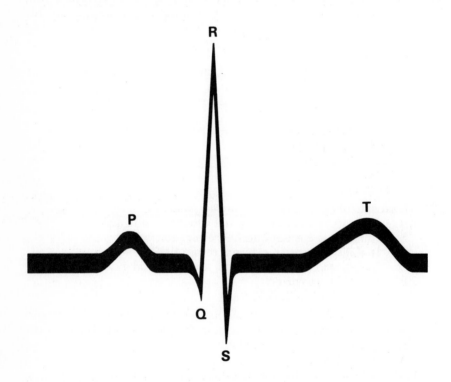

Figure 10.

176. The above illustration shows a normal cardiac cycle. If there were
no uniform atrial depolarization, what would disappear?
A.   P wave
B.   Q wave
C.   R wave
D.   T wave
E.   S wave
(25:Chap 6)

177. Which of the following are true statements regarding the Bird
Mark 7 ventilator when it is operating in the control mode?

I. It is time cycled into expiration.
II. Inspiration is initiated by a timing mechanism.
III. The I:E ratio is always constant.
IV. It is pressure cycled into expiration.
   A. I and IV
   B. II and IV
   C. I and III
   D. I and II
   E. III and IV
(4:249–262)

178. For which two of the following clinical conditions is acute alveolar hyperventilation with arterial hypoxemia a common clinical finding?
  I. Adult respiratory distress syndrome
  II. Acute bronchial asthma
  III. Myasthenia gravis
  IV. Drug overdose
   A. I and III
   B. II and IV
   C. III and IV
   D. II and III
   E. I and II
(5:199–203)

179. Recognized complications that may result from the use of a resuscitator bag, mask, and oral airway combinations include which of the following?
  I. Inadequate tidal volumes
  II. Hyperventilation
  III. Gastric distention
   A. II and III
   B. I and III
   C. I and II
   D. II only
   E. I only
(25:Chap 4, pp 6–7)

180. Which of the following ventilators is not capable of being volume cycled?
A. Bourns BP-200
B. Bennett MA-I
C. Baby Bird ventilator
D. Bourns Bear I
E. A and C are correct.
  (4:280)

181. The respiratory therapy practitioner is asked to set up a Baby Bird ventilator to deliver the following parameters:

Flow rate	10 L/min
Respiratory rate	30

Inspiratory time	0.8 second
Pressure limit	25 cm H_2O
PEEP	6 cm H_2O
FIo_2	0.75

If, after placing the patient on the ventilator, the pressure limit is reached during the inspiratory phase, which of the following will occur?

A. The inspiratory phase will be terminated.
B. The preset volume will continue to be delivered to the patient.
C. A time window will open and the ventilator will become an assister for 3 seconds.
D. Gas flow to the patient will cease for the remainder of the inspiratory time.
E. An inspiratory positive pressure plateau will be held for the remainder of the inspiratory time.
(4:28)

182. A patient is receiving continuous ventilatory support via a Bourns Bear I ventilator. The tidal volume is 900 cc, the peak pressure is consistent at 50 cm H_2O, and the patient is on 8 cm H_2O PEEP. Which of the following alarm settings would be *most* appropriate for this patient?

	High Pressure Limit	Low Inspiratory Pressure	Low PEEP Alarm
A.	55 cm H_2O	35 cm H_2O	3 cm H_2O
B.	60 cm H_2O	45 cm H_2O	4 cm H_2O
C.	65 cm H_2O	35 cm H_2O	4 cm H_2O
D.	60 cm H_2O	25 cm H_2O	6 cm H_2O
E.	60 cm H_2O	35 cm H_2O	7 cm H_2O

(60)

Directions: Each group of questions below concerns a certain situation. In each case, first study the description of the situation, then choose the one best answer to each question following it and mark the answer accordingly.

Questions 183–185
A 70-year-old patient with longstanding chronic obstructive pulmonary disease and cor pulmonale is admitted to the respiratory intensive care unit. Historical data reveals progressive deterioration despite an aggressive home respiratory care program.

183. Twelve hours post admission, the physician decides to intubate and begin continuous ventilatory support. Which of the following formulas should the respiratory therapy practitioner use to help determine this patient's tidal volume?

A. 5 cc/kg
B. 15 cc/lb.
C. 10 cc/kg

    D. 18 cc/kg
    E. 20 cc/kg
    (67) (25:Chap 15, p 2)

184. Which of the following is *least* likely to contribute to difficulties in weaning the patient with chronic obstructive pulmonary disease from continuous ventilatory support?
    A. Ventilatory muscle discoordination
    B. Psychologic dependence
    C. Sleep deprivation
    D. Use of IMV
    E. Electrolyte disturbances
    (2:599–601 and 664–666) (1:483)

185. Because a prolonged course of continuous ventilatory support is anticipated, this patient is intubated with an endotracheal tube using a low pressure, high residual volume type cuff. Also anticipated are the following complications of prolonged tracheal intubation. Which is *least* preventable?
    A. Tracheal necrosis
    B. Bacterial contamination of the airways
    C. Tracheal dilatation
    D. Tracheal stenosis
    E. Cuff malfunction
    (1:241)

Questions 186–188
A 31-year-old patient is admitted to the respiratory intensive care unit for intensive respiratory therapy. Fourteen months ago he sustained neurologic and spinal cord damage while in the line of duty as a police officer. Weaned after 4 weeks of continuous ventilatory support, his pulmonary rehabilitation was slow. Vigorous respiratory and physical therapy were required to increase his pulmonary reserves. Five months ago he was sent home with a tracheostomy button in place. However, despite the suction port, loss of upper airway reflexes has resulted in a chronic aspiration problem. Two weeks prior to admission, he developed a low-grade fever and began coughing productively. Symptoms have gradually increased in severity. At the time of admission a diagnosis of pulmonary abscess was made.

186. True statements about a tracheal button airway include:
    I.   It may facilitate suctioning.
    II. It is a type of fenestrated tracheostomy tube.
    III. It may be used to maintain a patent tracheal stoma.
    IV. It can be used to administer continuous ventilatory support.
    V. When "plugged," it may allow the patient to talk.
        A. I, II, and IV
        B. II, IV, and V
        C. III, IV, and V
        D. I, II, IV, and V
        E. I, III, and V
    (1:279–280)

187. The hallmark of anaerobic lung abscess is:
    A. Massive air trapping
    B. Pink frothy sputum
    C. "Currant jelly" sputum
    D. Copious amounts of foul-smelling sputum
    E. Rusty sputum
        (11:69)

188. Which of the following is (are) known to complicate the clinical picture of the patient with lung abscess?
    I.   Empyema
    II.   Pneumothorax
    III. Centrilobular emphysema
        A. I and III
        B. I and II
        C. I, II, and III
        D. III only
        E. II only
        (11:73 and 189–191) (46)

Questions 189–191
A 52-year-old woman is brought to the emergency department in respiratory distress. She is 4 feet, 6 inches tall and weighs approximately 40 kg. She has had kyphoscoliosis since late adolescence but has only become symptomatic in the past decade or so. This is her third admission in as many years. Each one has been precipitated by a respiratory infection. At present, she is in the intensive care unit where she is receiving supportive care.

189. Pulmonary laboratory tests on a patient with kyphoscoliosis generally reveal:
    I.   Restrictive defect
    II.   Decreased vital capacity
    III. Increased RV/TLC%
    IV.   Decreased FRC
        A. I, III, and IV
        B. II only
        C. I, II, and IV
        D. I only
        E. II, III, and IV
        (11:195–196) (2:212)

190. True statements regarding kyphoscoliosis include:
    I.   It is defined as lateral and posterior curvature of the spine.
    II.   Its incidence is higher in females.
    III. Primary pulmonary pathosis involves thickening of the alveolar-capillary membrane.
    IV.   Definitive treatment consists of performing a laminectomy.
        A. III and IV
        B. I, II, and IV
        C. I and II
        D. I and III

E.   II and IV
   (11:195–196)

191. Mechanical ventilation in the patient with marked kyphoscoliosis:
   A.   Is contraindicated
   B.   May worsen V/Q relationships
   C.   Should always be used in conjunction with PEEP
   D.   May result in pressure-related side effects
   E.   B and D are correct.
   (1:328–329) (49)

Questions 192–194
A 51-year-old woman is admitted to the intensive care unit after falling
at home. Admission roentgenograms show a compound fracture of the
pelvis. Physical examination reveals an extremely obese woman with a
complaint of shortness of breath and easy fatigability. She is only 62
inches tall and weighs 228 kg. Gross observation also reveals large and
pendulous breasts. Neck veins are distended, her respiratory rate is 32,
her pulse is 110, and her blood pressure is 170/130. Arterial blood is
analyzed, revealing the following data:

FI_{O_2}	0.21
Pa_{O_2}	53 mm Hg
Pa_{CO_2}	59 mm Hg
pH	7.37
Base excess	+8.3 mEq/L
HCO_3^-	32.9 mEq/L
Hb concentration	21.6 g/dL

Based on this information and the patient's relevant history, a diagnosis
of Pickwickian syndrome is made.

192. Which of the following is the correct interpretation of this
   patient's arterial blood gas data?
   A.   Fully compensated respiratory acidosis
   B.   Partially compensated metabolic alkalosis
   C.   Fully compensated metabolic alkalosis
   D.   Fully compensated metabolic acidosis
   E.   Acute respiratory acidosis
   (5:Chaps 12 and 13) (33:283)

193. The patient's hemoglobin concentration most likely represents:
   A.   Erythrocytopenia
   B.   Primary polycythemia
   C.   Idiopathic thrombocytopenic purpura
   D.   Secondary polycythemia
   E.   Polycythemia vera
   (11:197)

194. One hour postoperatively, the patient is in the recovery room on a
   Bennett MA-I ventilator. Arterial blood gas and other data

obtained on an FI_{O_2} of 0.6 with the patient in the control mode are as follows:

Pa_{O_2}	43 mm Hg
Pa_{CO_2}	26 mm Hg
pH	7.42
Base excess	-6.3 mEq/L
V_T	1200 cc

Based on the foregoing information, which of the following would be the most appropriate modification in the ventilator settings?
- A. Increase the FI_{O_2} to 0.8, decrease the tidal volume, and place on 20 cm H_2O PEEP
- B. Increase the tidal volume and add 5 cm H_2O PEEP
- C. Place on 5 cm H_2O PEEP, increase the FI_{O_2} to 0.8, and decrease the tidal volume
- D. Place on 15 cm H_2O PEEP and place on IMV
- E. Increase the FI_{O_2} to 1.0 and decrease the tidal volume

(46) (49)

Questions 195–197
A 68-year-old patient with a history of chronic bronchitis is admitted to the respiratory intensive care unit. This admission was preceded by a respiratory infection that did not respond to her home respiratory care program.

195. Which two of the following pathogens are most likely responsible for this patient's pulmonary infection?
  - I.   *Pseudomonas*
  - II. *Hemophilus influenzae*
  - III. *Streptococcus pneumoniae*
  - IV. *Klebsiella*
  - V.   *Escherichia coli*
      - A. I and II
      - B. I and V
      - C. IV and V
      - D. III and IV
      - E. II and III

(11:93)

196. Which of the following correctly describes the clinical picture of a patient with chronic bronchitis?
  - I.   Cough and sputum production is a chief complaint.
  - II. V/Q mismatching often leads to hypoxemia.
  - III. Dyspnea is the chief complaint.
  - IV. Polycythemia is not uncommon.
      - A. I, III, and IV
      - B. IV only
      - C. I, II, and IV
      - D. II, III, and IV
      - E. III only

(11:90–92)

197. While in the emergency department, the patient is placed on 3 L oxygen via nasal cannula. Arterial blood is sampled and the following results reported:

Pa_{O_2}	63 mm Hg
Pa_{CO_2}	72 mm Hg
pH	7.37
HCO_3^-	38 mEq/L

Based on the above information, the most appropriate recommendation for the respiratory therapy practitioner to make at this time would be:
A. Place on 35% heated aerosol mask
B. Increase oxygen liter flow to 5 L/min
C. Decrease oxygen liter flow to 2 L/min
D. Intubate and place on continuous ventilatory support with an FI_{O_2} of 0.4
E. No change in therapy is indicated.
    (49) (5:179–183)

Questions 198–200
The respiratory therapy practitioner is evaluating a patient who has become severely distressed while receiving continuous ventilatory support via a Bennett MA-I ventilator. On entering the room, the therapist immediately notes that the ventilator's peak cycling pressure has dropped from 45 cm H_2O to 15 cm H_2O.

198. Based on the available information, which of the following may have been responsible for the situation?
    I.   Right mainstem intubation
    II.   Exhalation valve malfunction
    III. Endotracheal tube cuff herniation
    IV.   Endotracheal tube cuff rupture
    V.   Leak in ventilator circuit
        A. I, III, and IV
        B. II, III, and IV
        C. II, IV, and V   *Same*
        D. II, III, and IV
        E. I and IV
    (57) (32:210–217)

199. Chest physical assessment is performed while the patient is being ventilated with 100% oxygen via a manual resuscitator. Pertinent findings include good aeration bilaterally and no signs of tracheal shift or consolidation. In addition, the patient's cardiac rate has dropped from 160 to 100 and she no longer appears distressed. Based on the above information, which of the following actions should the therapist take at this time?
A. Continue to assess the patient until a physician arrives
B. Inflate the endotracheal tube cuff
C. Check the ventilator for malfunction

    D.   Retract the tube several centimeters

    E.   Place the patient back on the ventilator

    (32:209)

200. Which of the following properly functioning alarms might the therapist have selected to have prevented this patient's life-threatening distress?

    I.   Apnea

    II.   Low source gas pressure

    III.   Low inspiratory pressure

    IV.   Low FI_{O_2}

        A.   I, II, and IV

        B.   III only

        C.   I, II, and III

        D.   I and IV

        E.   I only

    (1:357)

Answer Key and NBRC Examination Matrix Categories

1. A, III H	41. C, II B	81. B, I E	121. D, I C	161. A, III F
2. D, II A	42. A, III D	82. C, III I	122. B, III C	162. C, II A
3. B, II A	43. C, I E	83. D, III E	123. C, III B	163. D, III E
4. D, III D	44. A, III H	84. B, II A	124. C, II A	164. C, II A
5. D, I E	45. E, III F	85. C, I B	125. C, I B	165. D, I A
6. B, III H	46. E, II A	86. D, III E	126. A, III G	166. D, II A
7. B, I D	47. B, III C	87. A, II B	127. B, III I	167. D, III E
8. A, III G	48. A, I C	88. A, III D	128. E, I B	168. C, II B
9. E, II A	49. A, III J	89. A, III J	129. C, III D	169. C, II A
10. A, III B	50. D, III K	90. E, I B	130. E, III F	170. B, I D
11. C, II A	51. D, II A	91. C, III C	131. C, III J	171. C, III J
12. E, III D	52. A, III H	92. D, II B	132. C, III D	172. E, III G
13. A, I D	53. C, III I	93. B, III J	133. B, II A	173. C, I C
14. E, II A	54. E, III K	94. C, I B	134. D, III H	174. D, II A
15. D, III F	55. D, II A	95. A, III C	135. B, II A	175. B, III I
16. B, III J	56. E, I B	96. B, I B	136. D, II A	176. A, III G
17. D, I B	57. E, II A	97. C, III B	137. C, II A	177. B, II A
18. B, III G	58. E, III H	98. B, III A	138. B, I C	178. E, I D
19. E, III H	59. D, III G	99. C, II A	139. A, II A	179. B, III C
20. D, III D	60. D, I D	100. C, III C	140. C, I A	180. E, II A
21. B, III I	61. B, III J	101. E, I E	141. E, III E	181. E, II A
22. C, II A	62. E, II A	102. E, III A	142. C, III D	182. C, III H
23. D, III F	63. E, I B	103. B, I A	143. A, I B	183. C, III E
24. E, II A	64. E, III G	104. A, I E	144. A, II A	184. D, III E
25. D, II A	65. D, I B	105. B, I B	145. B, I D	185. B, I E
26. C, III G	66. D, III G	106. C, I B	146. C, I A	186. E, II A
27. B, II A	67. D, III J	107. A, I A	147. A, I B	187. D, I E
28. C, III K	68. E, III F	108. E, III F	148. B, I A	188. B, I E
29. C, II B	69. E, I C	109. E, III I	149. E, II B	189. C, I D
30. B, III C	70. B, I A	110. B, III J	150. A, II A	190. C, I E
31. A, II B	71. D, III E	111. A, II A	151. A, I D	191. E, III E
32. A, II A	72. D, III C	112. C, II A	152. A, III D	192. A, I D
33. B, I D	73. B, II A	113. D, III F	153. E, III G	193. D, I A
34. C, III B	74. D, I E	114. D, I B	154. C, III I	194. C, III H
35. D, III A	75. A, I B	115. C, III J	155. C, I B	195. E, I E
36. E, II A	76. C, III F	116. E, II A	156. D, I D	196. C, I B
37. B, I A	77. E, III E	117. A, I D	157. C, III E	197. E, III I
38. D, III F	78. B, I E	118. E, II A	158. A, II B	198. C, III G
39. C, I C	79. E, I B	119. B, III J	159. A, I B	199. C, III H
40. E, III H	80. B, III F	120. D, II A	160. D, II A	200. B, II A

UNIT II

Advanced Practitioner Examination Posttest

The following full-length Advanced Practitioner Examination posttest was constructed according to specifications outlined in the current NBRC Composite Examination Matrix (see reference 80). The examination categories and the number of questions allotted to each by the NBRC are listed in the table below. In addition, *the answer key at the end of this test is referenced to the examination matrix so the candidate may further identify his or her weak areas.* For a more thorough discussion of the NBRC Composite Examination Matrix, please refer to the Introduction of this book and to the Examination Category Review and Pretest.

Table 2. Advanced Practitioner Examination Content Matrix.

Examination Category	Number of Questions	Percentage of Questions
I. Clinical Data	25	25
A. Review patient records	10	10
B. Collect and evaluate clinical information	5	5
C. Perform and evaluate laboratory procedures	10	10
II. Equipment	10	10
A. Select, assemble, check, and correct malfunctions of equipment	6	6
B. Ensure cleanliness of equipment	1	1
C. Perform quality control and calibration procedures	3	3
III. Therapeutic Procedures	65	65
A. Maintain airway	3	3
B. Ensure ventilation	7	7
C. Ensure oxygenation	3	3
D. Assess patient response to therapy	20	20
E. Modify therapy	7	7
F. Recommend modifications in therapy	22	22
G. Assist physician with special procedures	3	3

Examination for Advanced Level Respiratory Therapy Practitioners

Time: 2 Hours

Directions: Each of the questions or incomplete statements below is followed by five suggested answers. Select the one that is best in each case and then mark accordingly.

1. A 79-year-old patient is seen in the intensive care unit while receiving continuous ventilatory support with an FIO_2 of 0.6 and 10 cm H_2O PEEP. The following data are noted at this time:

Pa_{O_2}	58 mm Hg
Pa_{CO_2}	42 mm Hg
pH	7.35
HCO_3^-	23 mEq/L
Colloidal osmotic pressure	14 mm Hg
Total serum proteins	3.0 g/dL
Na^+	140 mEq/L
Cl^-	103 mEq/L
K^+	5.0 mEq/L

The physician decides fluid administration is indicated. Which of the following should the therapist recommend?
A. 5% dextrose in H_2O
B. 5% albumin in H_2O
C. 0.45% NaCl
D. 40 mEq KCl in 100 mL D_5W
E. Lactated Ringer's solution
   (42) (1:436–437)

2. After breathing 100% oxygen for 15 minutes, which of the following patients would be *least* likely to have had all the nitrogen washed out of his lungs?
    A. An asthmatic patient in remission
    B. A patient in congestive heart failure
    C. A patient with normal lungs
    D. A patient with advanced stage emphysema
    E. A patient with alveolar proteinosis
    (16:12)

3. Following thoracocentesis, approximately 500 mL of a thick, milky-white fluid is drained from the pleural space. This fluid most likely represents a:
    A. Pleural transudate
    B. Chylothorax
    C. Hemothorax
    D. Empyema
    E. A and B are correct.
    (11:187–189)

4. Pulmonary function studies on a 60-year-old patient reveal an FEF_{25-75} of 0.3 L/min. Which of the following statements best describes this patient's pulmonary status?
    A. Mild restrictive lung disease exists.
    B. Mixed obstructive and restrictive lung disease exists.
    C. Mild obstructive disease exists.
    D. Severe obstructive disease exists.
    E. Severe restrictive lung disease exists.
    (16:33)

5. Following orthopaedic surgery, a 65-kg, 82-year-old woman develops respiratory failure. She is placed on a Bennett 7200 ventilator immediately after which depression in the arterial blood pressure is noted to occur. The following findings are charted at this time with the patient in the assist mode:

Respiratory rate	32/min
Tidal volume	900 mL
Peak flow rate	55 L/min
Peak pressure	48 cm H_2O

    The *least* appropriate therapeutic modification for the therapist to make at this time would be to:
    A. Recommend appropriate sedation
    B. Recommend fluid administration
    C. Decrease the tidal volume
    D. Decrease the flow rate
    E. Place the patient on SIMV
    (1:337–338) (6:182) (72)

6. Which of the following agents should the respiratory therapy practitioner recommend for sterilizing equipment used by a patient

who was being treated for a pulmonary infection caused by the microorganism *Mycobacterium tuberculosis?*
I. Glutaraldehyde solutions
II. Alcohols
III. Ethylene oxide
IV. Autoclaving
    A. I and III
    B. I, II, III, and IV
    C. I, II, and IV
    D. I, II, and III
    E. I, III, and IV
  (2:418–422)

7. The respiratory therapy practitioner is monitoring a 1250-g (30-week gestation) newborn in the neonatal intensive care unit who is receiving 70% oxygen via hood. The following information is charted at this time:

Pa_{O_2}	40 mm Hg
Pa_{CO_2}	36 mm Hg
pH	7.30
Respiratory rate	85
Appearance	Peripheral cyanosis noted
Heart rate	210/min

Which of the following would be the most correct recommendation for the therapist to make regarding the above information?
A. Initiate continuous ventilatory support with 4 cm H_2O PEEP and an FI_{O_2} of 0.5
B. Place on 15 cm H_2O CPAP with an FI_{O_2} of 1.0
C. Place on 4 cm H_2O CPAP with an FI_{O_2} of 0.8
D. Place on 100% oxygen via hood
E. Initiate continuous ventilatory support with 10 cm H_2O PEEP and an FI_{O_2} of 1.0
  (29:210–220)

8. A 54-year-old woman with a history of bronchiectasis dating back to her adolescence is brought to the hospital by paramedics. The patient is cyanotic and her respirations are labored, but she does not complain of dyspnea. Admission blood gases on 2 L oxygen via cannula are as follows:

Pa_{O_2}	45 mm Hg
Pa_{CO_2}	72 mm Hg
pH	7.36
HCO_3^-	38.7 mEq/L

Based on these data, the most appropriate modification in this patient's therapy would be to:
A. Intubate the patient and place on SIMV with an FI_{O_2} of 0.4
B. Decrease liter flow to 1 L/min

    C.   Intubate the patient and administer 40% oxygen via heated aerosol

    D.   Increase liter flow to 3 L/min

    E.   Make no modification at this time

    (49) (32:94–95) (50:180–183) (11:231–232) (63:102–121)

9.   Which of the following devices use(s) transducers as part of normal function and operation?

    I.   Fleisch pneumotachometer

    II.   Siemens Servo 900 C

    III. Pulmonary artery catheter

    IV. Heat transfer pneumotachometer

    A.   I and III

    B.   III only

    C.   I, II, III, and IV

    D.   II, III, and IV

    E.   I, II, and III

    (4:209–210) (16:114–115) (5:228–230)

10. An 80-kg, 30-year-old patient with flail chest and bilateral lung contusion is pharmacologically paralyzed and placed on a Bourns Bear II ventilator in the control mode with a tidal volume of 700 mL. Arterial blood gases drawn on an FIo_2 of 0.6 yield the following data:

Pao_2	40 mm Hg
$Paco_2$	23 mm Hg
pH	7.52
HCO_3^-	16 mEq/L
Base excess	−4 mEq/L

Which of the following therapeutic modifications should the respiratory therapy practitioner make at this time?

    A.   Place the patient on IMV mode and increase the FIo_2 to 0.8

    B.   Decrease the tidal volume, add 250 cc mechanical deadspace and 5 cm H_2O PEEP

    C.   Add 400 cc mechanical deadspace and increase the FIo_2 to 1.0

    D.   Decrease the respiratory rate and add 5 cm H_2O PEEP

    E.   Decrease the tidal volume and add 15 cm H_2O PEEP

    (1:349–352) (46)

11. A 2-point calibration of the Severinghaus Pco_2 electrode is most frequently performed using which of the following analyzed gas mixtures?

    A.   5% CO_2 and 80% CO_2

    B.   0% CO_2 and 10% CO_2

    C.   5% CO_2 and 20% CO_2

    D.   5% CO_2 and 10% CO_2

    E.   12% CO_2 and 20% CO_2

    (5:35)

12. Which of the following causes of hypoxemia is (are) believed to always be accompanied by an abnormal $P(A-a)o_2$ when the patient is breathing room air?
   I.   Shunting
   II. Low V/Q
   III. Hypoventilation
   IV. Diffusion defect
       A. I and IV
       B. II, III, and IV
       C. I, II, and IV
       D. IV only
       E. I, II, and III
   (2:193–194) (5:189–190)

13. Which of the following is *not* a recognized hazard of the use of negative pressure tank type ventilators (iron lung)?
   A. Venous pooling
   B. Patient inaccessibility
   C. Lack of patient assisting capability
   D. Airway patency not ensured
   E. Necrosis of tracheal mucosa
   (4:230–233)

14. Eight days post hepatic resection, the following blood gas and acid-base data are obtained on an alert patient who is on a Servo 900 C ventilator in the assist/control mode with 10 cm H_2O PEEP:

Pao_2	183 mm Hg
$Paco_2$	26 mm Hg
pH	7.59
HCO_3^-	24 mEq/L
Base excess	+4.0 mEq/L
FIo_2	0.7

   Which of the following would be the most acceptable modification of this patient's mechanical ventilatory therapy?
   A. Decrease the PEEP and place on SIMV
   B. Decrease the FIo_2 and add 300 cc mechanical deadspace
   C. Decrease the PEEP and decrease the minute volume
   D. Decrease the FIo_2 and pharmacologically paralyze the patient
   E. Decrease the FIo_2 and place on SIMV
   (46) (49)

15. Pulmonary function tests performed on a patient with pulmonary fibrosis would most likely reveal all of the following *except:*
   A. Decreased D_Lco
   B. Normal $\dfrac{FEV_1}{FVC}\%$
   C. Normal ERV

D.   Decreased TLC
E.   Decreased RV
(2:212)

16. Which of the following types of hypoxia is most frequently associated with elevations in mixed venous oxygen tensions? $\uparrow\uparrow \bar{v}O_2$
A.   Hypoxemic
B.   Anemic
C.   Circulatory
D.   Histotoxic
E.   A and C are correct.
(2:241)

17. Cough fractures are sometimes noted when viewing chest roentgenograms of patients with chronic obstructive pulmonary disease. These are known to involve which of the following ribs most frequently?
A.   First and second
B.   Second only
C.   Third and fourth
D.   Sixth through ninth
E.   Ninth through twelfth
(3:313)

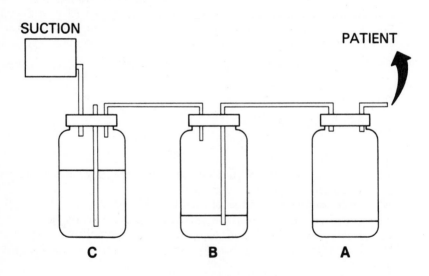

Figure 11.

18. Which of the following statements regarding three-chamber chest suction systems such as that pictured above is (are) true?
   I.   Constant bubbling in the suction control bottle indicates evacuation of air from the pleural space.
   II. The tube should be placed 15 cm to 20 cm below the surface in the water-seal chamber.

III.   The tube in the suction control bottle should be placed approximately 2 cm below the surface of the water.
IV.   Bottle *B* is the water-seal chamber.
    A.   I only
    B.   II and IV
    C.   III and IV
    D.   I and III
    E.   IV only
(7:351–357)

19. The respiratory therapy practitioner is monitoring a critically ill patient who has just received 12 units of stored ACD blood. Results of blood gas analysis are reported and show that the patient's P_{50} has dropped from 27 mm Hg to 20 mm Hg. Which of the following statements regarding this situation is (are) true?
I.   The patient's oxyhemoglobin dissociation curve has shifted to the left.
II.   The amount of oxygen available to the tissues has increased.
III.   2–3 DPG deficient blood may be responsible.
    A.   I only
    B.   I and III
    C.   II only
    D.   I and II
    E.   I, II, and III
(2:237–240)

20. Which of the following chest radiologic findings may be considered evidence of the presence of congestive heart failure?
I.   Cardiothoracic ratio less than 50%
II.   Presence of increased radiolucency
III.   Presence of Kerley-B lines
IV.   Evidence of mediastinal shift
    A.   I and III
    B.   III only
    C.   III and IV
    D.   I and IV
    E.   II and IV
(3:309–334)

21. All of the following are known complications of tracheotomy. Which are most frequently associated with a low tracheostomy incision?
I.   Tracheal stenosis
II.   Brachiocephalic (innominate artery) incision
III.   Vocal cord damage
IV.   Pneumothorax
    A.   I and III
    B.   II and III
    C.   II and IV
    D.   III and IV
    E.   I + IV

E.   I and IV
(36:91)

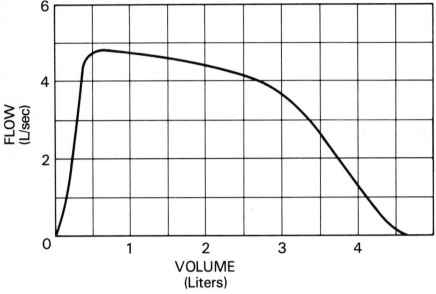

Figure 12.

22.   The preceding flow-volume loop was obtained from a 48-year-old, 62-kg patient. The best interpretation of this loop would be:
A.   Mild restrictive lung disease
B.   Severe chronic obstructive lung disease
C.   Combined obstructive-restrictive pulmonary disease
D.   Severe restrictive pulmonary disease
E.   Large airway obstruction
(2:221)

23.   The respiratory therapy practitioner is monitoring a patient who is receiving continuous ventilatory support. Pertinent data are listed below:

Time	9:00 AM	10:00 AM
PEEP	8 cm H_2O	12 cm H_2O
Peak pressure	38 cm H_2O	55 cm H_2O
Plateau pressure	31 cm H_2O	48 cm H_2O
Tidal volume	930 mL	980 mL
Inspiratory flow rate	0.67 L/sec	40 L/min

Which of the following assessments is (are) true regarding the above information?
I.   There is an increase in pulmonary elastance.
II.   There is an increase in effective static compliance.
III.   The airway resistance is unchanged.
IV.   The patient probably needs to be suctioned.

A. I and III
B. II and III
C. I and IV
D. II and IV
E. II only
(19:Chap 4) (34:122–126) (50)

24. Eight days after being placed on continuous mechanical ventilation, a patient who inhaled toxic gas in an industrial accident displays the following clinical data:

FIo_2	0.4
PEEP	15 cm H_2O
Pao_2	130 mm Hg
$Paco_2$	34 mm Hg
Ventilator mode	Assist/control

What ventilator change(s) should the respiratory therapist recommend at this time?
A. Decrease the PEEP to 10 cm H_2O
B. Decrease the PEEP to 5 cm H_2O and reduce the FIo_2 to 0.3
C. Decrease the FIo_2 to 0.35 and place on IMV
D. Add 100 cc mechanical deadspace and lower the FIo_2 to 0.3
E. Place the patient in the control mode and discontinue PEEP therapy
(46) (38:Chaps 4 through 6)

25. Following thoracotomy and chest tube placement, approximately 800 cc of a thick, yellowish liquid is drained. This fluid most likely represents:
A. Pleurisy
B. A pleural transudate
C. An empyema
D. Chylothorax
E. Hemothorax
(11:187–189)

26. An 1850-g newborn is seen in the nursery 4 hours post partum. The infant is evaluated by the respiratory therapy practitioner at this time and the following information is charted:

Pulse	185
Respiratory rate	78/min
Muscle tone	Good
Expiratory grunting	Audible with stethoscope
FIo_2	0.35

Based on the above information, which of the following is the most correct recommendation for the respiratory therapy practitioner to make at this time?
A. Increase FIo_2 to 0.5
B. Perform arterial blood gas analysis stat

    C. Place on 5 cm H_2O nasal CPAP
    D. Intubate and place on 5 cm H_2O CPAP
    E. Intubate and place on 5 cm H_2O PEEP
     (13:78–81) (29:179)

27. The quantity of oxygen being delivered to the peripheral tissue beds per minute can be calculated from which of the following formulas?

    A. $\dfrac{(Q_T)}{C(a\text{-}\bar{v})o_2}$

    B. $(Q_T)(Cao_2)$
    C. $(Q_T)(Pao_2)$
    D. $(Q_T) \times [C(a\text{-}\bar{v})o_2]$
    E. $(Vo_2) \div \dfrac{Q_T}{C(a\text{-}\bar{v})o_2}$

     (47)

28. In reviewing a patient's chart prior to performing pulmonary drainage techniques, the respiratory therapy practitioner notes that the patient's intracranial pressure is 10 mm Hg. This finding is most consistent with:
    A. Intracranial hypertension
    B. Normal intracranial pressure
    C. Cerebral anoxia
    D. Cerebral infarction
    E. Decreased cerebral perfusion pressure
     (25:Chap 15, p 13) (23)

29. A patient is seen in the intensive care unit following the development of severe oxygenation failure. He is currently on a Servo 900 C ventilator with an FIo_2 of 0.8 and 18 cm H_2O PEEP. A radiologic diagnosis of pulmonary edema is made. Pertinent data are as follows:

Pao_2	53 mm Hg
$S\bar{v}o_2$	45%
PWP	39 mm Hg
Oxygen consumption	250 mL/min
Serum albumin	5.0 g/dL
$C(a\text{-}\bar{v})o_2$	7.7 vol%
Total serum proteins	8.0 g/dL
Colloidal osmotic pressure	25 mm Hg

Based on the above information, the respiratory therapy practitioner can assess that the most probable cause of this patient's pulmonary edema is:
    A. Left ventricular failure
    B. Hypervolemia
    C. Hypoproteinemia
    D. Right ventricular failure

E.   Adult respiratory distress syndrome
(41) (42) (25:Chap 15, p 17) (1:Chaps 26 through 30)
(32:Chap 5) (5:Chap 20)

30. The respiratory care practitioner is asked to help set up a home
care program for a 74-year-old woman with advanced chronic
obstructive pulmonary disease. Which of the following daily activ-
ities could the therapist recommend to help this patient rebuild
her cardiopulmonary reserves?
  I.   Gardening
  II.   Sewing
  III. Walking
  IV.   Racquetball
  V.   Driving an automobile
  VI.   Household chores
      A.   I and II
      B.   I, II, III, V, and VI
      C.   I, III, and VI
      D.   II, III, IV, V, and VI
      E.   III only
    (2:688–691)

31. Which of the following patients have demonstrated an increased
incidence of gastrointestinal complications during continuous ven-
tilatory support?
  I.   Those receiving systemic corticosteroid therapy
  II.   Those with preexisting gastrointestinal disorders
  III. Those receiving prophylactic antacid therapy
      A.   II only
      B.   I and II
      C.   II and III
      D.   III only
      E.   I and III
    (1:388–389) (7:168–169)

32. A 45-year-old patient is seen in the intensive care unit by a respi-
ratory care practitioner. The patient's pulmonary wedge pressure
is 30 mm Hg. To determine whether left ventricular dysfunction
or hypervolemia is responsible for this abnormality, which of the
following should be measured?
  A. Q_T (cardiac output)
  B.   Pulmonary vascular resistance
  C. Pa_{O_2}
  D.   Effective static compliance
  E.   CVP
    (41) (25:Chap 15, p 17)

33. In reviewing a patient's chart prior to administering IPPB, the
respiratory therapy practitioner notes that the patient's "normal"
electrocardiogram is one of atrial fibrillation. While taking this
patient's pulse, the therapist will most likely note its:
  A.   Regularity

B.   Rapidity
C.   Strength
D.   Irregularity
E.   Absence
(25:Chap 6, p 14)

34. Which of the following would the respiratory therapy practitioner recommend as criteria for initiation of continuous ventilatory support in the newborn?
  I.   Hypoxemia on 60% oxygen and 2 cm H_2O CPAP
  II.   Hypoxemia on 60% oxygen via hood
  III. Hypoxemia on 100% oxygen and 12 cm H_2O CPAP
  IV. Pa_{CO_2} of 70 mm Hg on 30% oxygen
        A.   II and III
        B.   I and II
        C.   I and IV
        D.   I and III
        E.   III and IV
  (29:206 and 210)

35. Which of the following statements about the procedure of neonatal intubation is (are) true?
  I.   A curved laryngoscope blade is invariably preferred.
  II.   When a straight laryngoscope blade is used, the tip may be placed in the vallecula.
  III. Hyperextension of the head and neck should be avoided.
  IV.   The No. 2 laryngoscope blade is preferred for preterm newborns.
        A.   II only
        B.   II and III
        C.   II, III, and IV
        D.   I and IV
        E.   I and II
  (25:Chap 16, pp 4-6) (29:213-215)

36. True statements regarding pulmonary hypertension include:
  I.   It is defined as an abnormally high pulmonary wedge pressure.
  II.   It is generally believed to exist whenever the pressures in the pulmonary circuit (systolic/diastolic) rise above 35/15 (mm Hg).
  III. It is usually caused by right ventricular failure.
  IV.   It may be caused by increases in pulmonary vascular resistance.
        A.   I and IV
        B.   II and IV
        C.   II, III, and IV
        D.   I and III
        E.   I, II, and III
  (11:182-183)

37. In reading a patient's chart prior to therapy, the respiratory care practitioner notes that the patient's white blood cell count is 2000/ μL. This value is most consistent with:
   A. Leukocytosis
   B. Normal value
   C. Leukocytopenia
   D. Nosocomial infection
   E. Extrinsic asthma
      (7:392)

38. Venous return is believed to be impaired shortly after initiation of continuous ventilatory support on a 20-year-old man. The patient was admitted following hemorrhage sustained in a motorcycle accident. Which of the following should the respiratory therapist recommend to help lessen the severity of this side effect?
   I. Chronotropic stimulation
   II. Administration of propranolol
   III. Intravascular volume expansion
   IV. Administration of morphine
      A. III only
      B. II only
      C. II and IV
      D. II, III, and IV
      E. III and IV
      (1:Chap 27, pp 395–396 and 415) (2:600–603)

39. Which of the following is *not* associated with the formation of subcutaneous emphysema?
   A. Peripheral venipuncture
   B. Positive pressure ventilation
   C. Tracheotomy
   D. Traumatic intubation
   E. Central venipuncture
      (2:576) (1:281–286 and 386–387)

40. An unconscious patient is noted to become agitated, diaphoretic, and dusky while receiving continuous ventilatory support. Pertinent findings include the appearance of bibasal rales, an increase in the ventilator plateau pressure from 35 cm H_2O to 48 cm H_2O, and an increase in the PWP from 10 mm Hg to 38 mm Hg. Based on the above information, the most likely cause of this patient's distress is:
   A. Acute pulmonary embolus
   B. Cardiogenic pulmonary edema
   C. Upper airway secretions
   D. Intestinal rupture
   E. Adult respiratory distress syndrome
      (33:204) (32:215) (34:122–126)

41. Results of a single breath diffusion study reveal a D_{LCO} of 5 mL/ min/mm Hg. This value is most consistent with:
   A. Normal study
   B. Increased diffusion capacity

C. Decreased diffusion capacity
D. Small airways disease
E. Bronchiectasis
    (16:71) (2:705)

42. The physician asks the respiratory therapy practitioner to help evaluate the following pulmonary function data obtained on a 53-year-old patient with pneumonia who is in need of bronchial hygiene therapy:

	Before Bronchodilator	After Bronchodilator
FVC	2.43 L	2.48 L
$FEF_{200-1200}$	64% of normal	62% of normal
FEV_1	53%	55%
FEF_{25-75}	40%	43%

Based on the above information, which of the following should the therapist recommend?
A. IPPB four times a day with 0.5 cc metaproterenol
B. Aerosol therapy followed by postural drainage and percussion four times a day
C. 0.5 cc isoetharine four times a day via hand-held nebulizer
D. Breathing retraining every day
E. Incentive spirometry every hour while awake
    (16:94) (13:278–280)

43. Pharmacologic paralysis and sedation would most likely be recommended when continuous ventilatory support is required in the management of:
A. Guillain-Barré syndrome
B. Advanced stage emphysema
C. Narcotic overdose
D. Status asthmaticus
E. Myasthenia gravis
    (1:506)

44. A patient is seen in the intensive care unit. He is on a volume ventilator and is receiving an FIo_2 of 0.6 along with 12 cm H_2O PEEP. A diagnosis of pulmonary edema is made following review of clinical and radiologic data. Additional pertinent information is posted below:

Pao_2	44 mm Hg
$P\bar{v}o_2$	28 mm Hg
PWP	29 mm Hg
Oxygen consumption	250 mL/min
$C(a-\bar{v})o_2$	2.7 vol%
Colloidal osmotic pressure	25 mm Hg
Total proteins	8.0 g/dL

Based on the above information, the respiratory therapy practi-
tioner should assess that the most probable cause of this patient's
pulmonary edema is:
A. Adult respiratory distress syndrome
B. Right ventricular failure
C. Left ventricular failure
D. Hypervolemia
E. Hypoproteinemia
   (41) (42) (25:Chap 15, p 17) (1:Chap 25 through 30)
   (32:Chap 5) (5:Chap 20)

45. Which one of the following is *most* likely to be abnormal in a 45-
    year-old man who is free of cardiopulmonary symptoms but has
    smoked one pack of cigarettes daily for 20 years?
    A. FEF_{25-75}
    B. $FEF_{200-1200}$
    C. FEV_1
    D. Airway resistance (R_{AW})
    E. $\dfrac{FEV_1}{FVC}\%$
       (2:211)

46. A severely dyspneic and diaphoretic patient is seen in the emer-
    gency department. Following administration of edrophonium
    (Tensilon), a profound decrease in the patient's vital capacity is
    noted. Which of the following recommendations should the respi-
    ratory therapy practitioner make at this time?
    A. Administer 100% oxygen via nonrebreathing mask
    B. Obtain an arterial sample stat
    C. Administer succinylcholine stat
    D. Establish an airway and support ventilation
    E. Administer a second, larger dose of edrophonium stat
       (11:204) (2:761)

47. Which of the following are true statements regarding laryngo-
    scope devices?
    I.   The No. 0 and No. 1 blades are designed for neonatal use.
    II.   They are designed to be inserted in the right side of the
          mouth.
    III. The tip of the adult straight laryngoscope blade is designed
          to be placed under the epiglottis.
    IV.   Laryngoscopes with both adult and pediatric size handles
          are available.
          A. I, III, and IV
          B. II, III, and IV
          C. I and II
          D. I, II, III, and IV
          E. II and III
       (1:240–245) (25:Chap 4)

48. An 18-year-old woman is seen in the emergency department. She
    is deeply comatose and there are needle tracks on her arms.

Results of arterial blood gas analysis on room air are as follows:

Pa_{O_2}	45 mm Hg
Pa_{CO_2}	80 mm Hg
pH	7.10
Base excess	-6.3 mEq/L
HCO_3^-	22 mEq/L

Which of the following assessments is (are) true regarding this patient's status?
  I.   Low V/Q is responsible for the hypoxemia.
  II. The $P(A-a)_{O_2}$ is within normal limits. $69.73 - 45 = 24.73$
  III. The hypoxemia is due to hypoventilation.
  IV. Oxygen therapy would not be of benefit.
    A. I, III, and IV
    B. III only
    C. II and III
    D. II, III, and IV
    E. I and IV
  (2:394–395) (32:63–65) (5:Chaps 8 and 11)

49. The respiratory therapy practitioner is monitoring a hemodynamically stable 70-kg patient who is receiving controlled mechanical ventilation with a rate of 14 and a tidal volume of 700 mL. If the patient's tidal volume were increased to 1200 mL with other settings unchanged, which of the following would be most likely to occur?
  I.   An increase in alveolar ventilation
  II. A decrease in physiologic deadspace
  III. A decrease in Pa_{CO_2}
    A. I and III
    B. III only
    C. II only
    D. II and III
    E. I, II, and III
  (31:14–16)

50. An intern asks the respiratory therapy practitioner to help evaluate the following pulmonary function data obtained on a 64-year-old woman:

Weight	80 kg
FVC	3.6 L
$\dfrac{FEV_1}{FVC}\%$	48%
FEF_{25-75}	32% of normal
Slow vital capacity	2.1 L

The therapist's recommendation regarding the above data is:
A. Order a before and after bronchodilator test
B. Repeat study!

C. Intubate the patient and place on SIMV
D. Recommend that a home care program be set up
E. Obtain an arterial sample and a chest roentgenogram to confirm spirometric data
    (16:1 and 27) (2:211)

51. Transcutaneous oxygen monitoring devices use which of the following principles?
    I.   Polarographic principle
    II. Paramagnetism of oxygen
    III. Use of heat to "arterialize" capillary blood
    IV. Solubility and diffusibility of oxygen
         A. I and III
         B. II and IV
         C. I, III, and IV
         D. I, II, and III
         E. III and IV
    (5:39)

52. Large increases in intrathoracic pressure following initiation of positive pressure ventilation may typically result in:
    I.   Increased intracranial pressure
    II. Decreases in central venous pressure
    III. Reductions in venous return
    IV. Decreases in intrapleural pressure
         A. I and IV
         B. II and IV
         C. I and III
         D. I, II, and III
         E. II, III, and IV
    (1:321 and 328–329)

53. Which of the following statements about the clinical usage of Apgar scoring is (are) true?
    I.   The 5-minute score is generally lower than that at 1 minute.
    II. The last vital sign to deteriorate is the heart rate.
    III. A score of 0–3 represents severe asphyxia.
    IV. This system assesses the newborn's chances of having neurologic abnormalities.
         A. II and III
         B. I, II, and IV
         C. II and IV
         D. III only
         E. III and IV
    (13:51–55) (29:Chap 2)

54. An 18-year-old is seen in the emergency department following a near-drowning incident. The following data are charted at this time:

Pa_{O_2}	38 mm Hg
FI_{O_2}	10 L O_2 via simple oxygen mask
Pa_{CO_2}	28 mm Hg

pH	7.34
HCO_3^-	12 mEq/L
BP	170/110
Pulse	130
Appearance	Profound cyanosis noted

Which of the following assessments are true regarding this patient's presentation?

I.   Severe anemia is most likely responsible for the cyanosis.
II. PEEP or CPAP may be beneficial.
III. Refractory hypoxemia exists.
IV. Tachycardia and arterial hypotension exist.
   A.   IV only
   B.   II, III, and IV
   C.   II and IV
   D.   I and IV
   E.   II and III
   (30:128–129) (2:394–395) (50) (38:38–60)

55. In reading a patient's chart, the respiratory therapy practitioner notes that the patient's pulmonary wedge pressures are consistently in the range of 3 mm Hg to 4 mm Hg. These data are most consistent with:
   A.   Normal study
   B.   Left ventricular failure
   C.   Adult respiratory distress syndrome
   D.   Hypovolemia
   E.   Increased pulmonary vascular resistance
   (1:409)

56. The following pulmonary function data were obtained from a 61-year-old man as part of a routine preoperative screening program:

Test	Predicted	Observed
FVC	4.1 L	4.0 L
$\frac{FEV_1}{FVC}\%$	75%	70%
MEFR	8.1 L/sec	8.2 L/sec
FEF_{25-75}	3.4 L/sec	1.9 L/sec
Slow vital capacity	4.2 L	4.2 L

Which of the following is the most correct interpretation of the above data?
   A.   Moderate obstructive defect
   B.   Normal study
   C.   Small airways disease
   D.   Restrictive defect
   E.   Poor patient effort
   (20:197)

57. Intensive therapy is in progress for a 7-year-old boy who was admitted in severe status asthmaticus. The patient is receiving intravenous aminophylline, methylprednisolone, and isoproterenol. In addition, metaproterenol is being administered every 3 hours via unpressurized nebulizer. Current blood gas results with the patient receiving 4 L oxygen via simple oxygen mask are as follows:

pH	7.20
Pa_{O_2}	67 mm Hg
Pa_{CO_2}	43 mm Hg
HCO_3^-	16.6 mEq/L
Base excess	−8.9 mEq/L

The physician does not want to begin mechanical ventilation and asks for a recommendation. At this time, the practitioner should suggest which of the following?
A. Increasing the dosage of metaproterenol
B. Discontinuing the intravenously administered aminophylline
C. Correcting base deficit to enhance bronchodilator effectiveness
D. Administering a continuous ultrasonic aerosol
E. Postural drainage and percussion prior to metaproterenol administration
(23:168; Chap 8)

58. In reading the chart of a patient who is being treated for a pulmonary embolus, the respiratory therapy practitioner would be *least* likely to note documentation of which of the following signs and symptoms?
A. Dyspnea
B. Chest pain
C. Increased pulmonary wedge pressure
D. Hemoptysis
E. Neck vein distention
(11:180) (5:190–191)

59. A patient receiving continuous ventilatory support becomes distressed and exhibits diminished air entry over the left lung field. Other physical findings are nonspecific. Differential diagnosis can usually be accomplished rapidly by which of the following therapeutic modifications?
A. Advancing the endotracheal tube slightly
B. Stat chest roentgenogram
C. Inserting a 19-gauge needle into the chest wall
D. Arterial blood gas analysis
E. Retracting the endotracheal tube slightly
(29:222) (32:211)

60. A 63-year-old woman is in the intensive care unit on a volume ventilator. Because of severe hypoxemia, it is decided to add

PEEP in 5 cm H_2O increments. In so doing the following data were obtained:

	PEEP		
Parameter	5 cm H_2O	10 cm H_2O	15 cm H_2O
Temperature	38.1°C	38.1°C	38.1°C
Pa_{O_2}	51 mm Hg	73 mm Hg	82 mm Hg
Q_S/Q_T	24%	21%	18%
Q_T	6.2 L/min	6.5 L/min	5.1 L/min
$C(a-\bar{v})_{O_2}$	4.3 vol%	3.9 vol%	5.3 vol%
$S\bar{v}_{O_2}$	48%	53%	48%
Static effective compliance	20 cc/cm H_2O	25 cc/cm H_2O	20 cc/cm H_2O
FI_{O_2}	1.0	1.0	1.0
PWP (on ventilator)	8	9	12
Hb	12.3 g/dL	12.3 g/dL	12.3 g/dL

Which of the following assessments is (are) true regarding the above situation?

ARDS

I. Some cardiovascular depression is noted at 15 cm H_2O PEEP.
II. The increase in PWP indicates the presence of adult respiratory distress syndrome.
III. The Sv_{O_2} decreased at 15 cm H_2O PEEP because the Ca_{O_2} decreased.
IV. Tissue oxygenation is best at 10 cm H_2O PEEP.
  A. II, III, and IV
  B. I and IV
  C. I, II, III, and IV
  D. IV only
  E. I and II
  (46) (47) (25:Chap 15, p 17) (1:Chap 30)

61. In reading the chart of a patient who was admitted with advanced chronic bronchitis, the respiratory therapy practitioner would expect to see documentation of all of the following *except:*
  A. Cor pulmonale
  B. Cough and sputum production
  C. Cyanosis
  D. Pulmonary hypotension
  E. Clubbing of the digits
  (11:182–184) (2:705)

62. A 19-year-old patient with adult respiratory distress syndrome is receiving 8 cm H_2O PEEP with an FI_{O_2} of 0.7. Because of severe hypoxemia, the decision is made to increase the level of PEEP to 12 cm H_2O. The following data are collected at this time:

	8 cm H_2O PEEP	12 cm H_2O PEEP
$P(A-a)_{O_2}$	400 mm Hg	400 mm Hg
Sa_{O_2}	75%	75%
$S\bar{v}_{O_2}$	55%	47%
PWP (measured		
on ventilator)	7 mm Hg	8 mm Hg
Hb	15 g/dL	15 g/dL

The physician decides to leave the PEEP at 12 cm H_2O and asks the advanced respiratory care practitioner to recommend treatment for the decreased central venous oxygen content. The most appropriate response would be:

A.   Increase cardiac output
B.   Increase FI_{O_2}
C.   Decrease inspiratory flow rate
D.   Induce hypothermia
E.   Vigorous diuresis
   (65) (41) (46) (38:Chaps 4 through 6, p 63) (32:64–66 and 116–119)

63. A patient on a volume ventilator is noted to have both his peak and plateau pressures increase by 14 cm H_2O. Which of the following might have been responsible for this?
   I.   Atelectasis
   II.   Pneumothorax
   III. Bronchospasm
   IV.   Acute gastric distention
   V.   Herniation of the endotracheal tube cuff
       A.   I, II, and III
       B.   I, III, and IV
       C.   III and V
       D.   I, II, and IV
       E.   II and III
   (50) (34:122–126) (32:211)

64. The respiratory therapist is asked to collect appropriate weaning data on a comatose 20-year-old man who has a tracheostomy tube in place. The patient has been receiving continuous ventilatory support for the past 13 days following multisystem trauma sustained in a gang-related incident. He is currently on a Bennett 7200 ventilator in the assist/control mode with an FI_{O_2} of 0.4. The following information is presented to the physician by the therapist:

Pa_{O_2}	99 mm Hg
Pa_{CO_2}	33 mm Hg
pH	7.43
Vital capacity	Unable to obtain data
Negative inspiratory force	88 cm H_2O
Airway secretions	Minimal

Temperature	37.6°C
Resting minute volume	8.6 L/min
Pulse	80
BP	120/80

Based on the above information, which of the following is the most appropriate recommendation?
A.   Place on SIMV
B.   Place on T tube with FIo_2 of 0.5
C.   Do not attempt weaning until patient has regained consciousness
D.   Lower FIo_2 to 0.35 and obtain an arterial sample
E.   Insert a fenestrated tracheostomy tube and plug it for 1 hour every 4 hours
   (2:Chap 25, p 670) (62) (66)

65.   Which of the following is (are) known to cause metabolic alkalosis?
   I.   Lasix administration
   II.   Diarrhea
   III. Nasogastric suction
   IV.   Ileostomy loss
      A.   I and III
      B.   II and III
      C.   II and IV
      D.   I, III, and IV
      E.   II only
   (33:277–278)

66.   A 25-year-old automobile accident victim is seen in the emergency department after sustaining extensive trauma. The following pertinent data were obtained from blood gas analysis:

Pao_2	64 mm Hg
FIo_2	0.40
$Paco_2$	40 mm Hg
pH	7.33
HCO_3	19.6 mEq/L
V_D/V_T	0.78

Based on the above information, which of the following should the respiratory care practitioner recommend at this time?
A.   Stat IPPB with 0.25 cc metaproterenol
B.   Increase FIo_2 to 0.7
C.   Initiate continuous ventilatory support
D.   Repeat blood gas studies
E.   Insert a pulmonary artery catheter
   (38:60) (58) (31:136–138)

67.   The physician asks the respiratory therapy practitioner to modify all ventilator settings necessary to help keep a 1000-g newborn's

Pa_{CO_2} less than 60 mm Hg. Which of the following controls would the therapist be *least* likely to manipulate to help achieve this goal?
A.   I:E ratio
B.   PEEP/CPAP
C.   Inspiratory time
D.   Mandatory rate
E.   Pressure limit
   (29:217)

68.   When excessive levels of PEEP are administered, which of the following are commonly noted?
   I.   Decreases in $S\bar{v}_{O_2}$
   II.   Decreases in effective static compliance
   III.   Narrowing of the $C(a-\bar{v})_{O_2}$
   IV.   Decreases in PWP
      A.   I and IV
      B.   I and II
      C.   II and III
      D.   I and III
      E.   III and IV
   (1:373) (47)

69.   The occurrence of which of the following would most likely result in peripheral arterial hypertension?
   I.   Overadministraion of norepinephrine
   II.   Decrease in systemic vascular resistance
   III.   Hypervolemia
   IV.   Pharmacologic blockage of α-adrenergic receptors
      A.   I, II, and III
      B.   III and IV
      C.   I and IV
      D.   II and IV
      E.   I and III
   (25:Chap 9, pp 2–3) (1:45–46) (2:953)

70.   Which of the following size (I.D.) endotracheal tubes should be selected for a newborn who weighs 1500 g?
   A.   2.0 mm
   B.   3.0 mm
   C.   4.0 mm
   D.   5.0 mm
   E.   6.0 mm
   (25:Chap 16, p 2)

71.   Calibration of which of the following blood gas electrodes is usually achieved by using an analyzed gas with a concentration of 0% to establish the balance point?
   A.   pH electrode
   B. P_{O_2} electrode
   C. P_{CO_2} electrode
   D.   A and C are correct.
   E.   A, B, and C are correct.
   (5:158) P. 271

72. Which of the following would the respiratory therapy practitioner *not* recommend as a means of providing nutritional support to a 75-year-old patient with chronic obstructive pulmonary disease who is requiring prolonged, continuous ventilatory support?
   A. 5% dextrose in water
   B. 0.45% NaCl
   C. Intravenous lipids
   D. Nasogastric feeding
   E. Central vascular protein administration
   (31:Chap 8)

73. Which of the following is believed to be responsible for improvements in cardiovascular function reported after initiation of IMV and SIMV?
   A. Normalization of Pa_{CO_2} levels
   B. Decreased venous return
   C. Improved distribution of ventilation
   D. Decreased mean intrathoracic pressure
   E. Increased right ventricular filling pressure
   (2:600–602)

74. With a properly functioning, four-channel pulmonary artery catheter, it is possible to monitor which of the following parameters?
   I. Cardiac output
   II. Central venous pressure
   III. Pulmonary artery systolic and diastolic pressures
   IV. Mixed venous oxygen saturation
   V. Left ventricular systolic pressure
       A. I, III, and V
       B. II, III, IV, and V
       C. I, II, III, and IV
       D. I, II, and III
       E. II, III, and IV
   (5:228–230) (2:954–955)

75. Regarding the normal chest roentgenogram, which of the following statements is (are) true?
   I. The width of the heart should be greater than one half the distance across the lungs at the level of the diaphragm.
   II. The ribs should be an equal distance apart.
   III. The left diaphragm is usually about one half a rib interspace higher than the right.
   IV. The costophrenic angle should be considerably less than 90°.
       A. II and IV
       B. III and IV
       C. II only
       D. I, II, and IV
       E. I and III
   (3:309–334)

P. 136 ch 8 Shap. ABG Book

76. Clinical indications for pulmonary artery catheterization include:
    I.   Monitoring left ventricular function
    II. Monitoring cardiac output
    III. Monitoring mean peripheral venous pressure
    IV. Accessing true mixed venous blood
    A.   I, III, and IV
    B.   I, II, and IV
    C.   III and IV
    D.   II and III
    E.   I, II, III, and IV
    (2:954–955) (1:406–409)

77. Pulmonary function tests performed on a patient with chronic bronchitis would most likely reveal:
    I.   Severely decreased $D_{L_{CO}}$
    II. Decreased $\dfrac{FEV_1}{FVC}$ %
    III. Decreased expiratory flow rates
    IV. Dramatic response to bronchodilator therapy
    A.   I and III
    B.   II and III
    C.   II and IV
    D.   III and IV
    E.   I, II, and III
    (2)

78. A 71-year-old, 80-kg woman with a history of chronic obstructive pulmonary disease is found semiconscious at home. After being brought to the emergency department, she is intubated and placed on a volume ventilator in the assist/control mode. Subsequently, the following data are collected:

FI_{O_2}	0.4
Pa_{O_2}	54 mm Hg
Pa_{CO_2}	71 mm Hg
pH	7.47
Base excess	14 mEq/L
Pulse	120/min
ECG	Premature atrial contractions
BP	180/100
CVP	12 cm H_2O
HCO_3^-	40 mEq/L

Questioning the validity of the CVP measurement, the physician administers three successive 200-cc fluid challenges. The CVP, when measured following the third fluid challenge, is 13 cm H_2O. Based on the above information, the respiratory therapy practitioner should now recommend:
A. Another blood gas study
B. Pulmonary artery catheterization

C. Administration of an additional 200-cc fluid challenge
D. Switching the patient to SIMV
E. Measuring the patient's urine output
   (1:409–412) (61) (41)

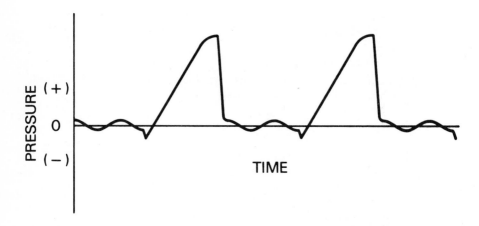

Figure 13.

79. The above pressure waveform is best described by which of the following terms?
    A. SIMV
    B. IMV
    C. EPAP
    D. CPAP
    E. Control mode ventilation
       (3:505)

80. In reviewing a patient's chart, the respiratory therapy practitioner notes that the patient's urine output has been dropping steadily and is now approximately 15 cc/hour. This value is most consistent with:
    A. Polyuria
    B. Oliguria
    C. Anuria
    D. Normal urine output
    E. Decreased antidiuretic hormone
       (89:977)

81. When excessive levels of PEEP are used, which of the following are most likely to result?
    I. Overdistention of pulmonary tissue
    II. Increased physiologic shunting
    III. Increases in airway resistance
    IV. Increases in oxygen tissue transport

A. I and III
B. I and II
C. II and IV
D. I, II, and III
E. I, III, and IV
(47) (1:373–374)

82. The respiratory therapy practitioner is monitoring a patient in the intensive care unit who is on a volume ventilator. The following parameters are noted at this time:

CVP	10 mm Hg
PWP	9 mm Hg
P.A. diastolic	31 mm Hg
P.A. systolic	48 mm Hg

These findings are most consistent with which of the following disorders?
I. Severe left ventricular failure
II. Pulmonary hypertension
III. Right ventricular failure
IV. Hypervolemia
V. Increased pulmonary vascular resistance
A. II and V
B. I, III, and V
C. I, II, and III
D. II, III, and IV
E. I and IV
(41) (33:203–204) (11:182–183) (32:Chap 5)

83. The respiratory therapy practitioner is assisting in a thoracotomy. On completion of the operation, chest tubes are connected to a three-bottle chest suction system. Subsequently, a large amount of bubbling is noted in the underwater seal chamber. What does this signify?
A. The chest tubes are leaking.
B. Too much suction has been applied to the unit.
C. Air is being evacuated from the pleural space.
D. The excess wall suction is being vented properly.
E. A and D are correct.
(7:351–355)

84. A 35-year-old patient received a vagotomy and partial pyloroplasty 8 days ago. Three days postoperatively he became septic and was taken back to the operating room to repair a perforated ileus. Since that time he has been on a volume ventilator with high levels of PEEP and FIo_2s of 0.7 or greater. Because of the danger of oxygen toxicity, the physician decides to raise this

patient's PEEP to 28 cm H_2O and at the same time lower the FIo_2 to 0.5. Concurrent and pertinent information is noted below:

	20 cm H_2O PEEP	28 cm H_2O PEEP
Pao_2	46 mm Hg	39 mm Hg
$P\bar{v}o_2$	32 mm Hg	24 mm Hg
$C(a-\bar{v})o_2$	3.5 vol%	5.8 vol%
Qs/QT	34%	28%
FIo_2	0.7	0.5
PWP (on ventilator)	7 mm Hg	9 mm Hg

Further orders are to leave the FIo_2 at the 0.5 level despite any cardiovascular depression noted at 28 cm H_2O PEEP. At this time, which of the following should the advanced respiratory care practitioner recommend to treat this patient's hypoxia?
A.   Decrease venous return
B.   Administer diuretics
C.   Induce hypothermia to lower metabolic demands
D.   Optimize cardiac performance by whatever means possible
E.   Apply inflation hold of 0.5 second
     (46) (47)

85.   A pulmonary function analyzing unit, when used to determine the functional residual capacity via the helium dilution method, must use which of the following in its circuit?
A.   Nitrogen meter
B.   Potentiometer
C.   Carbon dioxide absorbing mechanism
D.   Spectrophotometer
E.   Nonrebreathing valve
     (16:6–9)

86.   The respiratory therapist is monitoring a 48-year-old patient with bibasal viral pneumonia who is receiving continuous ventilatory support. The following data are obtained at this time with an FIo_2 of 0.5:

Pao_2	78 mm Hg
$Paco_2$	31 mm Hg
pH	7.48 mm Hg
HCO_3^-	22 mEq/L
PWP	26 mm Hg
Pulse	90
BP	150/100

Which of the following should the therapist recommend at this time?
A.   Add 5 cm H_2O PEEP
B.   Decrease the FIo_2 to 0.4
C.   Administer a diuretic

D. Administer $NaHCO_3$
E. Pharmacologically paralyze
   (41) (61) (58)

87. All five of the following patients are intubated and are receiving 100% oxygen via a volume ventilator. In addition, each one has a Pa_{O_2} of 50 mm Hg. The respiratory therapy practitioner would assess which one as having the largest intrapulmonary shunt fraction (assume an oxygen consumption of 250 mL/min for each patient)?
A. Patient A has a $C(a-\bar{v})_{O_2}$ of 2.5 vol%
B. Patient B has a $C(a-\bar{v})_{O_2}$ of 3.5 vol%
C. Patient C has a $C(a-\bar{v})_{O_2}$ of 5.0 vol%
D. Patient D has a $C(a-\bar{v})_{O_2}$ of 6.0 vol%
E. Patient E has a $C(a-\bar{v})_{O_2}$ of 8.0 vol%
   (46:3)

88. Which of the following chest radiologic findings would be noted in a patient with a massive right-sided atelectasis?
I.   Mediastinal shift to the right side
II. Increased opacification on the right side
III. Elevation of the left hemidiaphragm
IV. Rib spreading over the affected area
A. I only
B. II and IV
C. I, II, and III
D. I and III
E. I and II
   (3:309–334)

89. An 83-year-old patient is seen in the intensive care unit while receiving continuous ventilatory support with an FI_{O_2} of 0.7 and 8 cm H_2O PEEP. The following information is noted at this time:

Q_S/Q_T	18%
$C(a-\bar{v})_{O_2}$	8.2 vol%
PWP	3 mm Hg
$P(A-a)_{O_2}$	400 mm Hg
Oxygen consumption	250 mL/min

Which of the following should the respiratory therapist recommend to narrow the patient's $P(A-a)_{O_2}$?
A. Increase PEEP
B. Vigorously increase diuresis
C. Increase FI_{O_2}
D. Decrease PEEP
E. Administer fluids
   (41) (46:2–3) (1:Chap 27) (65)

90. Which of the following pulmonary function tests is believed to give the best information about the patency of the smaller airways?

A. FEF_{25-75}
B. $FEF_{200-1200}$
C. FEV_1
D. FEV_2
E. $\dfrac{FEV_{1\%}}{FVC}$
    (16:47) (2:221)

91. The respiratory therapy practitioner is asked to calibrate a spirometer to ensure accuracy of measured flow rates. To do so properly, the practitioner should employ:
    A. A potentiometer
    B. An ultrasonic transducer
    C. A rotometer device
    D. A calibrated "super" syringe
    E. A body plethysmograph
    (2:Chap 6)

92. For which of the following conditions would the respiratory therapy practitioner be *least* likely to recommend corticosteroid administration?
    A. Postextubation laryngeal edema
    B. Postoperative atelectasis
    C. Idiopathic pulmonary fibrosis (Hamman-Rich syndrome)
    D. Bronchial asthma
    E. Croup
    (25:Chap 9, pp 12–13) (31:55–56)

93. In which of the following types of hypoxemia will the sum of the Pa_{O_2} and the Pa_{CO_2} typically be greater than 110 mm Hg with the patient breathing room air?
    A. Hypoventilation
    B. Low V/Q
    C. Shunting
    D. Diffusion defect
    E. Decreased PI_{O_2}
    (2:242)

94. In reviewing a patient's chart prior to therapy, the respiratory care practitioner notes that the patient has a history of respiratory insufficiency due to neuromuscular blockade. The above is most consistent with which of the following disorders?
    A. Guillain-Barré syndrome
    B. Pickwickian syndrome
    C. Myasthenia gravis
    D. Narcotic overdose
    E. Upper cervical spine transection
    (11:202)

95. The physician wants the respiratory therapy practitioner to place a spontaneously breathing, 200-lb patient on a Bear I ventilator with an FI_{O_2} of 0.6. Which of the following are the most appropriate settings for this patient?

A. Tidal volume 1000 cc, backup rate 12, assist/control mode
B. SIMV mode, mandatory rate of 12, tidal volume 600 cc
C. Control mode with a rate of 20, tidal volume 1000 cc
D. A and B are correct.
E. All of the above are correct.
   (25:Chap 15, p 2) (49) (65) (1:336–342)

96. Which of the following is (are) true regarding the presence of large right-to-left intrapulmonary shunts (Q_s/Q_T)?
   I.   Results when alveoli are ventilated but not perfused
   II. Treatment includes application of PEEP therapy
   III. Can be differentiated from low V/Q by administration of high concentrations of oxygen
   IV. Treatment includes application of CPAP therapy
   V.   Generally leads to refractory hypoxemia
      A. I and III
      B. III and V
      C. II, III, and V
      D. II, III, IV, and V
      E. V only
   (2:394–395) (13:78) (5:Chap 16, p 19)

97. A 58-year-old, 80-kg patient is seen in the intensive care unit while receiving continuous ventilatory support with an FI_{O_2} of 1.0 and 6 cm H_2O PEEP. The following information is charted at this time with the patient in the assist/control mode:

$C(a-\bar{v})_{O_2}$	2.5 vol%
Q_s/Q_T	42%
Oxygen consumption	250 mL/min
PWP	15 mm Hg
$P(A-a)_{O_2}$	600 mm Hg

Which of the following should the respiratory therapy practitioner recommend to treat this patient's arterial hypoxemia?
A. Increase PEEP
B. Administer 500 cc lactated Ringer's solution
C. Administer dobutamine (Dobutrex)
D. Switch to control mode
E. Decrease the FI_{O_2}
   (46:2–3) (41) (1:Chap 27) (65)

98. In examining the chest roentgenogram of a critically ill patient, the respiratory therapy practitioner notes that the right costophrenic angle is considerably blunted. This finding is most consistent with which of the following disorders?
A. Noncardiogenic pulmonary edema
B. Idiopathic pulmonary fibrosis
C. Phrenic nerve paralysis
D. Pleural effusion
E. Chronic obstructive pulmonary emphysema
   (3:228)

99. True statements regarding the clinical use of an esophageal obtu-
     rator airway include:
     I.   Placement should be preceded by tracheal intubation.
     II.   Removal is often followed by regurgitation.
     III. Tracheal intubation with this airway may result in as-
           phyxia.
     IV.   It is contraindicated for use in small children.
           A. II, III, and IV
           B. II and III
           C. I, II, III, and IV
           D. I, III, and IV
           E. I and III
     (25:Chap 4, pp 2-3) (1:248-250)

100. A 54-year-old patient is admitted to the coronary care unit follow-
     ing a moderately severe left ventricular infarction. Important clin-
     ical data noted at this time with the patient receiving continuous
     ventilatory support are as follows:

Pa_{O_2}	48 mm Hg
FI_{O_2}	0.7
Pa_{CO_2}	31 mm Hg
Pulse	120
BP	180/130
PWP	30 mm Hg

     Which of the following therapeutic modalities would be *least* bene-
     ficial for the respiratory therapy practitioner to recommend at this
     time?
     A. Nitroprusside (Nipride)
     B. Furosemide (Lasix)
     C. Dobutamine (Dobutrex)
     D. Phenylephrine HCl
     E. Morphine sulfate
     (1:Chap 27) (25:Chap 3, pp 5-7)

Answer Key and NBRC Examination Matrix Categories

1. B, III F	21. C, III G	41. C, I C	61. D, I A	81. B, III C
2. D, I C	22. E, I C	42. B, III F	62. A, III F	82. A, III D
3. B, I A	23. A, III D	43. D, III B	63. D, III D	83. C, III G
4. D, I C	24. A, III F	44. D, III D	64. B, III F	84. D, III F
5. D, III E	25. C, I A	45. A, I C	65. A, I C	85. C, II A
6. B, III B	26. A, III F	46. D, III F	66. C, III F	86. C, III F
7. C, III F	27. B, III D	47. D, II A	67. B, III B	87. A, III D
8. D, III E	28. B, I A	48. C, III D	68. B, III C	88. E, I B
9. C, II A	29. A, III D	49. A, III B	69. E, III D	89. E, III F
10. D, III E	30. C, III F	50. B, III F	70. B, III A	90. A, I C
11. D, II B	31. B, III B	51. C, II A	71. B, II B	91. C, II B
12. C, III D	32. A, III D	52. C, III B	72. B, III F	92. B, III F
13. E, II A	33. D, I A	53. A, III D	73. D, III B	93. A, III D
14. E, III E	34. E, III F	54. E, III D	74. C, II A	94. C, I A
15. C, I C	35. B, III A	55. D, I A	75. A, I B	95. A, III E
16. D, III D	36. B, III D	56. C, I C	76. B, III D	96. D, III C
17. D, I B	37. C, I A	57. C, III F	77. B, I C	97. A, III F
18. E, III G	38. A, III F	58. C, I A	78. B, III F	98. D, I B
19. B, III D	39. A, III B	59. E, III E	79. A, III B	99. A, III A
20. B, I B	40. B, III D	60. B, III D	80. B, I A	100. D, III F

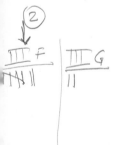